Ligament Reconstructions

World Scientific Series:
From Biomaterials Towards Medical Devices

ISSN: 2529-816X

Series Editors:

Roger Guilard
Université de Bourgogne
UFR Sciences et Techniques
Faculté des Sciences Mirande
ICMUB – UMR CNRS 6302
9 Avenue Alain Savary, BP 47870
21078 Dijon Cedex, France
Email: roger.guilard@u-bourgogne.fr

Karl M Kadish
Department of Chemistry
University of Houston
Houston, TX 77204-5003, USA
Email: kkadish@uh.edu

Vol. 3 *Ligament Reconstructions*
edited by L'Hocine Yahia (Université de Montréal, Canada)

Vol. 2 *Dental Biomaterials*
edited by Edward Sacher (École Polytechnique de Montréal, Canada) & Rodrigo França (University of Manitoba, Canada)

Vol. 1 *Drug Delivery Systems*
edited by Pieter Stroeve (UC Davis) & Morteza Mahmoudi (Tehran University of Medical Sciences, Iran & Harvard Medical School, USA)

Forthcoming

Biomaterials and Bioengineered Device Research for Ligament Reconstruction
edited by Véronique Migonney ((Université Paris 13, France) & L'Hocine Yahia (École Polytechnique de Montréal, Canada)

Biomaterials and Bioengineered Device Research for Joint Prostheses
edited by L'Hocine Yahia (École Polytechnique de Montréal, Canada) & Véronique Migonney (Université Paris 13, France)

Biomaterials and Bioengineered Device Research for Cardiovascular Applications
edited by Laurence Bordenave (Université de Bordeaux, France)

World Scientific Series in
From Biomaterials Towards Medical Devices – Vol. 3

Ligament Reconstructions

Editor

L'Hocine Yahia
Université de Montréal, Canada

Series Editors

Roger Guilard
Université de Bourgogne, France

Karl M. Kadish
University of Houston, USA

World Scientific

NEW JERSEY • LONDON • SINGAPORE • BEIJING • SHANGHAI • HONG KONG • TAIPEI • CHENNAI • TOKYO

Published by

World Scientific Publishing Co. Pte. Ltd.
5 Toh Tuck Link, Singapore 596224
USA office: 27 Warren Street, Suite 401-402, Hackensack, NJ 07601
UK office: 57 Shelton Street, Covent Garden, London WC2H 9HE

Library of Congress Cataloging-in-Publication Data
Names: Yahia, Hocine, 1952– editor.
Title: Ligament reconstructions / editor, L'Hocine Yahia, Université de Montréal, Canada ; series editors, Roger Guilard, Université de Bourgogne, France, Karl M. Kadish, University of Houston, USA.
Description: New Jersey : World Scientific, [2021] | Series: World scientific series: from biomaterials towards medical devices, 2529-816X ; vol. 3 | Includes bibliographical references and index.
Identifiers: LCCN 2020034111 (print) | LCCN 2020034112 (ebook) | ISBN 9789811204623 (hardcover) | ISBN 9789811204630 (ebook) | ISBN 9789811204647 (ebook other)
Subjects: LCSH: Anterior cruciate ligament. | Anterior cruciate ligament--Wounds and injuries. | Knee--Surgery. | Ligaments--Wounds and injuries.
Classification: LCC RD561 .L532 2021 (print) | LCC RD561 (ebook) | DDC 617.5/82059--dc23
LC record available at https://lccn.loc.gov/2020034111
LC ebook record available at https://lccn.loc.gov/2020034112

British Library Cataloguing-in-Publication Data
A catalogue record for this book is available from the British Library.

For any available supplementary material, please visit
https://www.worldscientific.com/worldscibooks/10.1142/11395#t=suppl

Desk Editors: Joy Quek/Aanand Jayaraman

Typeset by Stallion Press
Email: enquiries@stallionpress.com

https://doi.org/10.1142/9789811204630_fmatter

Preface

The anterior cruciate ligament (ACL) is one of the most vulnerable ligaments of the knee. ACL impairment results in episodic instability, chondral and meniscal injury and early osteoarthritis. It has been a long-held clinical belief that an ACL injury cannot heal spontaneously; therefore, this poor self-healing capacity makes surgical treatment inevitable. It is estimated that approximately 200,000 ACL reconstructions are performed each year in the USA alone, a number expected to increase further as a result of increased participation in athletic activities by adolescents and young adults. The ACL injury is the most common knee ligamentous injury in sports-related activities and a delay in returning to sports is enough to ruin a sportsman's career. Several areas of controversy exist in ACL tear management which has engaged surgeons and researchers in debates towards identifying an ideal approach for these patients.

During the past 20 years, an increasing body of work investigating the substitution of torn ACL via synthetic ligaments or biological grafts such as autograft, allograft, has been published. Autografts have shortcomings such as inadequate graft length or diameter and donor site morbidity while; allografts, on the other hand, have problems of allogenicity, insufficient supply of grafts, high costs, etc. A common disadvantage that both these grafts share is the requirement of integration of the graft in the osseous tunnels. The time required for this integration process is variable and subjective and is more for allografts than autografts. Extensive research has been done to overcome these problems associated with autografts and allografts and to develop a suitable synthetic substitute for ACL reconstruction. Ligament advanced reinforcement system (LARS) is the latest development in the synthetic ligament substitutes. Several studies showed good to excellent functional outcomes and good patient satisfaction. A few of the papers even rated LARS as better than the autograft ACL reconstructions and reported LARS enabling patients to go back to active sports-related activities within 2–3 months of the surgery.

In parallel, over the past 10 years, there has been increasing recognition that the lack of provisional scaffold in ACL injuries is the major reason for the absence of self-healing. In recent times, a bridge-enhanced ACL repair concept is gaining popularity. This concept is using biodegradable (e.g. polypropylene) suture as a guide and collagen-platelet rich plasma (PRP) hydrogel as a bridge (containing cells and growth factors). Platelet in plasma was identified as a source to be a provisional scaffold and initiate extracellular matrix protein production by fibroblast. Although biomechanical properties, yield load and stiffness of ACL repaired by collagen-PRP hydrogel, were found to be similar to that of human ACL, this bio-enhanced ACL reconstruction is not yet approved by the FDA.

This book provides an insight of ACL structure, orientation and properties followed by comparing the performance of various constructs that have been used for ACL replacement. New approaches, undertaken to induce ACL regeneration and fabricate biomimetic scaffolds, are also discussed. My goals for this new book on ligaments reconstruction were to produce a text that summarizes state of the art knowledge about cruciate ligament reconstruction, including recent advances in the past 10 years, to provide a useful reference for a broad audience, and to highlight areas for development of future work in this field. We have tried to make this book as pragmatic as possible. The approach is to include different schools of thought over the world — thanks to the German, French, Italian, Brazilian, Chinese, Australian and Canadian authors.

https://doi.org/10.1142/9789811204630_fmatter

About the Editor

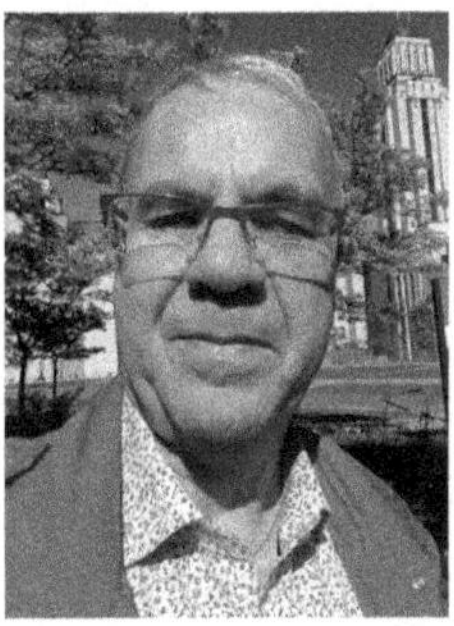

L'Hocine Yahia graduated from the University of Orleans (France) in 1977 in Mechanical Engineering and obtained his Ph.D. in Biomedical Engineering in 1980 from the Compiegne University of Technology (France). He then moved to Polytechnique Montreal to undertake training in Biomechanics and Biomaterials, obtaining a Ph.D. in Mechanical Engineering in 1984. He is a tenure track faculty member at Polytechnique Montreal (Canada) and associate professor at the Department of Surgery of Montreal University. Dr. Yahia is currently the director of the Innovation and Bioperformance Analysis Laboratory (LIAB).

His main interests varied from the musculoskeletal biomechanics, the properties of ligaments and fascia, the living systems from Prigogine's perspective, the redundancy problems in biomechanics and the biomimetics approach in biomaterials. Recent research topics include nanomaterials, antibacterial biomaterials, bioengineering thermodynamics for biosystems, biotensegrity and constructal approach in biomechanics and spinal biomechanics. He also serves as a Member of Scientific Advisory Board of Victhom Human Bionics and Begama Technologies Inc.

Dr. Yahia holds 10 patents, five books and speaks regularly at international meetings on his work. He has authored more than 200 peer-reviewed publications on biomaterials, cruciate ligaments, spinal ligaments, shape memory materials, nanoparticles and sterilization techniques.

https://doi.org/10.1142/9789811204630_fmatter

Acknowledgments

I would like to thank all the contributing authors for their time in meeting the manuscript deadlines and bringing their expertise to this project. I would also like to thank my research assistant, Ghislaine Bayade, for her untiring efforts, diligence in contacting authors, patience in compiling the manuscripts, and expertise in word-processing skills.

Finally, I would like to thank the staff at World Scientific for their patience and Prof. Roger Guilard for guidance in the preparation of this text.

https://doi.org/10.1142/9789811204630_fmatter

Contents

https://doi.org/10.1142/9789811204630_fmatter

Introduction

This book summarizes the experience gained by the Laboratory for Innovation and Bioperformance Analysis in dealing with cruciate ligaments reconstruction over the last three decades. The editor, L'H. Yahia, had collaborated with international authorities to produce this excellent work dealing with a great many aspects of knee surgery and especially the problems of the cruciate ligaments.

The idea of creating a comprehensive multi-author textbook exclusively devoted to cruciate ligaments reconstruction is motivated by two reasons. Firstly, the popularity and success of the book entitled *Ligaments and Ligamentoplasties* published in 1997 at Springer-Verlag has been an impetus to launch a new one on Ligament Reconstructions. On the other hand, this move is easily justifiable considering the immense clinical importance of the ligament injuries, and also the numerous advances that have been made in knowledge about the problem in the last few years. This book is arranged and organized the different chapters in a coherent manner that takes the reader from the basics of the injury and healing mechanisms, through the essence of reconstruction options, to a view of the future.

The book consists of 13 chapters. Chapter 1 deals with the ACL's injury and healing processes. The mechanism for ACL injuries is still misunderstood, and research continues to determine critical factors for prevention. Is the biological evolution of knee joint and ligament could explain why human ACL injuries are so common? Is it because Homo sapiens never fully completed human adaptation to bipedalism? This low capacity of the intra-articular ligaments to heal has long been attributed to the intrinsic differences in cell behavior and to the insufficient blood supply following injury. It was shown recently that the provisional scaffold (fibrin-platelet clot) found within the wound site of extra-articular ligaments was, in fact, missing in the ACL. A bio-active scaffold was then be developed as a carrier for cells, growth factors and enzymes required to optimize tissue healing. The two following chapters (Chapters 2–3) provide more details related to synthetic grafts. In the 1980s, several polymer materials such as poly(ethylene terephthalate) (PET), poly(tetrafluoroethylene) (PTFE), poly(amide) (PA) and poly(propylene) (PP) were used for the elaboration of ACL prosthesis. During the years 1990–2000, the second generation of the synthetic ligament was born and allowed to propose an innovative solution in this specific field. None of the first FDA approved artificial ligaments have demonstrated positive long-term results in vivo. It is important to mention that some synthetic ligaments, not approved by the FDA, have escaped recall and have survived in Europe and Asia until this day. This is particularly the case with LARS™, Trevira and LK ligaments, which are currently the most widely accepted synthetics; however, their use remains somewhat controversial. Regarding the biological grafts, there is no ideal graft for ACL reconstruction without any complications. The ideal graft for ACL reconstruction should reproduce the histological and the biomechanical characteristics of the native ligament, incorporate fully and quickly within bone tunnels, have no risk of rejection or disease transmission, have minimal donor site morbidity, be of sufficient length and diameter, and be cost-effective, as well as readily available. Further studies are necessary to standardize the processes involved in ACL reconstruction including the graft choice, the graft fixation methods, and the rehabilitation protocol. Chapter 4 presents potential animal models for the evaluation of human ACL reconstruction, may it be in the pathobiology or in the evaluation of new techniques or devices. Chapter 5 is devoted to the fibrocartilaginous ligament enthesis. This chapter begins describing the known development of native enthesis, and the biology and biomechanics of entheses. Clinically, strategies for re-attaching ligaments, attaching tendon grafts, and attempts to improve these attachments are discussed. The five following chapters (Chapters 6–8 and 10) treat in more details international clinical experiences, i.e. Italian, Chinese and Canadian respectively, using LARS synthetic ligament for ACL reconstruction. Promising results were obtained in the short, medium, and long term, but further studies (to be conducted with an even more accurate methodology) are necessary in order to provide additional and definitive evidence. Chapter 9 briefly introduces the "rediscovery" of the anterolateral ligament (ALL) and its role in anterolateral knee stability. The facts that the ALL is not a structure routinely described in MRI reports and that the reconstruction criteria are not fully established contribute to the misdiagnosis and undertreatment of this injury. In the last three chapters (Chapters 11–13) the authors present recent progress and challenges in designing biomimetic ligaments, understanding of "universal jolt" theory of human knee injuries, and development of in silico models for the design of tissue-engineered ligaments. We hope this book would serve as a bridge that covers the gap between biomaterials specialists and clinicians.

https://doi.org/10.1142/9789811204630_0001

Chapter 1

A Review of Cruciate Ligaments: ACL's Injury and Healing Processes

L'Hocine Yahia[*,‡], Ghislaine Bayade[*],
Werner Klingler[†], and Robert Schleip[†]

[*]*Laboratoire d'Innovation et d'Analyse de Bioperformance, Polytechnique Montréal, C.P. 6079, Succursale Centre-ville, Montréal, Québec, Canada*

[†]*Fascia Research Group, Division of Neurophysiology, Ulm University, Germany*

[‡]*lhocine.yahia@polymlt.ca*

Abbreviations

ACL	Anterior cruciate ligament
ACLD	Anterior cruciate ligament deficient
AM	Anteromedial bundle
BMAC	Bone marrow aspirate concentrate
CCL	Cranial cruciate ligament
ECM	Extracellular matrix
EDRF	Endothelium-derived relaxing factor
FDA	Food and drug administration
FKB	Functional knee braces
HITS	Head impact telemetry system
IM	Intermediate bundle
LCL	Lateral collateral ligament
MCL	Medial collateral ligament
MMP	Matrix metalloproteinase
MRI	Magnetic resonance imaging
NO	Nitric oxide
NOS	Nitric oxide synthase
OA	Osteoarthritis
PCL	Posterior cruciate ligament
PKB	Prophylactic knee braces
PL	Posterolateral bundle
PRP	Platelet-enriched plasma
ROS	Reactive oxygen species

1. Anterior Cruciate Ligament

1.1. *Anatomy and Function*

The knee joint is the largest and most complex joint in the human body. It is called a condylar joint because of the articulation between the femur and the tibia. The femur has two protrusions called condyles. These have a convex curvature in order to roll and to slide against the tibia. The tibia has two concave grooves that match the condyles of the femur. The two central ligaments that connect the tibia to the femur are called cruciate ligaments because of the way they form a cross. These cruciate ligaments fit neatly inside the space between the two condyles (Figure 1).

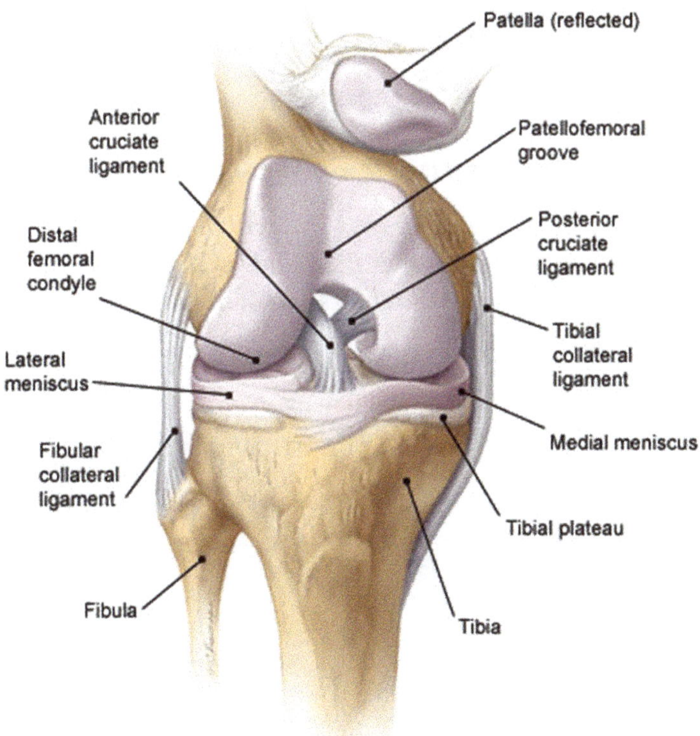

Figure 1. Anatomy of the human knee joint — Front view, straight knee.[38] The patellar tendon has been cut to allow observation of cruciate ligaments

Ligaments perform essential roles in body stabilization via maintaining bone alignments and guiding motions. They provide bone-to-bone connections in various parts of the body such as the knee. The primary function of the anterior cruciate ligament (*ACL*) is to control anterior translation of the tibia. The *ACL* also is a secondary restraint to tibial rotation as well as varus or valgus stress.[1] The *ACL* originates at the posteromedial aspect of the lateral femoral condyle. It courses distally in an anterior and a medial fashion to the anteromedial aspect of the tibia between the condyles. The position on the tibia is approximately 15 mm behind the anterior border of the tibial articular surface, and medial to the attachment of the anterior horn of the lateral meniscus.[2] It is said that the *ACL* includes two bundles: an anteromedial bundle (*AM*) that is tight in flexion and a posterolateral bundle (*PL*) that is tight in extension (Figure 2). The blood supply to the *ACL* comes from branches of the middle geniculate artery and its innervation comes from the posterior articular nerve, a branch of the tibial.

1.2. *Structure, Architecture and Organization*

ACL formation has been observed in fetal development as early as eight weeks. The *AM* and the *PL* bundles of the *ACL* begin to become apparent by week 16 of gestation. The fetal *ACL* is similar to

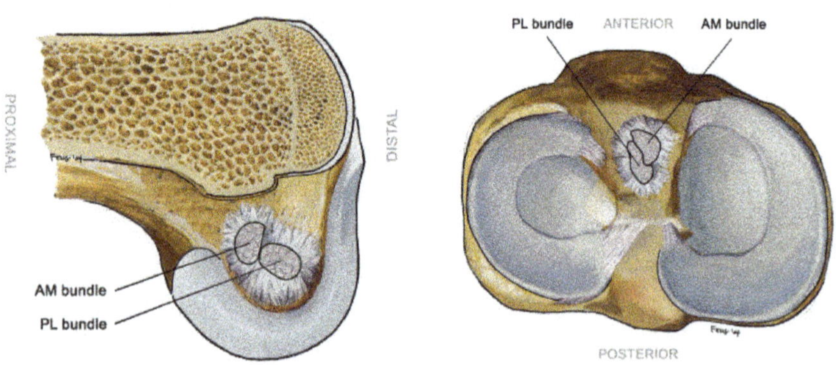

Figure 2. Attachment areas of the *ACL*[10]

the adult ligament but differs because the bundles are more parallel in orientation and the femoral origins are broader in size. Histologically, the fetal *ACL* is also more cellularized and vascularized. The *ACL* is an intra-articular, extra-synovial structure enveloped by two synovial layers. A septum of connective tissue-containing vascular-derived stem cells separates the *AM* and the *PL* bundles. This membrane contains periligamentous vessels that transversely penetrate the ligament and anastomose with a longitudinal network of endoligamentous vessels that vascularize the *ACL*.

ACL is mainly composed of water (>65%) and thus it is classified as a soft tissue. The dried *ACL* consists of mainly 70–80% fibrous collagen with the ratio of 9:1 of collagen type I to III.[4] Collagen constitutes the most abundant component of the extracellular matrix (*ECM*) of ligaments, where it provides tensile strength, regulates cell adhesion and migration, and directs tissue development.[5] Its basic building blocks consist of three alpha chains intertwined to form a triple helix, which further assembles into extended fibrillary structures with tissue-specific alignment and distribution.

A ligament consists of collagen fibrils of 30–250 nm diameter, which are responsible for the ligaments' resistance to elongation.[6] Collagen fibrils display unique crimp patterns every 45–60 μm to guide the motion passively. This crimp helps the *ACL* sustain a high range of loads throughout the motion of the knee. Therefore, the arrangement and the ultimate elongation of the collagen fibrils result in 8–9% ultimate elongation of the ligament.[7] Several fibrils form a fiber, which is organized into fascicles and surrounded by a thin sheath that allows slipping between adjacent fascicles.[8] Another useful observation of the natural ligament is that the ligament fans out near its ends and forms a "foot" region. This is believed to give the ligament a wide basis for torsional resistance. Furthermore, the merging of fascicles toward the middle of the natural ligament provides cross-linking. Any defects in the structure of *ACL*, therefore, lead to movement disability.[9]

As said above, the *ACL* comprises two main fiber bundles, the *AM* and the *PL* bundles[10,11] (Figures 2 and 3), which behave differently throughout the flexion-extension range.[12] *In vitro* studies have

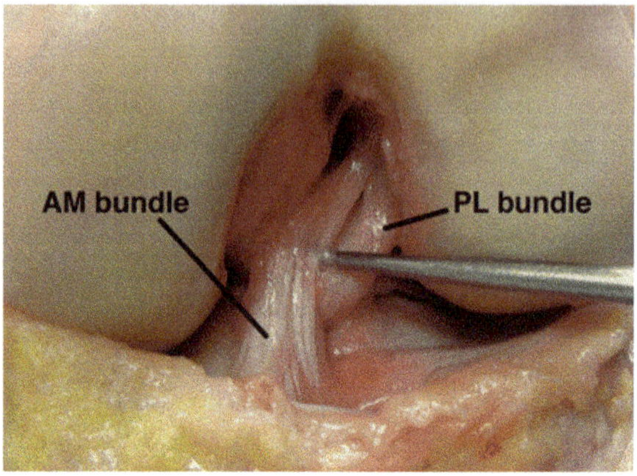

Figure 3. Bundles of the *ACL*[20]

shown that the *PL* bundle is taut in full extension, while the *AM* bundle is taut across the flexion-extension range.[13–15] The *PL* bundle relaxes during knee flexion, allowing the tibia to internally rotate during quadriceps muscles' contraction. This pattern supports the knee weight bearing in extension and allows movement during knee flexion.[16]

As the flexion angle increases, the axial rotation ("twisting") of the *ACL* bundles increases as well. At full extension, the *ACL* is internally twisted by approximately 10 degrees. This internal twist increases to approximately 40 degrees with the knee at 90 degrees of flexion.[17]

The *AM* and the *PL* bundles control the anterior translation of the tibia at any degree of knee flexion. At higher degrees of knee flexion, the *AM* bundle is more effective in controlling the anterior translation compared to the *PL* bundle. On the other hand, the *PL* bundle is more efficient from 0 to 20 degrees of knee flexion.[18]

The *ACL* bundles also play different roles in controlling rotational motion and stability of the knee joint due to the differences in their attachment areas and orientation.[19] The *AM* bundle is almost vertically oriented in the intercondylar notch in the coronal plane, thus having little ability to restrain tibial axial rotation.[20] On the other hand, the *PL* bundle slants across the intercondylar notch to a more distal-lateral femoral attachment. It has a more horizontal orientation, which suggests a further position from the axis of tibial axial rotation, implying by this a higher ability to control rotations of the tibia compared to the *AM* bundle.[21]

In 2016, Moewis *et al.* focused exclusively on the rotational laxity of the knee joint in the axial plane during passive conditions.[22] The fundament in this investigation is the clear role played by the *ACL* in the rotational stabilization of the knee joint in the axial plane, a role that — despite being considered secondary in the literature — seems crucial for the proper functioning of the knee joint. Evidence for this statement is found in the significant differences in axial rotational laxity between the *ACL*-injured and the contralateral healthy knees observed preoperatively, differences that surprisingly remained significant at higher flexion angles suggesting that the contribution in rotational stabilization by the *ACL* is not only limited between extension and low flexion as previously assumed. Moreover, despite the fact that the affected subject could theoretically be able to compensate and stabilize the knee joint through muscular contraction, the continuous post-operative recovery observed in the reduction of rotational laxity and energy dissipation as well as the increase in internal rotational stiffness strengthen the need of ligament reconstruction as the only way to achieve a proper recovery of functioning in the short term.

The *ACL* acts as the primary restraint to anterior translation of the tibia relative to the femur (i.e. prevents anterior "drawer" sign), while the posterior cruciate ligament (*PCL*) acts as the primary restraint to posterior translation of the tibia (posterior drawer sign). Additionally, the cruciate ligaments guide the tibia along a pathway of external rotation during extension (Figure 4). In the clinical literature, this conjoint axial rotation is often referred to as the "screw home" mechanism.[23] Bones, menisci and articular capsule structures act as static stabilizers of the knee, and the hamstrings and quadriceps act as dynamic muscle stabilizers.[23,24] The cruciate system has been described as a four-bar linkage system: A closed-chain linkage is composed of four bars, or rigid links, and four connections among these links. Each cruciate ligament represents a bar, and the remaining two bars are an imaginary line connecting the insertion points of the *ACL*

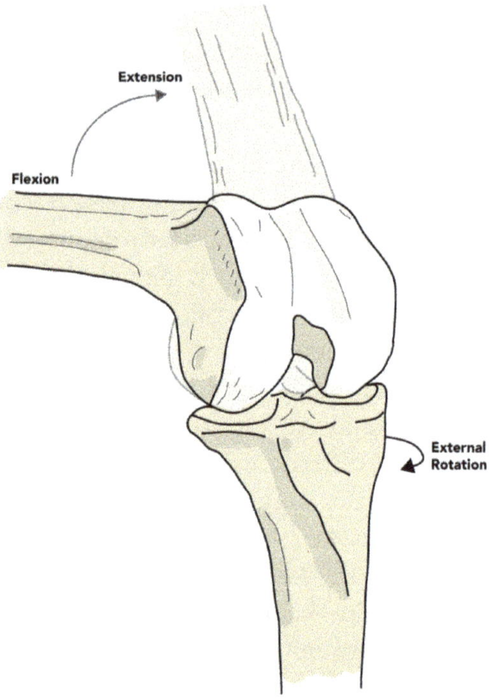

Figure 4. Upon extension, the knee rotates externally, guided by the cruciate ligaments[25]

and *PCL* on the femur, and one connecting the same imaginary line on the tibia. The pivoting connections are the femoral and tibial insertions of the *ACL* and of the *PCL*. The instant center of rotation lies at the overlap between *ACL* and *PCL*. During flexion, the ligaments roll and glide past one another, and this overlapping point moves posteriorly.[24]

The screw-home mechanism, considered to be a key element to knee stability for standing upright, is the rotation between the tibia and femur. It occurs at the end of the knee extension, between full extension (0 degrees) and 20 degrees of knee flexion. The tibia rotates internally during the swing phase and externally during the stance phase. The external rotation occurs during the terminal degrees of knee extension and results in tightening of both cruciate ligaments, which locks the knee. The tibia is then in the position of maximal stability with respect to the femur.[26]

Due to new trends, such as the concept of anatomical reconstruction, which gained power in the last decade, new motivation has been given to the study of this ligament, with important advances and innovations.[5] Therefore, this update on the *ACL* aimed to address some of the most interesting and current topics on the subject.

1.3. *Comparative Anatomy of the ACL: Animal Model*

The *ACL* is commonly injured in humans (i.e. torn *ACL*), but little is known about its comparative anatomy in other primates or mammals. As you will read in Chapter 4 of this book, large animals such as sheep, goats, pigs, monkeys, dogs and rabbits are used as models of the human knee to test *ACL* prosthetics or to discover determinants of disease progression.

Ruth *et al.*[25] recently found that humans are "typical" primates regarding bundle number, ligament circumference and fiber directionality. Results also indicate that animals with a greater range of motion have more coalescent bundles that are spatially closer to one another and may thus appear not to have many or any bundles at all. Conversely, animals with a more restricted range of motion have bundles that are apparently more distinct spatially but are very similar regarding collagen orientation and are easily divisible into bundles.

Each cruciate is structured in a "spiral" arrangement of fibers, so that each fiber twists along its path from femur to tibia and becomes taut or lax during knee flexion and extension somewhat independently of the rest of the ligament to which it belongs.

Since these observations were made, some investigators have described the human *ACL* with three bundles: *AM, PL* and intermediate bundle (*IM*). Each bundle has a different pattern of laxity and tension in concert with movement. For the human knee, the *AM* bundle is taut throughout the range of motion of the knee but reaches maximum tension between 45 and 60 degrees of extension.

The *AM* bundle of the *ACL* is the one that plays the classically described role of resisting anterior translation of the tibia upon the femur (i.e. "anterior drawer").[27,28] The *PL* bundle is taut during extension but lax during flexion[29] and most likely resists the internal rotation of the tibia.

The *IM* bundle has been reported to act in support of both *AM* and *PL* bundle functions, and especially in resisting rotation of the tibia.[28] The *IM* bundle was reportedly present in approximately 20.5% of a clinical sample of 73 patients when examined radiographically.[30]

While a consensus on the roles of each bundle of the *ACL* is fairly well-established, most data demonstrating these relationships are gathered on cadavers, and the biomechanics and the physiology of the cruciate ligament have been demonstrated to be different during physiological weight-bearing. Li and colleagues[31] have shown that the *AM* bundle demonstrates a constant length between full extension and flexion at 90 degrees, while the *PL* bundle decreases in length (i.e. experiences greater tension) with increased flexion.

Contraction of the quadriceps muscle may alter the motion of the cruciate ligaments, as the quadriceps tendon spans the knee joint and acts as a "dynamic stabilizer". Contraction of the quadriceps during flexion from 0 to 60 degrees results in the elongation of both bundles. Additionally, the "anterior drawer", or anterior-ward movement of the tibia relative to the femur, increases due to the contraction of the quadriceps when the knee is extended from 90 to 0 degrees.[29] However, the issue of bundle number and shape is currently debated, though in clinical practice the *ACL* is generally recognized to have only two primary bundles based on both function and anatomy: the *AM* and *PL* bundles.

The anatomy of the *ACL* has been described in domesticated animals and studied in pigs and goats — animals often used as models in *ACL* research. To find an animal "model" whose anatomy most closely resembles that of humans, Tantisricharoenkul and colleagues[32] conducted the widest assessment of *ACL* diversity in mammals to date, including humans, bears, lions, Diana monkeys, pigs, goats, and antelopes. They observed three bundles in all specimens and observed similar anatomy in all species (see Figure 5). They describe pig, goat and antelope as having an *AM* bundle that is separated from the *IM* and *PL* bundles by the anterior root of the lateral meniscus. Only the pig had a macroscopic synovial septum that separated *IM* and *PL*

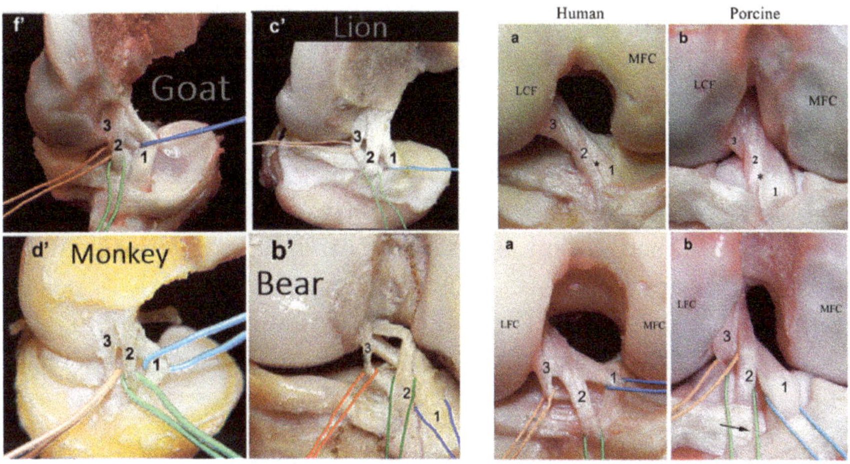

Figure 5. Comparison of knee bundles of five specimens: Porcine, human, goat, bear, monkey and lion. Comparative anterior view at 90° flexion with bundles separated (AM-1, IM-2, and PL-3)[32]

bundles from one another. In the remaining species, they describe the anterior root of the lateral meniscus as inserting lateral to the *ACL*, with all of the tibial insertions of the *ACL* being much closer together.

Tantisricharoenkul and colleagues[32] also describe the femoral and tibial insertions of the *ACL* in the same seven species: In all models, the *AM* bundle originates at the femur posterior to the *IM* and to the PL bundles and expands to the rim of the posterior articular cartilage. The *IM* bundle is posterior to the intercondylar ridge, which divides the *PL* bundle from the rest of the *ACL*. The *AM* bundle inserts tibially along the articular cartilage at the edge of the medial tibial plateau. The *PL* and *IM* bundles insert laterally, with the *PL* posterior to the *IM*.

In the basic quadruped, the knee is stabilized by the same four ligaments as well as in the bipedal knee. In humans, the *ACL* and *PCL* are typically described as resisting anterior and posterior translation of the femur on the tibia, but a more accurate description may be that they guide the tibia along its path of external rotation upon extension.[23] This role as a "guy-line" also likely applies to the quadrupedal knee but is rarely discussed in the literature. However, the cruciate ligaments likely have a greater role in preventing cranial tibial thrust ("cranial drawer") in the quadrupedal knee than they do in preventing anterior drawer in the bipedal knee. The quadrupedal tibia exhibits a caudally sloping tibial plateau, which results in cranio-dorsal translation of the tibia on the femur ("cranial tibial thrust") while bearing weight. Humans exhibit a relatively flat tibial plateau and thus do not experience tibial thrust during normal gait. However, humans are often described in clinical settings as exhibiting "anterior drawer" or "posterior drawer" in which the tibia can slide anteriorly or posteriorly against the femur. These clinical signs are manifestations of a torn *ACL* and *PCL*, respectively, and are the result of a derangement of normal knee kinematics and not a typical force present during normal gait.

During quadrupedal locomotion, propulsion occurs by way of elongation of the hindlimb as the limb contacts the ground and pushes the center of mass (which lies anterior to the limb) forward. Elongation of the hindlimb occurs at the foot, at the knee, and at the hip joints, as well as through flexion and extension of the vertebral column in many mammals.[23]

Whether an animal is digitigrade, plantigrade, or unguligrade may also influence the kinetics of the knee joint. Digitigrade animals bear their weight using only their digits. Unguligrade animals bear weight only on the distalmost tips of their digits, which are surmounted by a specialized structure such as a hoof. These animals have a suite of adaptations that increase stride length as well as elongation of limb elements and fusion of the most distal limb ones. In some species in which the total range of knee motion is limited, the distal femur has distinctly separate contact surfaces for the patella and tibia, allowing each portion of the joint that contacts the femur to have its own developmental and kinetic patterns.[23]

Plantigrade animals such as bears as well as animals with grasping hands and feet such as primates share an increased range of motion in the knee joint[23] This is because the entire foot is fixed to the substrate and is therefore eliminated from the chain of limb elements involved in limb elongation during propulsion. This is especially true with primates, who also require a great deal of pliancy in their limbs to account for inhabiting a more mobile, arboreal environment. In some hominoids, the vertebral column is also essentially inflexible, further contributing to the need for an increased range of motion in the knee and other joints. As a result of this expanded range of motion, the same portion of the distal femur contacts both the patella (in flexion) and the tibia (in extension).[23]

1.3.1. *Tibial Rotation and ACL Complexity*

Ruth *et al.*[25] found that *ACL* circumference is not larger in animals with a greater range of motion, i.e. *ACL* circumference is not the target of natural selection in any of the animals studied, but is instead a trait based on body size. It seems that animals with a greater range of motion have more variation in collagen fiber orientation than do those with a more restricted range of motion.

Additionally, when compared within a species, the eigenvectors representing collagen orientation were highly variable. This variability could be the result of age, body size, developmental or life history differences, or genetic. Ferretti *et al.*[33] demonstrated that fetal *ACL* bundles are distinct from one another. They appear to coalesce by adulthood, when the bundles can be distinguished but are not as separated from one another as they were in fetal life. Connective tissue and collagen are repaired and are remodeled in a manner similar to bone. Such repair may alter the appearance and the organization of the *ACL* during life.

Furthermore, these ligaments were "harvested" from specimens and were fixed without regard for physiological tension or anatomical position. The degree to which a knee is flexed or is extended may change the orientation of the collagen fibers within the ligament. Future studies comparing ligament orientation throughout development would illuminate the understanding of ligament remodeling and structure.

1.3.2. *Organization of ACL Bundles*

Ruth *et al.*[25] suggest that animals with greater external tibial rotation have more coalescent, rope-like bundles that are spatially closer to one another. Based on the samples, animals with less tibial rotation tend to exhibit bundles with distinct separations. One explanation could be that animals with more tibial rotation require a greater variety of fiber orientations in order to accommodate their greater range of rotation. As the tibia rotates, the *ACL* is thought to act as a kinematic guide.[23] If this is the case, different groups of collagen fibers will be sequentially taut or lax throughout the flexion–extension cycle. In animals with less rotation of the knee, less variation in the orientation of these fibers is required. Likewise, less variation in the length of fibers would be required as well. The separation of fibers may be the result of the existence of two distinct populations of fibers of two significantly different lengths, which are taut or lax during different periods of the flexion–extension cycle, much like the major portions of the *ACL* and *PCL*.

Conversely, in animals with a greater range of motion at the knee, greater variation in the orientation of collagen fibers is required. Instead of displaying two distinct populations of fibers that are taut or lax at different times, these animals may display one large population with numerous subpopulations of fibers, oriented in different directions and presumably taut or lax at different times.

Translational animal models including mouse, rabbit, goat and sheep, pig, dog and horse are used to study the human knee structures.

1.3.3. *Dog*

From Gregory *et al.*'s group, the dog model is thought to be the closest to a gold-standard animal model for knee osteoarthritis (*OA*) currently available.[34] The canine stifle (knee) joint is remarkably similar to the human knee.

Apart from size, the macroscopic and microscopic anatomical structures are very similar.[35] As in the human knee joint, the canine stifle joint consists of a medial and a lateral femorotibial compartment as well as a patellofemoral compartment. The canine stifle joint also contains similar structures such as the *ACL*, the *PCL*, the menisci, the meniscal ligament, the fat pad and the patellar tendon to the human knee joint (see Figure 6).[35] The major anatomical difference is that

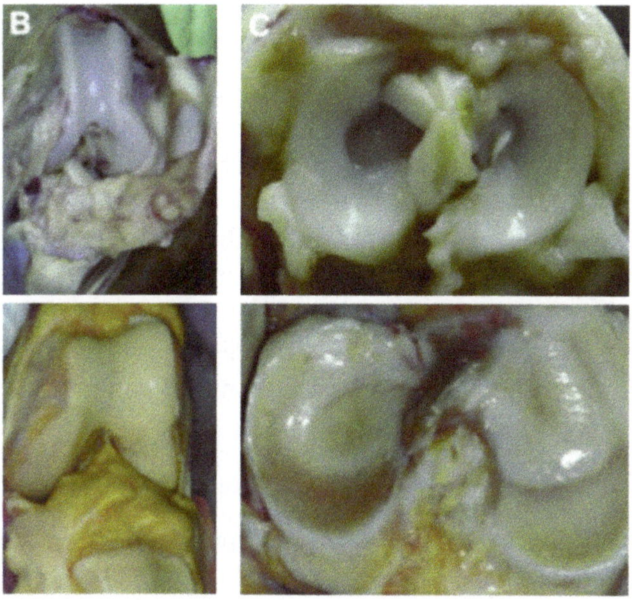

Figure 6. Comparative gross images of a canine knee (top) and a human knee (bottom). The figures show normal patellofemoral joints (B) and normal tibial plateaus (C)[36]

the canine stifle joint consists of sesamoid bones in the popliteus and lateral and medial heads of the gastrocnemius muscles and a long digital extensor tendon that is intra-articularly located. In the canine stifle joint the *ACL* is referred to as the cranial cruciate ligament (*CCL*) and is comparable to the human *ACL*.[12]

1.3.4. *Ostrich*

A wide range of joint motion allows humans to climb trees or to ballet dance, but this flexibility has a cost. When running, muscle power is used for propulsion but also to prevent sideways joint movement, thereby increasing energy requirements over a given distance. The researchers suspected that ostriches had a more efficient approach. Unlike energy-consuming muscles and tendons, their ligaments can act as a "joint corset", limiting sideways motion without consuming energy.

The surprising yet obvious statement that "birds and humans are the only true bipeds" introduces the account of the research that Nina Schaller has been doing for nearly a decade. In 2011, Nina Schaller[37] studied the outstanding speed and endurance of the ostrich — investigating the biomechanics and efficiency of the bird's performance by means of anatomy (dissection) and physiology (functional study). Her measurements showed that ligaments are the main elements that guide an ostrich leg through the stride, allowing muscle power to be devoted almost exclusively to forward propulsion. This experiment showed that saving metabolic energy by using ligaments as a passive leg-stabilizing mechanism is an excellent locomotor endurance strategy.

1.3.5. *Elephant*

The kinematics of the elephant knee joint matches the human knee.[38–41] Any deviation of the helical axis from the horizontal flexion–extension axis indicates a compulsory rotation. This is true for the helical axis in extension, which runs from proximal–medial to distal–lateral and represents the screw-home motion. The only difference between the elephant and human knee is that the human screw-home motion is smaller, i.e. 10 degrees instead of 16 degrees during flexion from 60 degrees until maximal extension.[39,40] The cause of the screw-home motion is the oblique path of the *PCL* isometric bundle, which is attached to the inner side of the medial femoral condyle.[26] In higher mammals, the most anterior (cranial) *PCL* fibers usually originate from the roof of the intercondylar fossa, and hence are purely aligned in the sagittal plane. These fibers, however, are missing in the elephant knee. Thus, all *PCL* fibers are oblique, which explains the greater extent of screw-home rotation.

1.3.6. *Pigs*

Porcine models are rarely used to study ligament reconstructions, probably due to the high costs associated with those experiments. Nevertheless, Fuss *et al.*[42] found that the porcine *AM* bundle exhibits more torque than the human's knee.

To summarize, large animal models are a very valuable tool for developing and testing new surgical procedures. Choosing an appropriate large animal model for a certain surgical procedure, or development of an *ACL* substitute, is essential for the correct interpretation of the outcome and the translation into the human model. However, regarding the evaluation of the bio-functionality of *ACL* substitutes, the quadruped model could be inappropriate.

2. ACL Injury

Injury to the *ACL* of the knee is potentially devastating for the patient and can result in both acute and long-term clinical problems. *ACL* injuries create disruptions in the balance between joint mobility and joint stability, which can lead to abnormal transmission of forces throughout the joint, resulting in damage to other structures in and around the joint.

Understanding the structure and function of injured ligaments becomes more complicated due to the variability and unpredictable nature of ligament healing. This may be due to the dramatic physiological and structural changes that ligaments sustain as a result of injury, as well as the complex and the dynamic cellular processes that occur during healing. Consequently, the *ACL* has always been and continues to be the subject of great interest to orthopedic scientists and to clinicians worldwide. In terms of biomechanics, there are two types of *ACL* injury: Contact or trauma *ACL* injury together with a non-contact *ACL* injury. Contact/trauma injury occurs when excessive tension is applied on the *ACL* due to an exterior force, while non-contact injury appears when a person generates excessive loading or momentum on the *ACL* without external contact.

2.1. *Epidemiology*

ACL injuries are extremely common, with estimates as high as 400,000 patients each year in the United States sustaining this injury (in comparison with 120,000 patients undergoing hip replacement surgery).[43]

The great majority of *ACL* tears occur from non-contact athletic injuries. According to the National Collegiate Athletic Association injury surveillance system, which has tracked all injuries associated with United States college athletics since 1988, American football players sustain the greatest number of *ACL* tears, but these are predominately contact injuries. Female athletes sustain higher rates of *ACL* injury per athletic exposure across sports.[44,45] One athlete participating in a single game or in a practice equals one exposure. Among skiers, recreational alpine skiers have the highest incidence of *ACL* rupture, while expert recreational skiers the lowest.[46] Competitive alpine skiers sustain *ACL* injuries at a high rate.[47] It is reported that participants in women's ice hockey and men's baseball have a low incidence.[48] In a retrospective study of *ACL* injuries in professional hockey players, the incidence of this injury has been shown to be infrequent compared with other professional sports.[49]

2.2. *Clinical Needs*

The acute *ACL* injuries further lead to instability and to degenerative diseases including *OA*, meniscus and knee cartilage tears.[50] Lacking significant vascularization and envelopment by synovial tissue cause poor intrinsic healing capacity for *ACL*.[51]

With the recognition of *ACL* injury, came the realization that untreated *ACL* tears often caused progressive deterioration of the knee with instability and damage to the menisci and cartilage.[52,53] Surgical treatments are, therefore, crucial to substitute the symptomatic unstable ligament with various grafts.[54] With the current state of the art in *ACL* reconstruction, multiple techniques have been presented but none has shown clearly defined and improved results.

2.3. *Sport ACL Injuries*

Acute injuries are more frequently related to sports injuries, with the *ACL* the most affected to rupture in the knee joint. Probably most common in football, torn *ACLs* also occur in baseball, soccer, basketball, track and field, tennis ... basically all high-impact, fast-paced sports. Repetitive trauma, traumatic or chemically induced injury and disuse have been described as major causes for pathogenic conditions. Internal rotation of the hip may contribute to knee valgus and internal rotation of the tibia causes significant increases in the *ACL* strain. Current knowledge of *ACL* injury mechanisms in male football players is limited. The *ACL* injury in professional athletes can cause long lay-offs from sports and may be career-threatening.[55] On average, one player suffers an *ACL* injury every second season in a professional men's football team squad.[56]

Recently, Walden *et al.*[57] described the *ACL* injury mechanisms, particularly the playing situation, the player–opponent behavior and the biomechanics in male professional football players based on systematic video analysis. Around 85% of the *ACL* injuries resulted from non-contact or from indirect contact mechanisms. These authors identified three main playing situations for these injuries: (1) pressing, (2) re-gaining balance after kicking, and (3) landing after heading. Regardless of the playing situation, the professionals frequently observed knee valgus, but they rarely saw an overt dynamic valgus collapse. In contrast, a dynamic valgus collapse was obvious in all three tackling-induced direct contact *ACL* injuries.

Thus, it seems that a majority of *ACL* injured athletes are likely to have a relatively straight knee at the time of injury. Vertical compression at a straight knee has previously been shown to load the *ACL* through the anterior tibial drawer and internal rotation.[58]

Running is one of the most common sports that gives rise to overuse injuries of lower back and the leg.[59] The predominant site of leg injuries is the knee, for which the location-specific incidence ranged from 7.2% to 50.0%.[60] Poorly perfused tissues, such as ligaments, tendons and cartilage, are particularly at risk because they adapt more slowly than muscles to increased mechanical load.[61] Hreljac *et al.*[59] suggested that injury should be avoided not by minimizing the stress applied to a biological structure, but by optimizing the amount and the frequency of loading stress. Given the dynamic nature of the relationship between applied stress and injury, there must be an optimal level of applied stress for any biological structure.

Overuse injuries of the musculoskeletal system generally occur when a structure is repeatedly exposed to loading forces. Forces lower than the threshold associated with acute injury ultimately lead to fatigue of that specific structure.[62,63] There is no standard definition of overuse running injury,[59,64] but it should minimally include a musculoskeletal ailment that can be attributed to running and that causes a restriction of running speed, distance, duration or frequency for at least a week.[59]

Olsen *et al.*[65] identified two main injury mechanisms for *ACL* injuries in team handball. The most common (12 of 20 injuries), a plant-and-cut movement, occurred in every case with a forceful valgus and external or internal rotation with the knee close to full extension. The other main injury mechanism (4 of 20 injuries), a 1-legged jump shot landing, occurred with a forceful valgus and external rotation with the knee close to full extension. The results from the video analysis and questionnaire data were similar.

ACL injury caused by trauma or by contact sport only accounts for about 30% of *ACL* injuries. The remaining 70% of *ACL* tears are from non-contact injuries.[66,67] Risk factors such as age,[67] gender,[68,69] bodyweight,[70] and genetics[71] are involved in the pathogenesis of non-contact ligament ruptures. Histological examination of degenerative *ACL* has been shown to be associated with an increase in cell number, in the disorientation of collagen fibers, with inflammation and with glycosaminoglycans accumulation and chondroid metaplasia.[67] Chondroid metaplasia is characterized by cells becoming more rounded with the chondroid transformation that is being arranged in chains.[72–74]

3. Injury Mechanism

The mechanism for *ACL* injuries is still misunderstood, and research continues to determine critical factors for prevention. As mentioned in the previous section, it can be direct (trauma or physical contact) or indirect. Commonly, *ACL* tears occur with an abrupt landing, associated with a rapid change of direction with the knee in a semi-flexed position with valgus and varus stress and internal to external rotation. The mechanisms of ligament injuries depend on both intrinsic and extrinsic factors. Contact or direct trauma, structural vulnerability, and rapid growth are some intrinsic factors that lead to *ACL* injuries, subsequent instability, abnormal loading patterns and the development of *OA*.[75]

Neuromuscular control deficit during dynamic movements has been hypothesized to be the primary cause for both primary and secondary *ACL* injury risks (re-injury following *ACL* reconstruction). The deficit in dynamic active neuromuscular control manifests as excessive joint loads and leads to detrimental *ACL* stress/strains and ultimate failure. Non-contact *ACL* injury mechanisms are multiplanar in nature, involving the tibiofemoral joint articulation in all three anatomical planes. Previous studies have identified combined multi-planar loading, including anterior tibial shear, knee valgus and internal tibial rotation, to be the worst-case scenario and primary mechanism of non-contact *ACL* injury.[76]

Female athletes sustain a twofold to an eightfold greater rate of injury than their male counterparts.[77] Recent videotape analyses demonstrate significant differences in average leg and trunk positions during injury compared with control subjects. These findings as well as cadaveric and *MRI* studies indicate that axial compressive forces are a critical component in non-contact *ACL* injury. A complete understanding of the forces and risk factors associated with non-contact *ACL* injury should lead to the development of improved preventive strategies for this devastating injury.

Serious injuries have not decreased in men's professional football in the past decade, and prevention of *ACL* injury is a priority area within sports medicine/physiotherapy research.[78] Understanding the injury mechanisms is a key factor in injury prevention research.[79]

To better understand the mechanisms of *ACL* injury, some authors have examined the evolution of ligaments, the animal model and the biomechanical modeling. Understanding a biomechanical system as complex as the human knee may be made easier by studying the structure of the analogues in the limbs of other animals.

Can the biological evolution of the knee joint and ligament explain why human *ACL* injuries are so common? Is it because Homo sapiens never fully completed human adaptation to bipedalism? One of the reasons the *ACL* is so vulnerable to tearing is that it is forced to endure much more strain than it is really designed for. However, Alexander[80] argued that the low safety factor of ligaments and tendons is compensated by the ligament-muscles reflexes protection since mechanoreceptors were found in all knee ligaments including *ACLs*.[81]

In quadrupeds, the strain of running and jumping is spread among four limbs and the muscles absorb most of it. When human ancestors transitioned to walking on just two feet, however, the strain placed on the legs doubled, since it was being spread over half as many limbs. This was too much for the muscles by themselves, so human bodies recruited the bones to help with the strain. As a result, the legs became straightened so that the bones could bear most of the impact and strain. Compare a standing human to a standing ape: human legs are fairly straight, while apes' legs are bow-legged and usually bent. For weight-bearing, they use their muscles more, and humans use their bones more.

This straight-leg arrangement works out okay for normal walking and running. The problem comes in when one tries to make sudden shifts in the weight strain on one's knees. When one stops suddenly while running, or when one makes a sharp turn at high speed, the human knee must bear the force of this sudden, intense strain.

Sometimes, the *ACL* is simply not strong to hold the leg bones together as it twists or it pulls away from the bones under the force of body momentum, and so frequently it tears.

Making matters much worse, humans as a species are getting heavier, making their momentum even greater during those sudden shifts. This is especially true for athletes, who now weigh more than ever before, and who also make lots of sudden high-speed weight shifts. It seems that the knee is less than perfectly adapted for a bipedal posture and lifestyle, and the *ACL* frequently tears as a result.

In humans, the tibial plateau is perpendicular to the long axis of the tibia and is essentially a flat surface. In quadrupeds, the tibial plateau slopes downward anteriorly. Gravity pulls the femur down this slope, a motion discussed in veterinary literature as "tibial thrust". The *CCL* is reported to prevent this tibial thrust. In dogs, a steeper tibial plateau is correlated with an increased risk of *CCL* rupture.[82]

3.1. *New Universal Theory of Injury Prediction and Prevention*

The prediction and prevention of traumatic brain injury, spinal injury and musculo-skeletal injury is a very important aspect of preventive medical science. Recently, the Ivancevics[83] have proposed a new coupled loading-rate hypothesis as a unique cause of all above injuries. This new hypothesis states that the main cause of all mechanical injuries is the Euclidean Jolt, or SE(3)-jolt, which is an impulsive loading that strikes any part of the human body (head, spine or any bone/joint) — in several coupled degrees-of-freedom simultaneously. Remember that in dynamical systems in general, the coupling of variables may cause chaotic behavior. Indeed, without coupling, there is no chaos; with chaos meaning unpredictability and uncontrollability. This is related to the coupling of jerks and masses which causes injuries. Hence, it never goes in a single direction only. Also, it is never a static force. It is always an impulsive translational and/or rotational force coupled to some mass eccentricity. This is, in a nutshell, the Ivancevics' universal Jolt theory of all mechanical injuries.

To show this, based on the previously defined covariant force law, the Ivancevics have firstly formulated the fully coupled Newton–Euler dynamics of:

1. Brain's micro-motions within the cerebrospinal fluid inside the cranial cavity;
2. Any local intervertebral motions along the spine; and
3. Any local joint motions in the human musculo-skeletal system.

Then, from this, the Ivancevics have defined the essential concept of Euclidean Jolt, which is the main cause of all mechanical injuries. The Euclidean Jolt has two main components:

1. Sudden motion, caused either by an accidental impact or slightly distorted human movement.
2. Unnatural mass distribution of the human body (possibly with some added masses), which causes some mass eccentricity from the natural physiological body state.

3.2. *The Significance of the Jolt Theory for Ligament Injury*

As we live in a 3D space, one could think that motion of any part of the human body, either caused by an accidental impact or by voluntary human movement, "just obeys classical mechanics in six degrees-of-freedom: three translations and three rotations". However, these six degrees-of-freedom are not independent motions as it is suggested by the standard term "degrees-of-freedom" (DOF). These six motions of anybody in space are coupled. Firstly, three rotations are coupled in the so-called rotation group (or matrix, or quaternion). Secondly, three translations are coupled with the rotation group to give the full Euclidean group of rigid body motions in space. A simple way to see this is to observe someone throwing an object in the air or hitting a tennis ball: how far and where it will fly depends not only on the standard "projectile" mechanics, but also on its local "spin" around all three axes simultaneously. Every golf or tennis player knows this simple fact. Once the spin is properly defined, a "fully coupled Newton–Euler dynamics" is set — to start with.

The covariant force law for any biodynamical system (which was introduced earlier by Vladimir Ivancevic in his biodynamics books and papers) goes one step beyond the Newton–Euler dynamics and it states:

Euclidean Force co-vector field =
Body mass distribution × Euclidean Acceleration vector field

This is a nontrivial biomechanical generalization of Newton's fundamental definition of the force acting on a single particle. Unlike classical engineering mechanics of multi-body systems, this fundamental law of biomechanics proposes that forces acting on a multibody system and causing its motions are fundamentally different physical quantities from the resulting accelerations. In simple words, forces are massive quantities while accelerations are massless quantities. More precisely, the acceleration vector field includes all linear and angular accelerations of individual body segments. When coupling them all with the body's mass-distribution matrix of all body segments (including all masses and inertia moments), the force co-vector field, comprising all the forces and torques acting on the individual body segments can be obtained. In this way, the 6-dimensional Euclidean force for an arbitrary biomechanical system is defined.

Now, for prediction of injuries, it takes the rate-of-change (with respect to time) of the Euclidean biomechanical force defined above. In this way, the Euclidean Jolt will be obtained, which is the sudden change (in time) of the 6-dimensional Euclidean force:

Euclidean Jolt co-vector field =
Body mass distribution × Euclidean Jerk vector field

And again, it consists of two components: (i) massless linear and angular jerks (of all included body segments), and (ii) their mass distribution.

For the sake of simplicity, the mass distribution matrix includes all involved segmental masses and inertia moments, as well as "eccentricities" or "pathological leverages" from the normal physiological state. Therefore, the cause of all brain, spine and musculo-skeletal injuries has two components:

1. Coupled linear and angular jerks; and
2. Mass distribution with "eccentricities".

The Ivancevics have claimed that there are no injuries in static conditions without any mass eccentricities. All injuries are caused by coupled linear and angular jerks, which are also all coupled with the involved mass distribution. The Euclidean Jolt causes two forms of discontinuous brain, spine or musculo-skeletal injury:

1. Mild rotational disclinations; and
2. Severe translational dislocations (or, fractures).

The Ivancevics have developed the soft-body dynamics of biomechanical disclinations and dislocations, caused by the Euclidean Jolt, using the Cosserat multipolar viscoelastic continuum model.

According to this new universal theory, the main causes of knee injuries are the knee SE(3)–jolts, the sharp and sudden "delta" (forces + torques) combined. These knee SE(3)–jolts do not belong to the standard Newton–Euler dynamics. The only way to monitor them would be to measure "*in vivo*" the rate of the combined (forces + torques) rise in the knee joint.

In other words, a Euclidean jolt is the time derivative of the Euclidean force (three-dimensional force + three-dimensional torque). In the case of the knee, it happens when all the body mass is resting on one leg while the knee is semi-flexed and then, caused by some external shock, the knee "jerks"; this often happens in running, in skiing, in sports games (e.g. soccer, rugby) and in various crashes or impacts. The reason why this happens in this scenario is the following: in a semi-flexed position, the knee joint has all six DOF (Figure 7); if a sudden jerk with the full body mass hits the knee in this position, it will happen in all six DOF simultaneously, tearing apart the soft tissue.[83]

If the resulting jolt is of high intensity, then even the hard tissue will be damaged. To demonstrate this formally, based on the

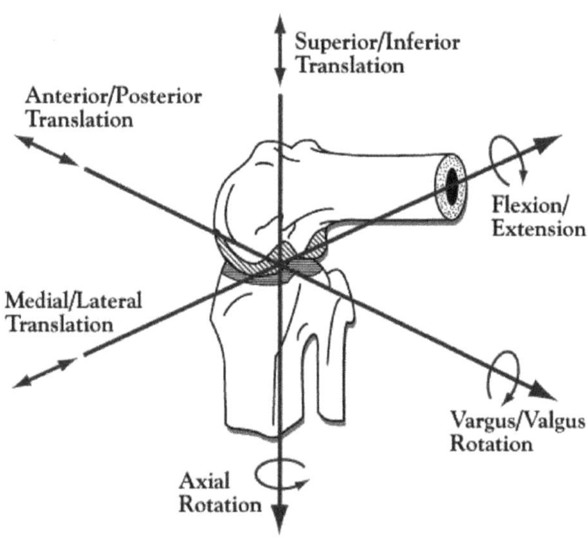

Figure 7. Six degrees of freedom (DOF) of knee flexion[84]

previously defined covariant force law, the coupled Newton–Euler dynamics of the knee motions was formulated and the corresponding coupled SE(3)-jolt dynamics derived from it. The effect of SE(3)-jolt can be seen in two forms of discontinuous knee injury: (i) mild rotational disclinations and (ii) severe translational dislocations. Both the knee disclinations and dislocations, as caused by the SE(3)-jolt, are described using the Cosserat multipolar viscoelastic continuum model. While we can intuitively visualize the knee SE(3)-jolt, for the purpose of whole human musculo-skeletal dynamics simulation, to avoid deterministic chaos caused by nonlinear coupling, it is necessary to use a simplified, decoupled approach (neglecting the 3D-torque matrix and its coupling to the 3D force vector). In this decoupled framework of reduced complexity, the following can be defined: the cause of knee dislocations is a linear 3D–jolt vector, the time rate-of-change of a 3D-force vector (linear jolt = mass × linear jerk). The cause of knee disclinations is an angular 3-axial jolt, the time rate-of-change of a 3-axial torque (angular jolt = inertia moment × angular jerk). This decoupled framework has been implemented in the Human Biodynamics Engine,[85] a high-resolution neuro–musculo–skeletal dynamics simulator (with 270 DOFs, the same number of equivalent muscular actuators and two-level neural reflex control), developed by Ivancevic at Defence Science and Technology Organization, Australia. This kinematically validated human motion simulator has been described in a series of papers and books.[86,87]

Using 35 players equipped with the *HITS*, linear acceleration, rotational acceleration, maximum jerk, impact duration and impact force were collected during practices and games. Overall, these athletes experienced maximum head jerks of 10.38 ± 9.92 m/s,[3] impact durations of 8.99 ± 3.01 ms, and impact force of 1314.88 ± 1023.36 N.[88]

In summary, using as an example a human knee joint, Ivancevic proposed a new coupled-loading-rate hypothesis, which states that a generic cause of any musculo-skeletal injury is a Euclidean jolt, or SE(3)-jolt, an impulsive loading that hits a joint in several coupled degrees-of-freedom simultaneously.

To prevent these injuries, professionals need to develop musculoskeletal jolt awareness. For example, never overload a flexed knee and avoid any kind of uncontrolled motions (like slipping) or collisions with external objects.

For example, it is common for soccer players to injure their knees and even tear a ligament. These injuries are not surprising considering all the footwork, cutting, jumping, sliding and running required on the soccer field, all of which put human bodies in vulnerable positions. Doing specific exercises to strengthen the thighs and wearing a soccer knee brace are ways to help reduce the chances of the soccer knee injury. The soccer knee brace should have the ability to control all possible impulsive knee loadings as well as external shocks.

3.3. *Injury Prevention: Braces*

Knee braces have been used by the sports medicine community to treat instability of the knee due to an *ACL* disruption, to protect an *ACL* graft, and to prevent knee ligament injuries during sport. Both functional and prophylactic braces are designed with the objective of allowing normal joint kinematics while limiting unwanted displacements and rotations between the tibia and the femur that might detrimentally strain a healing ligament or a graft or produce intra-articular injury. Subjective studies have shown that braces help most subjects with knee ligament injuries feel better and even improve athletic performance in those with torn knee ligaments; however, many athletes report that knee bracing hinders their performance and that braces migrate and slide out of position on the leg during activity.[89] Knee braces can be classified into three types: rehabilitation, prophylactic and functional knee braces:

1. Rehabilitation braces are designed to allow a protected range of motion of injured knees post-operatively.
2. Prophylactic knee braces (*PKBs*) are designed to prevent or to reduce the severity of knee injuries in the uninjured population. Their aim is to restrict excessive movement that might be harmful, complementing or reinforcing present ligaments.

3. Functional knee braces (*FKBs*) are braces designed to provide stability for unstable knees by reducing translation and rotation of the knee in patients who have already suffered an injury.

It was claimed that knee braces provide around 30% more resistance to forces applied to the knee ligaments during sporting activities. They offer extra support to previously injured knees and help prevent knee ligament injury and knee pain. Some studies suggest that braces can reduce the strain on the *ACL* during various movements, which may mean they can prevent *ACL* tear, but it is still very unclear if knee braces can prevent injuries. Many athletes wonder if wearing braces can prevent knee injuries. Therefore, there is a need for additional biomechanical and clinical research into the efficacy of knee bracing.

The current literature indicates that much more is known about *FKBs* than *PKBs*, likely due to the widespread use of functional knee bracing in post-operative care. *FKBs* are recommended in Anterior Cruciate Ligament Deficient (*ACLD*) patients and are biomechanically effective under low-loading conditions. They may not be as effective in high-loading conditions, such as athletic activity. Perhaps the most significant changes due to the application of the functional brace were altered muscle timing and activation patterns in *ACLD* knees during dynamic activities. *FKBs* may not mechanically stabilize the knee but instead alter proprioception and motor patterns of the lower-limb muscles, reducing the variability of tibial rotation and of the anterior tibial translation of the *ACLD* knee.

The use of *PKBs* to prevent knee injuries has long been a contentious area of research. Two published review articles on *PKBs* for prevention of knee injuries in football players concluded that data were not clear enough to make a recommendation for or against *PKBs*.[90,91] The best study to date of *PKBs* and *ACL* injury remains a prospective, randomized study of 1396 cadets playing intramural tackle football at the U.S. Military Academy.[92] This study showed that use of *PKBs* did not significantly decrease the severity of *ACL* and Medial Collateral Ligament (*MCL)* injuries. There was, however, a trend toward a reduced rate of less severe *ACL* and *MCL* injuries in athletes who used braces.[92] Based on the data published in that paper, the rate of *ACL* injury in the non-braced cadets was 3.0 times higher (95% CI: 1.0–9.2) than in braced cadets. Other large epidemiologic studies conducted to date have focused on the effectiveness of *PKBs* in reducing *MCL* injuries in the sport of football; however, these investigations have not dealt with the effect of bracing on the reduction of *ACL* injuries.[93–96] The efficacy of *PKBs* in preventing *ACL* disruptions remains an unanswered question.[97]

In conclusion, more research is needed to determine the effectiveness of both *PKBs* and *FKBs*. Although there are many kinds of knee braces in the market, there are very few serious studies demonstrating their performance. This situation is a strange reminder of the case of running shoes. Until 1972, when the modern athletic shoe was invented by Nike, people ran in very thin-soled shoes, had strong feet, and had a much lower incidence of knee injuries. In fact, there is no evidence that running shoes are any help at all in injury prevention. Recently, it has been reported that the very expensive running shoes sold (Nike earns 19 trillion dollars/year) have not been seriously studied. No scientific studies showing their benefits or performances, and that running barefoot is safer and more efficient.[98]

4. Healing of Ligaments

The *ACL* and the *PCL* have a central location inside the intra-articular joint while the *MCL* and Lateral Collateral Ligament (*LCL*) are located on the inner and outer sides of the knee joint (extra-articular). The two main intra-articular ligaments in the knee joint, *ACL* and *PCL*, connect the femur to the tibia. The *ACL* prevents too much forward movement of the leg (that is, the tibia sliding in front of the femur) and resists rotation of the tibia. The *PCL* prevents too much backward movement of the leg. Of these two ligaments, the *PCL* is stronger and is less susceptible to injury.

4.1. *Poor Healing Capacity of Intra-articular Ligaments*

The basic mechanisms of ligament healing, including the growth factor expression and cell line recruitment, are poorly understood.

The *ACL* has long been thought to have a poor healing capacity, with a substantially high rate of failure (40–100%), even after surgical repair using suture.[76] The hypovascular and the hypocellular nature of ligaments retard their self-regeneration capacities.[9] Ligament healing is characterized by the fibro-vascular scar that never attains the mechanical properties of the normal ligament, leading to a relatively high failure rate after the repair, especially in the setting of the *ACL* repair.

Following *ACL* injury, disruption of the thin synovial sheath of *ACL* causes blood dissipation in the synovial fluid. This dissipation hardens formation of localized hematoma and further provision of cytokines, growth factors and reparative cells at the injury site.[99] These cells, however, exhibit low mobility, proliferation, metabolic activities and matrix production tendency.[100] The higher matrix metalloproteinase activities and the poor adhesive strength of these cells diminish ligament self-healing.[101] The synovial fluid that surrounds the *ACL* washes away the blood clot that forms as an early bridge between the two torn ends of the ligament.

The unsatisfactory outcomes of the *ACL* primary repair have led to unanimous abandonment of suture repair and widespread adoption of *ACL* reconstruction. *ACL* reconstruction has remained the gold standard of care for *ACL* injuries, especially for young individuals and for athletes who aim to return to high-level sporting activities.[102,103] The injured *ACL* is typically reconstructed using different biological or synthetic grafts as discussed in Chapter 2 of this book.

The healing potential of the intra-articular and extra-articular knee ligaments is different. The intra-articular ligaments (*ACL* and *PCL*) are not known to heal when they are torn, while the extra-articular ligaments (*MCL* and *LCL*) usually heal spontaneously. This low capacity of the intra-articular ligaments to heal has long been attributed to the intrinsic differences in cell behavior and to the insufficient blood supply following injury. However, Kiapour and Murray (2014)[76] showed recently that the provisional scaffold (fibrin-platelet clot) found within the wound site of extra-articular ligaments was, in fact, missing in the *ACL*.[99] The prevention of clot formation is mainly due to the continuous flow of the synovial fluid within the knee joint, dispersing the blood as a hemarthrosis.[76] Kiapour and Murray further demonstrated that this lack of provisional scaffold leads to a decreased presence of critical *ECM* proteins and cytokines such as fibrinogen, fibronectin, *PDGF-A, TGF-β1, FGF-2* and von Willebrand's factor within the *ACL* wound site.

In order to test the hypothesis that the missing provisional scaffold was a key mechanism behind the failure of the *ACL* to heal, Kiapour and Murray (2014)[76] used a collagen-based scaffold to fill the gap between the two ends of the torn ligament. This bio-active scaffold was then used as a carrier for cells, growth factors and enzymes required to optimize tissue healing. In the first *in vivo* studies, platelets maintained with their physiological plasma were placed within the collagen-based scaffold, and the loaded scaffold was used to repair torn *ACL* using multiple established large animal models. These studies further demonstrated the improved biological and mechanical healing of the *ACL* using this novel bio-enhanced technique.[76]

In a 2012 randomized trial in a large animal model, the biomechanical outcome of bio-enhanced *ACL* repair was found to be equal to that of *ACL* reconstruction.[104] More importantly, while 80% of the knees treated with *ACL* reconstruction developed post-traumatic *OA* by one year post-operatively, *OA* was not seen in those knees treated with bio-enhanced repair within the same time period.[105]

4.2. *A New Paradigm in ACL Repair and Healing*

4.2.1. *Platelet-enriched Plasma (PRP)*

Platelet-enriched plasma (*PRP*), which was first used by oral surgeons to help regenerate bone and soft tissue in the jaw, is simple to produce and to deploy: the procedure includes extracting some blood from the patient, spinning it in a centrifuge to concentrate the platelets, and then injecting the resulting fluid into an injured joint or using it in combination with surgery. *PRP* is replete with growth factors and other substances that promote healing. Studies have so far shown that it can help heal inflamed tendons, such as "tennis elbow", and relieve pain in an arthritic joint; but whether it can effectively address the wide variety of problems for which it is used is not yet clear.

A newer biologic is made of bone marrow instead of blood and is richer in stem cells than *PRP*. It is similarly extracted from the patient (through a thin needle in the hip, under local anesthesia) and concentrated using a centrifuge. Bone marrow aspirate concentrate (*BMAC*) can be turned into a dense clot that serves as a blood-red spackle, which surgeons use to fill gaps in cartilage and to surround and to nurture grafted tissue.

Because *PRP* and *BMAC* come from the patient and go right back into the patient, they did not need to be approved by the Food and Drug Administration (*FDA*), and their use has spread rapidly without a lot of testing.

When the *MCL* tears, the two ends bleed, and the blood forms a provisional scaffold between the two torn ends where the tissue then grows into and heals itself. In the *ACL*, the ends bleed when it gets injured, but the blood can't solidify. It can't clot between the two ends of the ligament because of the fluid in the knee joint. So, basically, these two torn ends are washing around in this liquid instead of getting reconnected by a solidified blood clot.

Although the biologics (*PRP* and *BMAC*) appear to promote healing, they cannot generate a sturdy enough scaffold to repair a torn meniscus or an *ACL*. That is why researchers are trying out 3D printing and other innovations.[106] Murray *et al.* (2014)[106] developed a scaffold, basically like a sponge, that can be used to hold the blood between the two torn ends of the *ACL* long enough for the cells around and the tissue around to grow into it and reunite. The sponge-like material was made of proteins such as collagen that are found in connective tissue. The sponge is soaked in the patient's blood and then sutured between the two torn ends of the ligament, creating a temporary bridge for healing, much the way a blood clot would. It has worked so well in pigs that Murray *et al.*[106] have recently received *FDA* approval to try this in the first set of 10 patients. One especially hopeful finding comes from pigs: those treated with the new technique developed far less arthritis than those given traditional *ACL* reconstruction.

4.2.2. *Scarless Healing*

Given that ligament has so little regenerative capacity, the concept of scarless healing is very compelling. If mechanisms of true regenerative, scarless healing can be elucidated and applied to ligament tissue and to its attachment sites, many hope that this would be an answer to the current challenge of poor healing.

As discussed above, *PRP* is a sample of autologous blood with a concentration of platelets three to four times greater than the baseline. Its use is compelling, as platelets contain alpha granules which contain a multitude of growth factors that have a role in cell recruitment, proliferation and angiogenesis. There are several different preparations commercially available.[107]

One of the barriers to the usefulness of *PRP* may be the timing of delivery of the growth factors. Once the *PRP* is activated, the alpha granules release the factors within an hour. Most of these growth factors have a half-life of only a few minutes.[108] Most studies of tendon healing show a spike in cell proliferation, growth factor production and extracellular matrix production from seven to 14 days after injury and repair.[109]

Delivering the growth factors at the appropriate peak in metabolic activity is likely critical for success. Therefore, sustained delivery with the use of platelet-rich fibrin matrix is compelling[110] as this product contains the platelets in an absorbable fibrin matrix, providing a slow, and controlled a release of factors as the fibrin matrix absorbs. Nevertheless, further research is necessary to optimize the *PRP* used for ligament therapy. Indeed, challenging questions remain to be answered as raised by Buschmann and Bürgisser (2017).[111] Which growth factor is the most effective during natural wound healing; is it one or a cocktail of growth factors that control this healing? Moreover, the choice of the appropriate scaffold/delivery system with the sustained release kinetics and dose should be determined.

In these regards, a better understanding of the mechanisms underlying scarless fetal wound healing could stimulate a bio-inspired approach. It is well known that the early-gestation fetus of mammals can heal skin wounds by tissue regeneration without scar formation.

It has long been thought that the absence of an inflammatory response during early gestation is an important factor that allows tissue regeneration ("scarless healing"). However, once a functioning immune system develops in later gestation, the inflammatory response to wounding leads to healing via a scar-mediated pathway. Although there are other factors that govern the response to wounding in the fetus and lead to scarless healing, the absence of inflammatory response appears to play an important role.[112]

It would be instructive to understand the temporal and the spatial signals that recruit ligament stem cells, as well as the morphogenetic signals that direct embryonic ligament development in order to compare these processes to those that take place during the post-natal repair.

It is important at this point to remind that the healing process is a complex system that is difficult to understand by only experimental studies using the trial-and-error method. Biological processes, like living systems, are dynamic and open, exchanging matter and energy with the surroundings, and they undergo continuous metabolic activity, consisting of a multitude of interdependent biochemical reactions taking place, not at equilibrium, but rather in the vicinity, often exhibiting a steady-state behavior.

Cell metabolism consists of thousands of individual chemical and enzyme-catalyzed chemical reactions. These chemical reactions in living organisms occur in characteristically organized sequences, called metabolic pathways. There are two main types of metabolic pathways: (i) pathways which lead from large molecules (low oxidative state) to smaller molecules (high oxidative state); they are called catabolic pathways or catabolism; (ii) pathways which lead from small molecules (high oxidative state) to large molecules (low oxidative state) that are essential for the formation of cellular material and which are referred to as anabolic or as biosynthetic pathways, or anabolism. The main concept of catabolism is, therefore, to provide the cell with small molecules or precursors suitable for the biosynthesis of all major chemical constituents of the living cell with reductant and energy to carry out these endergonic and reducing reactions leading towards compounds of low oxidative state. Whereas all catabolic pathways are oxidative and thus energy-producing, the biosynthetic pathways are reductive and energy-consuming. Metabolism consists therefore entirely of energy transformation and transfer mechanisms, which are based on thermodynamics.

The exact nature of the catabolic processes and tissue remodeling that occur during soft tissue repair and the mechanism of tissue remodeling that are essential to appropriate regeneration of the injured ligaments are only partially understood. Recent studies have shown that the attenuation of early phases of initial tissue remodeling by matrix metalloproteinase-9 (*MMP9*) leads to fewer adhesions and scar tissue development in a murine model of the flexor digitorum longus tendon injury. It was speculated that the continued presence of *MMP9* promotes the uncontrolled synthesis of fibrotic tissue.[112] Thus, *MMP9* not only has direct effects on the accumulation of extracellular matrix, but also has effects on mediating inflammatory response and local stem cell differentiation. *MMP2* and *MMP14* are also seen during fracture healing and are sequentially expressed as cartilage is resorbed. They also appear to be expressed late in tendon healing during the subsequent active remodeling, and reorganization phase of healing, after around 21 days.[112] This suggests that *MMP2* and *MMP14* were involved in the transition from fibroblastic granulation tissue to a more organized collagen structure.

4.2.3. *Nitric Oxide*

Nitric oxide (*NO*) is a short-lived free radical with an unpaired electron. Although a factor released by vascular endothelial cells that relaxes the surrounding smooth muscle cells was initially termed endothelium-derived relaxing factor (*EDRF*), in 1987 Murad F., Ignarro L.J., and Furchgott R.F. discovered that *EDRF* was *NO*.[113] *NO* is a tasteless and odorless gas that is capable of penetrating the cell membrane, and exerts its effects without the use of a receptor, thereby representing a new signaling pathway for intercellular communication. The Nobel Prize (1998) was awarded to Murad F., Ignarro L.J., and Furchgott R.F. for the discovery that *NO* is a signaling molecule.[114,115] Since *NO* is a gas, difficulties were associated with determining its localization and its production in the body; however, the discovery of nitric oxide synthase (*NOS*), which plays a role in the synthesis of *NO* from l-arginine, accelerated understanding of the expression and function of *NOS* in the body. Using purification and cloning methods, three *NOS* isoforms have been identified to date: *nNOS*, *iNOS*, and *eNOS*.[116]

NO is believed to be mainly a catabolic player in joint physiology.[117] In pathological situations such as *OA*, additional reactive molecules, so-called reactive oxygen species (*ROS*), are abnormally produced and contribute directly or indirectly to cartilage degradation, *MMP* activation and cell death induction. *MMPs* play a key role in the progression of various joint diseases and they influence joint inflammation as well as matrix degradation. Most actions of *MMPs* in joints are catabolic in nature. Various studies have detected *MMPs* in *CCL* tissue during aging, degeneration, or in torn *CCLs*. *CCL* has been shown to produce more *NO* compared to other ligaments. *In vitro* experiments have demonstrated that different *NO* donors induce apoptosis in *CCL* cells.

Ligament fibroblasts are actively involved in *ECM* homeostasis. *CCL* fibroblasts produce substantial amounts of *NO* under a specific stimulus.[134] Interestingly, normal *CCL* produces more *NO* compared to torn *CCL*, to normal cartilage or to normal *MCL* of the stifle in dogs.[118]

Recent findings of a study using a novel canine model revealed that synovial debridement of *CCL* has detrimental effects on clinical signs such as pain, and on effusion function, as well as histology.[119] High *NO* concentrations could, therefore, be a reason for the insufficient healing capacities of ruptured *CCL* in humans and in dogs. Moreover, high *NO* concentrations in canine *CCL* may contribute to matrix homeostasis disturbance such as inhibition of normal collagen synthesis, leading to an intrinsic weakness of the ligament. *In vitro* experiments have demonstrated that different *NO* donors induce apoptosis in *CCL* cells.[120] *CCL* apoptosis is influenced by inhibition of caspase-3 and is attenuated by treatment with *ROS* scavengers or a tyrosine kinase inhibitor.[121]

All the above-described observations correspond with the theory that an initial event leads to inflammation of the cruciate ligament complex.[122] Ligament fibroblasts develop a dysregulation of matrix homeostasis as a reaction in the inflammatory stimulus, including upregulation of matrix production, and peroxynitrite-induced premature ligament fibroblast death.

Mounting evidence indicates that an appropriate concentration of *NO* at the injury site is favorable for tissue repair, while deficient endogenous *NO* production could hamper the recovery process.[123] Exogenous supplementation of *NO* could be the best way to cope with the problem of *NO* deficiency. Curative effects showed that localized and well-timed *NO* replenishing in an on-demand manner could be a superior strategy to promote tissue repair compared to spontaneous *NO* release.

In tendon healing, experiments performed during the last 20 years showed similar effects as in ligament, i.e. that *NO* is induced by all three isoforms of *NOS* after tendon injury and that *NOS* activity is upregulated in tendinopathy. Though *NO* is found only sparingly in healthy tendon tissue, its production is ramped up significantly following an injury, either an acute tendon injury, like a rupture, or an overuse injury like tendonitis.

Innovative research by Bokhari and Murrell (2012)[124] has demonstrated that, when rats with tendon injuries are fed a drug which inhibits *NO* production, their tendons heal worse than rats healing naturally. And when injured rats are fed a drug that increases *NO* production, their tendons heal stronger and better-organized than rats who are not. Further, the role of *NO* in tendon injury extends to humans as well. Bokhari and Murrell (2012)[124] evaluated samples of torn rotator cuff tendons that were to be discarded following surgical repair and found that *NO* was very common in these injured tendons, too. Bokhari and Murrell (2012)[124] instigated human trials using nitroglycerin patches to deliver *NO* to injured tendons. The patches were ideal because they can be positioned over the most painful area of the tendon, and because they deliver a continuous amount of the drug throughout the course of a day. Bokhari and Murrell (2012)[124] tested nitroglycerin patches as a supplemental treatment to normal physical therapy for lateral epicondylitis (tennis elbow), supraspinatus tendinopathy (shoulder tendonitis) and Achilles tendonitis over a period of six months. All three trials used control groups with placebo patches, and all three found significant benefits several weeks after the patients began to use the nitroglycerin patches. Results a few years out were varied; the Achilles tendonitis patients who had used the nitroglycerin patches for six months continued to be better off than the placebo group at three years out, but there were no differences between the lateral epicondylitis groups five years out.

However, the major problem with its application in clinical settings is the high reactivity of *NO*, which makes it difficult to supply *NO* with spatiotemporal accuracy while maintaining its bioactivity. To deliver *NO* at a specified rate to a preferred location for a precise period is highly demanded. The significant technological advancements in controlled release make it possible to manage *NO* delivery at the target site with a sustained release rate and an optimum concentration, and then to provide a longer therapeutic duration of *NO*. Recently, the authors of this chapter developed Fe_3O_4/silica core/shell nanoparticles in their laboratory and their functionalization with S-nitrosothiols capable to deliver exogenous *NO* into human alveolar epithelial cells.[125] Moreover, these nanoparticles act as large storage reservoirs of *NO* that can be targeted magnetically to the specific site with a sustainable release of *NO* for up to 50 h. Such nanoparticles provide an enhancement of the biocompatibility with released *NO*, while allowing intracellular accumulation ascribed to their small size.

5. Concluding Remarks

The primary function of the *ACL* is to control anterior translation of the tibia. The *ACL* bundles also play different roles in controlling rotational motion and stability of the knee joint due to the differences in their attachment areas and orientation. The screw-home mechanism, considered to be a key element to knee stability for standing upright, is the rotation between the tibia and femur.

Due to new trends, such as the concept of anatomical reconstruction, which gained power in the last decade, new motivation has been given to the study of this ligament, with important advances and innovations. Therefore, this update on the *ACL* highlighted some of the most interesting and current topics on the subject.

Choosing an appropriate large animal model for a certain surgical procedure, or development of an *ACL* substitute, is essential for the correct interpretation of the outcome and for the translation into the human model. Translational animal models including mouse, rabbit, goat, sheep, pig, dog and horse, have been used to study the human knee structures. However, regarding the evaluation of the bio-functionality of *ACL* substitutes, the quadruped model could be inappropriate.

Injury to the *ACL* of the knee is potentially devastating for the patient and can result in both acute and long-term clinical problems. *ACL* injury caused by trauma or by contact sport only accounts for about 30% of *ACL* injuries. The remaining 70% of *ACL* tears are from non-contact injuries. The mechanism for *ACL* injuries is still misunderstood, and research continues to determine critical factors for prevention. Can the biological evolution of the knee joint and ligament explain why human *ACL* injuries are so common? Is it because Homo sapiens never fully completed human adaptation to bipedalism? One of the reasons the *ACL* is so vulnerable to tearing is that it is forced to endure much more strain than it is really designed for. Is it because intense physical activities overload our capacity, i.e. supra-physiological activities?

Recently, a new coupled-loading-rate hypothesis states that a generic cause of any musculo-skeletal injury is a Euclidean jolt, an impulsive loading that hits a joint in several coupled DOF simultaneously. Informally, it is a rate-of-change of joint acceleration in all six DOF simultaneously, times the corresponding portion of the body mass. In the case of a human knee, this happens when most of the body mass is on one leg with a semi-flexed knee — and then, caused by some external shock, the knee suddenly “jerks”; this can happen in running, in skiing, in sports games (e.g. soccer, rugby) and in various crashes/impacts.

To prevent these injuries, professionals need to develop musculo-skeletal jolt awareness. Although there are many kinds of knee braces in the market, there are very few serious studies demonstrating their performance. More research is needed to determine the effectiveness of both *PKBs* and *FKBs*.

The basic mechanisms of ligament healing, including the growth factor expression and cell line recruitment, are poorly understood. Ligament regeneration most often ends up in poor fibrous scar-like tissue lacking the collagen organization seen in normal healthy tissues. Given that ligament has so little regenerative capacity, the concept of scarless healing is very compelling. If mechanisms of true regenerative and scarless healing can be elucidated and can be applied to ligament tissue and its attachment sites, that would be an answer to the current challenge of poor healing. Substantial research is necessary before this can be achieved.

A sponge-like material made of proteins such as collagen that are found in connective tissue is suggested to promote the healing. The sponge is soaked in the patient's blood and then sutured between the two torn ends of the ligament, creating a temporary bridge for healing, as a blood clot would.

Finally, mounting evidence indicates that an appropriate concentration of *NO* at the injury site is favorable for tissue repair, while deficient endogenous *NO* production could hamper the recovery process. Exogenous supplementation of *NO* could be the best way to cope with the problem of *NO* deficiency. The role of *NO*, however, is less simple and needs to be further elucidated.

Acknowledgments

The authors would like to acknowledge the financial support from the Natural Sciences and Engineering Research Council of Canada (NSERC). Authors are also grateful to Ms. Amel Belhaoua for the encouragement and Ms. Sandrine Ypperciel for suggesting valuable corrections.

References

1. Markolf, K. L.; Mensch, J. S.; Amstutz, H. C. *J. Bone. Joint. Surg. Am.* **1976**, *58*(5), 583.

2. Fu, F. H.; Bennett, C. H.; Lattermann, C.; Ma, C. B. *Am. J. Sports. Med.* **1999**, *27*(6), 821.
3. Kennedy, J. C.; Alexander, I. J.; Hayes, K. C. *Am. J. Sports. Med.* **1982,** *10*(6), 329.
4. Riechert, K.; Labs, K.; Lindenhayn, K.; Sinha, P. *J. Orthop. Sci.* **2001**, *6*(1), 68–74.
5. Luzo, M. V. M. *et al. Rev. Bras. Ortop.* **2016**, *51*(4), 385–395.
6. Yahia, L. H.; Drouin, G. *J. Mater. Sci.* **1988**, *23*, 3750–3755.
7. Woo, S. L.-Y.; Young, E. P.; Kwan, M. K. Fundamental studies in knee ligament mechanics. In: Daniel, D. *et al.* eds., *Knee Ligaments: Structure, Function, Injury and Repair* (New York, NY: Raven Press, **1990**).
8. Yahia, L. H.; Drouin, G. *J. Orthopaed. Res.* **1989**, *7*, 243–251.
9. Shirazi, A. N.; Chrzanowski, W.; Khademhosseini, A.; Dehghani, F. Anterior cruciate ligament: Structure, injuries and regenerative treatments. In: Bertassoni, L. E.; Coelho, P. G., eds., *Engineering Mineralized and Load Bearing Tissues* (Switzerland: Springer International Publishing, **2015**) pp. 161–186.
10. Beasley, L. *et al. Oper. Tech. Orthop.* **2004**, *15*, 5–19.
11. Girgis, F. G.; Marshall, J. L.; Monajem, A. *Clin. Orthop. Relat. Res.* **1975**, *Jan–Feb*(106): 216–231.
12. Arnoczky, S. P., *Clin. Orthop. Relat. Res.* **1983**(172), 19–25.
13. Amis, A. A.; Dawkins, G. P. *J. Bone. Joint. Surg. Br.* **1991**, *73*(2), 260–267.
14. Kurosawa, H. *et al. Clin. Orthop. Relat. Res.* **1991**, *265*, 233–240.
15. Sapega, A. A. *et al. J. Bone. Joint. Surg. Am.* **1990**, *72*(2), 259–267.
16. Palmer, I. *Clin. Orthop. Relat. Res.* **2007**, *454*, 17–22; discussion 14.
17. Prodromos, C. *et al. The Anterior Cruciate Ligament: Reconstruction and Basic Science.* 2nd Edition (Elsevier, **2018**).
18. Colombet, P. *et al. Orthop. Traumatol. Surg. Res.* **2012**, *98*(8 Suppl), S201–S210.
19. Zantop, T. *et al. Am. J. Sports. Med.* **2007**, *35*(2), 223–227.
20. Ziegler, C. G. *et al. Am. J. Sports. Med.* **2011**, *39*(4), 743–752.
21. Amis, A. A. *Knee Surg. Sports Traumatol. Arthrosc.* **2012**, *20*(4), 613–620.
22. Moewis P. *Understanding Rotational Joint Laxity in the Human Knee.* Thesis (Berlin, **2016**).

23. Lovejoy, C. O. *Gait Posture.* **2007**, *25*(3), 325–341.
24. Fu, F. H.; Harner, C. D.; Johnson, D. L.; Miller, M. D.; Woo, S. L.-Y. *J. Bone. Joint. Surg. Am.* **1993**, *75*-A, 1–12.
25. Ruth, A. A. *Comparative Anatomy of the Anterior Cruciate Ligament and Its Associated Structures in Primates: A Study of Body Size, Bundle Number, and Bipedality* (Kent State University, **2016**).
26. Fuss, F. *J. Anat.* **1992**, *180*(2), 297–304.
27. Zantop, T.; Herbort, M.; Raschke, M. J.; Fu, F. H.; Petersen, W. *Am. J. Sports Med.* **2006**, *35*, 223–227.
28. Kato, Y.; Ingham, S. J. M.; Maeyama, A.; Lertwanich, P.; Wang, J. H.; Mifune, Y.; Kramer, S.; Smolinski, P.; Fu, F. H.; *YJARS* **2012**, *28*, 247–254.
29. Yasuda, K.; van Eck, C. F.; Hoshino, Y.; Fu, F. H.; Tashman, S. *Am. J. Sports Med.* 2011, *39*, 1789–1799.
30. MacKay, J. W.; Whitehead, H.; Toms, A. P. *Clin. Anat.* **2014**, *27*, 1097–1102.
31. Li, G.; DeFrate, L. E.; Rubash, H. E.; Gill, T. J. *J. Ortho. Res.* **2006**, *23*, 340–344.
32. Tantisricharoenkul, G.; Linde-Rosen, M.; Araujo, P.; Zhou, J.; Smolinski, P.; Fu, F. H. *Knee Surg. Sports Traumatol. Arthrosc.* **2014**, *22*, 961–971.
33. Ferretti, M.; Levicoff, E. A.; Macpherson, T. A.; Moreland, M. S.; Cohen, M.; Fu, F. H. *Arthroscopy* **2007**, *23*(3), 278–283. https://doi.org/10.1016/j.arthro.2006.11.006.
34. Gregory, M. H.; Capito, N.; Kuroki, K.; Stoker, A. M.; Cook, J. L.; Sherman, S. L. *Arthritis* **2012**, *2012*, 1–14.
35. Cook, J. L.; Kuroki, K.; Visco, D.; Pelletier, J.P.; Schulz, L.; Lafeber, F. P. *Osteoarthr. Cartilage* **2010**, *18*(3), S66–S79.
36. Calmbach, W. L.; Hutchens, M. *Am. Fam. Physician* **2003**, *68*(5), 907–912.
37. Schaller, N. *Science in School* **2011**, *I*(21), Winter, 12–17.
38. Fuss, F. K. Helical axis surface of the knee joint. In: Bouisset, S.; Métral, S.; Monod, H., eds. Proceedings of the XIVth Congress of the International Society for Biomechanics Paris, International Society of Biomechanics, **1993a**, pp. 438–439.
39. Fuss, F. K. Helical axes – kinematic analysis, interpretation, and application. In: Magjarevic, R.; Tonkovic, S.; Bilas, V.; Lackovic, I., eds.

IFMBE Proceedings (Proceedings of the International Federation for Medical and Biological Engineering, vol. 1, Part II, **2001**) pp. 620–623. Zagreb: Croatian Medical and Biological Engineering Society.

40. Fuss, F. K. Kinematics of the knee after isometric single-bundle PCL reconstruction. Proceedings of the 2002 Combined Orthopaedic Meeting (25th Singapore Orthopaedic Association Meeting, 22nd Asean Orthopaedic Association Meeting, 5th Combined Meeting of Spinal and Pediatric Sections APOA, 7th Meeting of Knee and Sports Medicine Section APOA, 3rd Meeting of Asia Pacific Orthopaedic Society for Sports Medicine, Singapore: National University of Singapore, CDROM edition, **2002**).
41. Fuss, F. K.; Hamel, G.; Duval, N.; DeGuise, J.; Yahia, L. H. Altered knee kinematics after posterior cruciate ligament rupture and replacement by means of a ligament prosthesis. In: Yahia, L. H., ed. Proceedings of the 1st International Symposium on Advanced Biomaterials (SIBA 1997) *Montréal: École Polytechnique*, **1997**, 136.
42. Fuss, F. K. *J. Anat.* **1991**, *178*, 11–20.
43. Junkin, D. M.; Johnson, D. L.; Fu, F. H.; *et al.* Knee ligament injuries. In: Kibler W. B., ed. *Orthopedic Knowledge Update: Sports Medicine. Rosemont: American Academy of Orthopedic Surgeons*, **2009**. p. 136.
44. National Collegiate Athletic Association. NCAA Injury Surveillance System Summary. Indianapolis, Ind: National Collegiate Athletic Association; **2002**.
45. Agel, J.; Rockwood, T.; Klossner, D. *Clin. J. Sports Med.* **2016**, *26*, 518.
46. Prodromos, C. C.; Han, Y.; Rogowski, J. *et al. Arthroscopy* **2007**, *23*, 1320.
47. Pujol, N.; Blanchi, M. P.; Chambat, P. *Am. J. Sports Med.* **2007**, *35*, 1070.
48. Hootman, J. M.; Dick, R.; Agel, J. *J. Athl. Train* **2007**, *42*, 311.
49. Sikka, A. P. A.; Robby, S.; Dhami, R. B. S.; Dunlay, R.; Boyd, J. L. *Sports Med. Arthrosc.* **2015**, *23*(1), 17–21. doi: 10.1097/JSA.0000000000000044.
50. Petrigliano, F. A.; McAllister, D. R.; Wu, B. M. *Arthroscopy* **2006**, *22*(4), 441–451.

51. Mousavizadeh, R.; Backman, L.; McCormack, R. G.; Scott, A. *Rheumatology* **2015**, *54*, 318–323.
52. Waldén, M.; Krosshaug, T.; Bjørneboe, J.; Andersen, T. E.; Faul, O.; Hägglund, M. *Br. J. Sports Med.* **2015**, 1–10.
53. Niyibizi, C. *et al. Knee. Surg. Sports Traumatol. Arthrosc.* **2000**, *8*(5), 281–285.
54. Rice, R. S.; Waterman, B. R.; Lubowitz, J. H. *Arthroscopy* **2012**, *28*(4), 539–547.
55. Shah, V. M.; Andrews, J. R.; Fleisig, G. S. *et al. Am. J. Sports. Med.* **2010**, *38*, 2233–2239.
56. Waldén, M.; Hägglund, M.; Werner, J. *et al. Knee. Surg. Sports Traumatol. Arthrosc.* **2011**, *19*, 3–10. https://doi.org/10.1007/s00167-010-1172-7.
57. Thomeé, R.; Waldén, M.; Hägglund, M. *Br. J. Sports Med.* **2015**, *49*, 1422.
58. Meyer, E. G.; Haut, R. C. *J. Biomech.* **2008**, *41*, 3377–3383.
59. Hreljac, A. *Med. Sci. Sports Exerc.* **2004**, *36*, 845–849.
60. Van Gent, R.; Siem, D.; van Middelkoop, M.; van Os, A.; Bierma-Zeinstra, S. *et al. Br. J. Sports Med.* **2007**, *41*: 469–480
61. Walther, M.; Reuter, I.; Leonhard, T.; Engelhardt, M. *Orthopäde* **2005**, *34*, 3999.
62. Hreljac, A.; Marshall, R. N.; Hume, P. A. *Med. Sci. Sports Exerc.* **2000**, *32*, 1635–1641.
63. Stanish, W. D. *Med. Sci. Sports Exerc.* **1984**, 16, 1–7.
64. Rolf, C. *Scand. J. Med. Sci. Sports* **1995**, *5*, 181–190.
65. Olsen, O. E.; Myklebust, G.; Engebretsen, L.; Bahr, R. *Am J Sports Med.* **2004**, *32*(4), 1002–1012.
66. Cimino, F.; Volk, B. S.; Setter, D. *Am. Fam. Physician* **2010**, *82*(8), 917–922.
67. Hasegawa, A.; S. Otsuki, S.; C. Pauli, C.; Miyaki, S.; Patil, S.; Steklov, N.; Kinoshita, M.; Koziol, J.; D'Lima, D. D.; Lotz, M. K. *Arthritis & Rheumatism* **2012**, *64*(3), 696–704.
68. Harmon, K. G.; Ireland, M. L. *Clin. Sports Med.* **2000**, *19*(2), 287–302.
69. Posthumus, M.; September, A. V.; Keegan, M.; O'Cuinneagain, D.; Van der Merwe, W.; Schwellnus M. P.; Toth, A.; F. Cordasco (2000).

J. Gend. Specif. Med.: JGSM: the official journal of the Partnership for Women's Health at Columbia, **2000**, *4*(4), 25–34.

70. Uhorchak, J. M.; Scoville, C. R.; Williams, G. N.; Arciero, R. A.; Pierre, P. S.; Taylor, D. C. (2003). *Am. J. Sports Med.* **2003,** *31*(6), 831–842.
71. Posthumus, M.; September, A.V.; Keegan, M. *et al. Br. J. Sports Med.* **2009**, *43*, 352–356.
72. Vasseur, P. B.; Pool, R. R.; Arnoczky, S. P.; Lau, R. E. 1985, *Am. J. Vet. Res. 46*(9), 1842–1854.
73. Narama, I.; Masuoka-Nishiyama, M.; Matsuura, T.; Ozaki, K.; Nagatani, M.; Morishima, T. *J. Vet. Med. Sci.* **1996**, *58*(11), 1091–1097.
74. Comerford, E. J.; Tarlton, J. F.; Wales, A.; Bailey, A. J.; Innes, J. F. *J. Comp. Pathol.* **2006,** *134*(1), 8–16.
75. Rodrigues, M. T. *et al. J. Tissue Eng. Regen. Med.* **2012**, *7*(9), 673–686.
76. Kiapour, A. M.; Murray, M. M. *Bone Joint Res.* **2014,** *3*, 20–31.
77. Boden, B. P. *et al. J. Am. Acad. Orthop. Surg.* **2010,** *18*(9), 520–527.
78. Engebretsen, L.; Bahr, R.; Cook, J. L. *et al. Br. J. Sports Med.* **2014,** *48*, 1270–1275.
79. Bahr R.; Krosshaug, T. *Br. J. Sports Med.* **2005**, *39*, 324–329.
80. Alexander, R. M. *Sci. Prog.* **1981**, *67*(265), 109–130.
81. Yahia, L. H.;Newman, N. *Anat. Anz. Jena.* **1991**, *173*, 233–238.
82. Morris, E.; Lipowitz, A. J. *J. Am. Vet. Med. Assoc.* **2001**, *218*, 363–366.
83. Ivancevic, V.; Ivancevic, T. *Human-Like Biomechanics.* (Springer, Dordrecht, **2005**).
84. Komdeur, P.; Pollo, F. E.; Jackson, R. W. *Proc. (Bayl. Univ. Med. Cent.)* **2002**, *15*(3), 257–259.
85. Ivancevic, V.; Snoswell, M. *IEEE Trans. Sys. Man Cyber.B* **2001**, *31* (3), 319–330.
86. Ivancevic, V.; Beagley, N. *New Sci.* **2003**, p. 15, 9th August.
87. Ivancevic, V.; Ivancevic, T. *Geometrical Dynamics of Complex Systems.* (Springer, Dordrecht, **2006**).
88. Berliner, D. L.; Nabors, C. J. Jr. *J. Reticuloendothel. Soc.* **1967**, *4*, 284–313.
89. Greene, D. L.; Hamson, K. R.; Bay, R. C.; Bryce, C. D. *Am. J. Sport Med.* **2000**, *28*(4), 453–459. https://doi.org/10.1177/03635465000280040301.

90. Salata, M. J.; Gibbs, A. E.; Sekiya, J. K. *Sports Health* **2010**; 2(5): 375–379.
91. Pietrosimone, B. G.; Grindstaff, T. L. *et al. J. Athl. Train.* **2008**, *43*, 409–415.
92. Sitler, M.; Ryan, C. J.; Hopkinson, L. W.; Wheeler, L. J.; Santomier, J.; Kolb, L. R.; Polley, C. D. *Am. J. Sport Med.* **1990**, *18*(3), 310–315. https://doi.org/10.1177/036354659001800315.
93. Albright, J. P.; Powell, J. W.; Smith, W.; Martindale, A.; Crowley, E.; Monroe, J.; ... Marshall, J. *Am. J. Sport. Med.* 1994, *22*(1), 12–18. https://doi.org/10.1177/036354659402200103.
94. Albright, J. P.; Powell, J. W.; Smith, W.; Martindale, A.; Crowley, E.; Monroe, J.; ... Marshall, J. (1994). *Am. J. Sport Med.* 1994, **22**(1), 2–11. https://doi.org/10.1177/036354659402200102.
95. Hewson, G. F.; Mendini, R. A.; Wang, J. B.; *Am. J. Sport Med.* **1986**, *14*(4), 262–266. https://doi.org/10.1177/036354658601400403.
96. Teitz, C. C.; Hermanson, B. K.; Kronmal, R. A.; Diehr, P. H. *J. Bone. Joint Surg. Am.* **1987**, *69*(1), 2–9.
97. Najibi, S.; Albright, J. P. *Am. J. Sport. Med.* **2005**, *33*(4), 602–611. https://doi.org/10.1177/0363546505275128.
98. McDougall, C. *Born to Run* (New York: Vintage Books, A Division of Random House, Inc., **2011**).
99. Murray, M. M. *et al. J. Bone Joint Surg. Ser. A.* **2000**, *82*(10), 1387–1397.
100. Bray, R. C.; Leonard, C. A.; Salo, P. T. *J. Orthop. Res.* **2002**, *20*(5), 984–989.
101. Zhou, D. *et al. J. Orthop. Res.* **2005**, *23*(4), 949–957.
102. Hewett, T. E.; Di Stasi, S. L.; Myer, G. D. *Am. J. Sports Med.* **2013**, *41*, 216–224.
103. Musahl, V.; Becker, R.; Fu, F. H.; Karlsson, J. *Knee Surg. Sports Traumatol. Arthrosc.* **2011**, *19*(Suppl 1), S1–S3.
104. Vavken, P.; Fleming, B. C.; Mastrangelo, A. N.; Machan, J. T.; Murray, M. M. *Arthroscopy.* **2012**, *28*, 672–680.
105. Murray, M. M.; Fleming, B. C. *Am. J. Sports Med.* **2013**, *41*, 1762–1770.
106. Haslauer, C. M.; Proffen, B. L.; Johnson, V. M.; Murray, M. M.; *Wound Repair Regen.* **2014**, *22*, 103–110. doi:10.1111/wrr.12130.

107. Galatz, L. M.; Gerstenfeld, L.; Heber-Katz, E.; Rodeo, S. A. *J. Orthop. Res.* **2015**, *33*, 823–831.
108. Foster, T. E.; Puskas, B. L.; Mandelbaum, B. R. *et al. Am. J. Sports Med.* **2009**, *37*, 2259–2272.
109. Galatz, L. M.; Sandell, L. J.; Rothermich, S. Y. *et al. J. Orthop. Res.* **2006**, *24*, 541–550.
110. Rodeo, S. A.; Delos, D.; Williams, R. J. *et al. Am. J. Sports Med.* **2012**, *40*, 1234–1241.
111. Buschmann, J.; Bürgisser, G. M. *Biomechanics of Tendons and Ligaments.* (Woodhead Publishing, Elsevier Ltd, **2017**).
112. Loiselle, A. E.; Frisch, B. J.; Wolenski, M. *et al. PloS One.* **2012**, *7*(7), e40602.
113. Ignarro, L. J.; Buga, G. M.; Wood, K. S.; Byrns, R. E.; Chaudhuri, G. *Proc. Natl. Acad. Sci.* **1987**, *84* (24), 9265–9269. doi:10.1073/pnas. 84.24.9265.
114. Arnold, W. P.; Mittal, C. K.; Katsuki, S.; Murad, F. *Proc. Natl. Acad. Sci. USA.* **1977**, *74*, 3203–3207.
115. Ambea, K.; Watanabea, H.; Takahashib, S. *Jpn. Dent. Sci. Rev.* **2016**, *52*, 14–21.
116. Muir, P. D. *Advances in the Canine Cranial Cruciate Ligament.* 2nd ed. (Hoboken: Wiley Blackwell, **2018**).
117. Louis, E. *et al.* Vet. J. **2006**, *172*, 466–472.
118. Spreng, D.; Sigrist, N.; Jungi, T. *et al. Am. J. Vet. Res.* **2000**, *61*(5), 530–536. doi:10.2460/ajvr.2000.61.530.
119. Bozynski, C. *et al. J. Knee. Surg.* **2015**, *28*, 404–410.
120. Murakami, H.; Shinomiya, N.; Kikuchi, T.; Fujikawa, K.; Nemoto, K. *J. Orthop. Sci.* **2005**, *10*(1), 84–90.
121. Forterre, S.; Zurbriggen, A.; Spreng, D. *BMC Vet. Res.* **2012**, *8*, 40. https://doi.org/10.1186/1746-6148-8-40.
122. Hayashi, K. *et al. J. Am. Anim. Hosp. Assoc.* **2004**, *40*, 385–390.
123. Oplander, C.; Muller, T.; Baschin, M.; Bozkurt, A.; Grieb, G.; Windolf, J.; Pallua, N.; Suschek, C. V. *Nitric Oxide-Biol. Ch.* **2013**, *28*, 24–32.
124. Bokhari, A. R.; Murrell, G. A. C. *J. Shoulder. Elbow. Surg.* **2012**, Feb, *21*(2), 238–244.
125. Zhang, X. F.; Mansouri, S.; Mbeh, D. A.; Yahia, L.; Sacher, E.; Veres, T. *Langmuir.* **2012,** Sep 4, *28*(35), 12879–12885.

https://doi.org/10.1142/9789811204630_0002

Chapter 2

History of the Anterior Cruciate Ligament Prosthesis

Véronique Migonney

LBPS/CSPBAT, Institut Galilée, Université Paris 13 Sorbonne Paris Cité, 99 Avenue Jean Baptiste Clément 93430 Villetaneuse
veronique.migonney@univ-paris13.fr

Abbreviations

ACL	Anterior cruciate ligament
PA	Poly(amide)
PCL	Posterior cruciate ligament
PET	Poly(ethylene terephthalate)
pNaSS	Polystyrene sodium sulfonate
PP	Poly(propylene)
PTFE	Poly(tetrafluoroethylene)

1. Introduction

The history of anterior cruciate ligament (ACL) repair breaks down into stages that have been marked by significant advances. It can be presented in different ways depending on whether you are a surgeon, a chemist, a biomechanic or a biologist. Logically and by obviousness, orthopedic surgeons started this story, on which they have been working for more than a century. However, for the development of ligament prostheses, the contribution of biomaterials specialists is essential. Indeed, it will allow the development of new generations of synthetic ligament prostheses, which would be perfectly tolerated and bio-integrated. Biomaterials science proposed innovative solutions by roughing together the skills of surgeons, chemists, biologists and industrial partners to led advances in that field of research. Today biomaterial solutions such as ligament prostheses carry many hopes for patients who suffer from ligament rupture. This chapter is devoted to explain and summarize this peculiar history.

In the surgery point of view, the ACL reconstruction is today considered as a common act of the knee surgery. It can be carried out either by autologous ligamentoplasty or in the particular case of high-level athletes requiring a very fast recovering, by the implantation of a synthetic ligament prosthesis. However, despite the fact that the reconstruction of the ligament by autologous tissues still represents the "gold standard", ideas have abound to propose less invasive, less restrictive and less deleterious solutions for the knee stability after the ACL rupture. Indeed, the choice between the different ACL repair solutions has strongly evolved along time history of the ACL repair. This is partly explained by the mistakes and resounding failures that have stirred and marked the minds of the community of orthopedic surgeons and of the patients slowing down the innovations and progresses. This history is unique because it is strewn with more or less successful trials, but also with innovations that have had a hard time convincing surgeons and patients alike.

For a long time, solutions such as ACL reconstruction or replacement were not even considered but since the middle of the 19th to the beginning of 20th century surgeons have been highly interested in that pathology and started to improve the diagnosis and to propose solutions and practice to this knee surgery. Solutions to "repair" a broken ligament have evolved slowly for more than a century and in the recent years, we are witnessing a race towards the most innovative solution but it is it the most suitable? Then, it appeared interesting to go back to the first steps of the ACL repairing and follow its evolution that has been considerably agitated to finish by the latest innovations.

2. Context of the Anterior Cruciate Ligament Rupture

2.1. *The Major Role of the ACL in the Knee Joint*

Located in the center of the knee, the ACL opposes the tibia move forwards as well as an excessive internal rotation of the tibia relative to the femur. Almost concomitantly, the posterior cruciate ligament (*PCL*) opposes the tibia moving backwards. ACL and *PCL* play together a fundamental role in the knee stabilization and act as the "central pivot" of the knee articulation. Then, any damage or even partial rupture of one of the ACL or *PCL* ligament will compromise the stability of the knee joint.

2.2. *The Causes of ACL Rupture*

An ACL injury is usually caused by sudden hyperextension or torsion applied to the joint. Its frequency varies according to the practiced sport, the age and the sex of the patient: (i) the incidence may be particularly high in sports such as football and ski then affecting young people (ii) the incidence of rupture is 2–8 times higher in women than in men. Despite sports that represent around 70% of the ACL ruptures, 10% may be attributed to accidents at work and 20% to traffic and to everyday life accidents. Today, the ACL rupture is the most common pathology of the knee — especially in the context of sports practice — and the most commonly that requires clinical treatment. In USA and Europe, the prevalence of ACL rupture is 0.5–1 per 1000 inhabitants. The annual cost of such pathologies increases quickly and can become very high if we take into account that these ruptures are frequently associated to meniscus injuries. As an example, in the USA, for 25,0000 cases, the annual cost of ACL rupture treatments has been evaluated around 1 billion US dollars.

2.3. *The Particularity of the ACL and the Need to Find Repairing Solutions*

It is worthy to note that one of the peculiarities of the ACL, when compared to the other ligaments and tendons, is that it cannot regenerate itself when injured. Therefore, in addition to the problems of knee joint instability and generated pains and in the absence of clinical treatment, the progression to knee arthritis becomes inevitable. The functional sequelae make it almost obligatory, the use of repair solutions as ligamentoplasty, which is generally performed by tendon autograft. The use of auto-tendon is not without drawbacks and it induces important recovery times for professional and sports activities. In fact, the duration of hospitalization and rehabilitation may be evaluated to 6 to 9–12 months with a cost that critically depends on the country concerned.

Faced with the medical, economic and societal challenges represented by rupture of the ACL, the development of ligament prostheses appeared to offer the ideal solution reducing the rehabilitation to 3 weeks. The first generation of ligament prostheses appeared in the 1980s but unfortunately, it was a disaster that could have been avoided if knowledge in materials chemistry and biological response to biomaterials had been taken into account. This frustrating story contributed to slowdown and even stopped their use. In the recent years, innovative solutions led to second and third generations of ligament prostheses to make the artificial ligament returning to the front of the stage.

Today, ligamentoplasty remains the gold standard solution and many improvements in surgical techniques have and go on yielding excellent results. On the other side, the solutions provided by the ligament prostheses of the last generations would be able to make the minds move and bring progresses for the good of the patient. The history of the ligament prosthesis is amazing and interesting because it shows that at the beginning of the 20th century, one surgeon yet tried to implant the first ligament prosthesis, made of silk. At that time, the biomaterials knowledge was not born, and the host response not well understood. The first innovative implantation could not have been a success. It was no yet the time for ligament prostheses. It was not until more than a century before ligament prostheses were accepted.

3. The Different Stages of the Repairing Solutions

3.1. *Introduction*

As mentioned previously, the surgery of ACL reconstruction had a hard time winning. Indeed, when looking at the past, it is surprising to see how diagnostics and technics have struggled to impose themselves. Unfortunately, and despite the evolution of mentalities, the tremendous improvements of surgical techniques, the investment of researchers from the different domains such as chemistry, biology, biomechanics, it is almost still true today. Moreover, the proposed repairing solutions strongly vary from country to country. At the beginning of the 20th century, surgeons have been interested in ACL reconstruction and repair and their enthusiasm gave rise to many works of which some were as original as innovative. Mayo Robson,[1] Lange[2] and Hey Groes,[3] to name just a few, made extraordinary advances, which were not all exploited. Prior to them, the research work of surgeons focused more on the description of ligament rupture than its repair. Colombet *et al.*[4] in the *History of ACL Surgery* perfectly and precisely described this historical description. It was devoted to the different steps and progressions of the surgery of ACL rupture and repair from the surgeon point of view.[1] The step after concerns the development of ligament prostheses. The hopes they have generated and as much as the bitter defeats and the successes observed. This can be summarized in four generations of ligament prostheses.

3.2. *Early Stage: The Basics of Surgery*

The history of the ACL rupture and repair started in the middle of the 19th century when surgeons Bonnet[5] analyzed and precisely described the clinical signs of the ACL rupture. Thirty years after Noulis[6] precised the role of the ACL in the knee stability and proposed a test used today and known as "the Lachman test" which yet described how to assess the ACL integrity on the knee extension.

Between 1920 and 1940, the ACL surgery was mainly marked by the works of:

(i) **Hey Groes**[3,7] who described the anatomy and physiology of cruciate ligaments, their rupture and their repair based on the results from an interest number of operated patients;
(ii) **Campbell**[8] who was the first to use auto or allografts on patients — he yet reported nine operated patients with a very good result, i.e. returning to football 6–10 months after;
(iii) **Macey**[9] who described an innovative surgical technique using the semi-tendinous with a new approach where patients were allowed to practice physical activities after 8 weeks.

3.3. *Second Stage: Stabilization Technics and Diagnosis*

From 1940 to 1950, the development of the ACL surgery focused on the knee stabilization technics. Lindemann and Augustine[10,11] were the first to use lateral ligaments and semi-tendinous tendons in association with metallic wires and screws. In the same time, the diagnosis was more and more improved. Trillat from the School of Lyon taught the knee exam in the extended position and described the dry click when tibia moved slightly forward and receded. Ritchey precisely described the laxity test further named it the "Lachman test".[12]

Between 1960 and 1980 new techniques using the patellar tendon were developed and in particular the technics of Jones,[13,14] which is not the technique used today however. In 1969, it is noteworthy that Franke[15] was the first to use a free transplant made of patellar tendon and two patellar and tibial bone patches. In 1976, he reported over 100 cases of ACL and he recommended this operation early to prevent the occurrence of cartilage lesions. He also limited to 50 years the maximum age for an intervention. The 1970s plunged us back into doubt with the use of non-anatomic extra-articular replacement techniques: Lemaire[16] published only extra-articular ligament reconstruction techniques with discussed results.

4. First Generation of Ligament Prostheses

Despite the obvious progresses of the diagnosis of ACL rupture and of the techniques to replace the ruptured ligament, the surgical gesture stayed aggressive, the recovering was still long, the pain was frequent and the results were not enough reliable. From 1980, a new generation of surgeons decided to come back to some studies that proposed the use of reinforcement materials, interference screws as well as prosthesis and associate them with the arthroscopy technic to set up innovative solutions of ACL repair. To remember, Lange[2] started in the early 1900s the use of silk reinforcement, Corner in 1914 used silver wire and Rubin and Marschall implanted polyester prostheses.[17,18]

The idea of using synthetic ligament prostheses was relatively consecutive or parallel to the birth of the era of biomaterials and the success of different prostheses or implants such as total hip prosthesis, intra-ocular implants, and vascular prostheses. In the same time, the introduction of arthroscopy for ACL prosthesis implantation promised to revolutionize and to achieve a fast and minimally invasive surgery. These enthusiastic bets should have brought a renewal of ligament repair. Nevertheless, the lack of knowledge of the mechanical and physico-chemical properties of the materials used to weave, to braid or to knit fibers and to elaborate ACL prostheses led to disastrous choices and prostheses of poor quality. The resounding failures strongly marked orthopedic surgeons for decades. The worst choice remained that of using carbon fibers: Dandy[19] was the first to carry out the implantation of carbon fibers ACL prostheses under arthroscopy and these assays were associated to synovial and hepatitis carbon deposits.

In the 1980s, several polymer materials such as poly(ethylene terephthalate) (PET), poly(tetrafluoroethylene) (PTFE), poly(amide) (PA) and poly(propylene) (PP) were used for the elaboration of ACL prosthesis. Once again, the ignorance of these semi-crystalline polymers and their behavior in the form of fibers led to very disappointing results — an unacceptable rate of synovitis and ruptures — which condemned for a time the synthetic ligaments. During the same period, a number of surgeons remained faithful to autografts and began to use increasingly arthroscopy.[20,21]

Today, the usual surgical techniques rely on the replacement of ACL by an autologous transplant: the patellar tendon (Kenneth Jones technique) or the tendons of the internal and of the semi-tendinous right muscles (DIDT technique).

However, the use of an autograft is not without its drawbacks (morbidity due to tissue sampling, lack of anchorage of the graft to the bone level and failure rate still too high with an estimated failure rate of about 15%) and it results in significant recovery times for the resumption of sports activities (>6 months).

5. Second Generation of Ligament Prostheses

As the lesions of the cruciate ligaments represent a considerable public health issue, especially as they reach a young and active population and despite the failures of the first ligament prostheses, the need of ACL prostheses that reduces the iatrogenesis of the surgical procedure and provides immediate mechanical support was expected. This last solution had been proposed to high-performance athletes for whom the functional recovery must be fast and to patients with less frequent but more severe multilevel ligament lesions. In the latter case, the absence of a sufficient transplant can lead to the use of allografts presenting a risk of viral transmission or to the use of a synthetic ligament prosthesis as a healing tutor for the PCL. At the end, the development of a new generation of ACL prosthesis being able to reduce indirect costs associated with periods of functional re-adaptation and cessation of work was also an economic benefit.

During the years 1990–2000, a second generation of synthetic ligament was born and allowed to propose an innovative solution in this specific field. LARS society (Arc sur Tille, France) developed the LARS ligament prosthesis made of PET and constituted by an innovative and patented structure which perfectly mimic the natural ligament fibers in the intra-articular part of the prosthesis.[22,23] LARS still represents the second generation of the ligament prostheses and it is one of the most used artificial ligaments during the last 15 years. Cerulli *et al.*[24] and Lavoie *et al.*[25] published follow-up studies with excellent scores proving the reliability of the LARS ACL prosthesis.

6. Third Generation of Ligament Prostheses

The tremendous progresses in the understanding of the *in vitro* and *in vivo* biological responses to synthetic materials and implants opened the era of biocompatible, bioactive and smart biomaterials. It was not enough to get the required mechanical properties of one material to use it as an implant, the control of the interactions at the interface between a (bio) material and the living system was necessary.

LARS ligament made of PET gives good results and belongs to the family of PET artificial ligaments that have attracted the attention from the orthopedic surgeons wanting to find an attractive prosthesis solution. Nevertheless, despite the positive results of some PET ligaments as the LARS and its excellent mechanical properties, PET remains a hydrophobic polymer and it cannot allow the desired adhesion and controlled regrowth of fibroblast ligament cells along the fibers of the ACL prosthesis — thus, it is not biointegrated. Several advances to improve the performance of ACL ligaments on the ligament "biointegration" were proposed but the main part of them focused on the mineralization in the bone channel and not in the recolonization of the intra-articular part.

The improvement of the cell recolonization of the ligament fibers has not been studied — Migonney and — Brulez met this challenge and developed a surface chemical treatment of the PET fibers allowing the control of the biologic responses at the PET/protein/cell interface.[26,27] The covalent radical grafting of a bioactive polymer, the polystyrene sodium sulfonate (pNaSS) was set up and shown to induce the biointegration of the ACL prosthesis in the surrounding tissues.[28–33] The pNaSS grafted ligament prosthesis also called "LIGART" represent the third generation of ACL ligament: it is made of "bioactive" and "bio-integrable" PET.[34]

LIGART synthetic ligament is obtained by functionalizing the surface of the ligament prosthesis by radical grafting "from" process of pNaSS and it is characterized by the following elements:

- the improvement and control of the biological response *in vitro* and *in vivo*;
- the control of the inflammatory response;
- the improvement of the *in vivo* biomechanical behavior.

These very positive results obtained after more than 10 years of intensive research development were demonstrated *in vitro* and were validated *in vivo* in the large animal, the sheep (60 animals), in an experimental model of replacement of the ACL and in the dog in the framework of a clinical study at the Ecole Vétérinaire of Alfort (ENVA) by Viateau, in a model of spontaneous rupture of the ACL.[35] The first implantations in humans in a clinical trial are in progress by the team of Cerulli.

Although the "bioactive" and "biointegrable" ligament LIGART represents an advantageous and a rapidly functional solution for the replacement of the LARS ligament prosthesis, it can be considered as an "intermediate" solution for a particular patient population such as young patients due to the non-resorbable nature of the material.

7. Fourth Generation of Ligament Prostheses

In the recent years, ligament prosthesis has been of increasing interest to both the surgeon community and the research community. It is as if the story of the ligament would accelerate abruptly.

The first synthetic ligaments appearing in the 1980s had a very brief craze, quickly stopped by resounding failures due to the types of materials used. The LARS prosthesis appeared in the middle of the 1990s stopped much of the reluctance with regard to the ligament prosthesis.

LIGART ACL prosthesis aimed to propose a new generation of "bioactive and biointegrable" artificial ligaments and upset the concept of ligament prostheses by providing a perfectly integrated and accepted structure by the surrounding host tissues. However, it took more than a decade to develop and to start the clinical trial.

In light of this short history, the aim of the LIGA2BIO project is to propose the development of a bioactive and a biodegradable ligament of fourth generation, which combines the interests brought:

- by grafting the "bioactive" polymer, poly (sodium styrene sulfonate) onto a synthetic surface[36,37] to enhance the biological response and cell colonization[38];
- by the controlled biodegradability of the scaffolding which ensures the gradual replacement of the synthetic structure by a healthy, "regenerated" natural tissue[39];

- by improving the bone anchorage for a better integration in the bone tissue.

Through this approach, this project aims to lay a solid foundation for the creation of an implantable biodegradable medical device that takes into account the requirements of biocompatibility, sterilization, integrity that are essential for CE marking.

The challenge of offering "ligament prosthesis" able to be bioactive, LIGA2BIO project started in 2015 through a consortium headed by B. Brulez (LARS), V. Migonney (University Paris 13) and J. Tankere (MDB Texinov). This new prosthesis will allow (i) a rapid recovery of the patient's physical activities, (ii) avoiding hostile reactions from the host, (iii) removing the permanent character of the prosthesis.

8. Conflict of Interest Statement

Prof. Migonney is collaborating with LARS company since 2000.

Acknowledgments

The author thanks B. Brulez from LARS Company for the long and fruitful collaboration, V. Viateau and M. Manassero for the *in vivo* experiments they carried out with LIGART and LIGA2BIO prostheses on sheep, rat and dogs, G. Cerulli for his constructive discussions and his precious advices and all the colleagues who participated to the LIGART challenge.

References

1. Mayo Robson, A. W. *Ann. Surg.* **1903**, *37*, 716–718.
2. Lange, F. About the tendon plastic. *Verh. Dtsch. Orthop. Ges.* **1903**, *2*, 10–12.
3. Hey Groes, E. W. *Lancet* **1917**, *2*, 674–675.
4. Colombet, Ph.; Allard, M.; Bousquet, V.; Delavigne, C.; Flurin, P. H. *The History of ACL Surgery*, In *Orthopedic Mastery* No. 87, **1999**.

5. Bonnet, A. *Traité des maladies articulaires*, Vols 1&2 (Ed Baillère Paris, **1845**), pp. 354–357.
6. Noulis, G. *Sprained Knee. Doctoral Thesis n°* 142. Faculty of Medicine of Paris, **1875**, pp 1–53.
7. Hey Groes, E. W. *Br. J. Surg.* **1920**, *7*, 505–515.
8. Campbell, W. C. *Surg. Gynecol. Obstet.* **1936**, *62*, 964–968.
9. Macey, H. B. *Surg. Gynecol. Obstet.* **1939**, *69*, 108–109.
10. Lindeman, K. *Z. Orthop.* **1950**, *79*, 316–334,
11. Augustine, R. W. *Am. J. Surg.* **1956**, *92*, 380–388.
12. Ritchey, S. J. *Armed. Forces. Med. J.* **1960**, *11*, 167–176.
13. Jones, K. G. *J. Bone Join Surg.* **1963**, *45A*, 925–932.
14. Jones, K. G. *J. Bone Join Surg.* **1970**, *52A*, 1302–1308.
15. Franke, K. *Orthop. Clin. N. Am.* **1976**, *7*, 191–193.
16. Lemaire, M. *J. Chir.* **1975**, *110*, 281–294.
17. Marshall, J. L., Warren, R. F., Wickiewicz, T. L. *Clin. Orthop.* **1979**, *143*, 97–106.
18. Rubin, R. M.; Marshall, J. L.; Wang, J. *Clin. Orthop.* **1975**, *113*, 212–236.
19. Dandy, D. J. *Arthroscopic Surgery of the Knee.* (Churchill Livingstone, Edinburgh, **1981**).
20. Dandy, D. J.; Flanagan, J. P.; Steemeyer, V. *Clin. Orthop.* **1982**, *167*, 43–49.
21. Johnson, L. L. *Arthroscopy* **1993**, *9*(2), 131–142.
22. Laboureau, J. P.; Brulez, B. Pre-adjusted prosthetic ligament and method of manufacture, 1996, US Patent 6,866,681, **2005**.
23. Brulez, B.; Laboureau, J. P. Method for fixing traction threads to ends of a prosthetic ligament, US Patent 7,494,506, **2009** — Google Patents.
24. Cerulli, G.; Caraffa, A.; Cerulli, G.; Projetti, M.; Aisa, G.; Rizz, A. *Arthroscopy* **1996**, *4*(1), 19–21.
25. Lavoie, P.; Fletcher, J.; Duval, N. *The Knee* **2000**, *7*(3), 157–163.
26. Brulez, B.; Laboureau, J. P.; Migonney, V.; Pavon, G. Siove polymer surface treatment process, French Patent n° 0300495, **2003**.
27. Brulez, B.; Laboureau, J. P.; Migonney, V.; Pavon, G.; Siove biomimetic prosthetic ligament and production method thereof, French patent n° 0300497, **2003**, European patent n° EP Patent 1,599,238, **2006**, Brevet US n° 7,700,147, **2010**, WO Patent n° 2,004,067,051.
28. Ciobanu, M.; Pavon-Djavid, G.; Gueguen, V.; Siove, A.; Gamble, L.; Castner, D.; Migonney, V. *Biomacromolecules* **2006**, *7*(3), 755–760.

29. Pavon-Djavid, G.; Gamble, L. J.; Ciobanu, M.; Gueguen, V.; Castner, D. G.; Migonney, V. *Biomacromolecules* **2007**, *8*(11), 3317–3325.
30. Vaquette, C.; Viateau, V.; Guérard, S.; Anagnostou, F.; Manassero, M.; Castner, D. G.; Migonney, V. *Biomaterials* **2013**, *34*(29), 7048–7063.
31. Zhou, J.; Ciobanu, M.; Pavon-Djavid, G.; Gueguen, V.; Migonney, V. *IEEE Eng. Med. Biol. Soc.* **2007**, *1*, 5115–5118.
32. Viateau, V.; Manassero, M.; Anagnostou, F.; Guérard, S.; Mitton, D.; Migonney, V. *Arthroscopy* **2013**, *29*(6), 1079–1088.
33. Guerard, S.; Manassero, M.; Viateau, V.; Migonney, V.; Skalli, W.; Mitton, D. *Adv. Biomech. Appl.* **2014**, *1*(4), 239–252.
34. Viateau, V.; Zhou, J.; Guérard, S.; Manassero, M. *IRBM.* **2011**, *32*(5), 118–122.
35. Viateau, V.; Manassero, M.; Anagnostou, F.; Guérard, S.; Mitton, D.; Migonney, V. *Veterinary Surg.* **2012**, *41*(5), E1.
36. Brulez, B.; Guilard, R.; Migonney, V. Ligament *prothétique biomimétique* resorbable, PCT/FR2014/052992, Resorbable Biomimetic Prosthetic Ligament, WO2015/075397.
37. Huot, S.; Rohman, G.; Riffault, M.; Pinzano, A.; Grossin, L.; Migonney, V. *Biomed. Mater. Eng.* **2013**, *23*(4), 281–288.
38. Rohman, G.; Huot, S.; Vilas-Boas, M.; Radu-Bostan, G.; Castner, D. G.; Migonney, V. *J. Mater. Sci. Mater. Med.* **2015**, *26*(7), 206.
39. Djaker, N.; Brustlein, S.; Rohman, G.; Huot, S.; de la Chapelle, M. L.; Migonney, V. *Biomed. Opt. Exp.* **2014**, *5*(1), 149–157.

https://doi.org/10.1142/9789811204630_0003

Chapter 3

Recent Evolution of the ACL Reconstruction

L'Hocine Yahia[*,‡], Ghislaine Bayade[*],
Werner Klingler[†], and Robert Schleip[†]

[*]*Laboratoire d'Innovation et d'Analyse de Bioperformance, Polytechnique Montréal, C.P. 6079, Succursale Centre-ville, Montréal, Québec, Canada H3C 3A7*
[†]*Fascia Research Group, Division of Neurophysiology, Ulm University, Germany*
[‡]*lhocine.yahia@polymlt.ca*

Abbreviations

AAOS	American Academy of Orthopedic Surgeons
ACL	Anterior cruciate ligament
ACLR	ACL reconstruction
BPTB	Bone-patellar tendon-bone
FDA	Food and Drug Administration
FE	Finite element
HT	Hamstring tendon
IDE	Investigational device exemption
LAD	Ligament augmentation devices
LARS	Ligament advanced reinforcement system
LK	Leeds-Keio
NiTi	Nickel–titanium
OA	Osteoarthritis
PCL	Polycaprolactone
PET	Polyethylene terephthalate
PMA	Premarket approval
PolyNASS	Polystyrene sodium sulfonate
PTFE	Polytetrafluoroethylene
STT	Semitendinosus tendon

1. Introduction

Anterior cruciate ligament reconstruction (ACLR) is a standard care procedure with an average of more than 200,000 operations performed in the United States of America per year.[1] While the rates of ACL injuries are variable, ACLR is in fact, very costly for the society due to the huge quantity of surgeries done every year. These reconstructions increase the health care cost to more than $1 billion.[2] The alternative graft is passed through the tunnels made in the femur and in the tibia and it is secured using fixatives.[3] The tendons of the same patient (autograft) or donor tissues (allograft), non-degradable synthetic grafts are alternative approaches that have been attempted for ACLR.[4] Here, various types of autogeneic, allogeneic, and synthetic grafts for ACLR are reviewed by comparing their advantages and disadvantages.

2. History of Synthetic Replacement of the ACL

2.1. *Early History*

In 1903, Lange of Munich performed for the first time a reconstruction of the ACL using braided silk constructs associated with the half-tendinous ligament prosthesis. The result was a failure and his compatriot, Herr Herz, concluded in 1906 that the use of silk was a good idea but that the attempt to copy nature had failed. They were perhaps not far from the right path.[5] The procedure did not work and eventually set the stage for the next few decades. In 1914, Dr. Corner first made many attempts to reconstruct a ruptured ACL using a synthetic graft, which was just a piece of silver filament. Afterwards in 1918, Smith tried to repair the ACL using a silk ligament, but his attempt ended in failure 3 months later. It is interesting to note that, some decades later; this natural biomaterial is now reintroduced.[6] Despite enormous efforts, the difficulties involved in providing successful ligament repair remain an important challenge to this day.

2.2. *Development During the Last 40 Years*

As early as 1903, Lange from Munich had used silk as a reinforcement of the semi-tendinous without success and Corner in 1914 of the silver threads. In 1975 Rubin, Marschall[7] had made an experimental model of a Dacron® prosthesis. Then, after being silenced for nearly

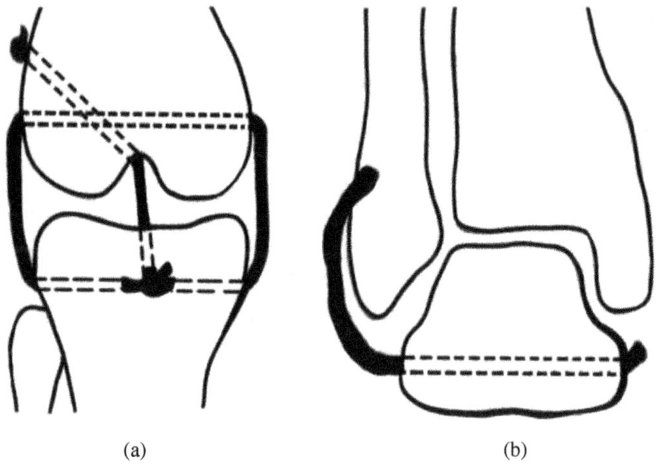

Figure 1. A carbon-fiber strand used for the replacement of ACL, medial and collateral ligaments (a). Correction of the collateral instability (b)[13]

1980 years, synthetic grafts became popular in the 1980s and in the 1990s. A first wave in the early 1980s was launched with reinforcements made of carbon, which was the material of fashion at that time.

Benson suggested the potential biological and biomechanical significance of pure carbon in 1971.[8] During the 1970s and the early 1980s, a group from Cardiff experimented extensively the use of carbon implants as an agent for the induction of new tendon synthesis in animal models.[9–12] Jenkins argued that "since a high proportion of the tissues of living organisms is composed of carbon compounds, it would not perhaps be surprising that implants of the pure element should be well tolerated by these tissues"[10] (see Figure 1). Initial results were promising with new tendon being formed around the carbon grafts at 3 months after implantation and no obvious clinical dysfunction in an ovine model.[10] Jenkins *et al.* concluded that filamentous carbon is recognized in living tissues with virtually no adverse reaction and that it can be used to induce the formation of new tendon or ligament with a physical strength equal to the original structure.[10] The implants were extremely well tolerated in the ovine model regarding foreign body response, and this encouraged the

Cardiff group to progress to clinical trials in the human lower limb.[11] This study included two ACLRs in isolation and 31 combined knee ligament procedures. The two ACLRs were reviewed yearly post-operatively (maximum 3 years) and both reported a significant improvement in the function of their knees. The only complication documented in this preliminary report was sinus formation overlying graft material in two ankles at the position of the graft, but it was considered too superficial. No complications were reported in the knee group.

In 1983, Rushton *et al.* reported the clinical, arthroscopic, and histological findings in 10 knees that had undergone ACLR using a carbon-fiber graft.[14] Carbon-fiber ACL grafts had been implanted into 39 patients and the 10 reported cases had experienced pain and discomfort post-operatively. All 10 patients had synovitis with evidence of carbon fiber in the joint. Occasionally, the fiber stained the articular surface and the menisci. The femoral notch of some patients contained inflamed synovium. Such synovium was stained black. In some patients, a "new ligament" appeared to have formed but gentle probing with a blunt hook revealed this to be a thin, fibrous sheath covering unchanged carbon-fiber graft. Histologically two patients demonstrated a fibroblastic response to the carbon fiber. Five patients showed evidence of chronic synovial inflammation and papillary proliferation of the synovium was present in all 10 knees. A mild foreign-body giant-cell reaction to the carbon-fiber filaments and hemosiderin was seen in surface cells of the synovium, in macrophages, and around some fragments of carbon fiber. Other complications included ulceration of the skin over subcutaneous carbon-fiber knots used to secure the graft, similar to the findings of the Jenkins study 3 years earlier.[13]

In the 1980s, intra-articular ACLR began to come to the forefront. John Insall is often given credit for the early intra-articular reconstructions — he reported a technique where a band of fascia Lata was passed through the knee and sutured to the front of the tibia.[15]

ACLR has evolved considerably over the past 30 years. Artificial ligaments were proposed using one biocompatible material. However, because of the high strength and large elastic deformation required, a single material cannot mimic the mechanical behavior of the ligament. For a single material, the deformation and the strength are related through the modulus of elasticity. Several types of prostheses have been implanted in the human knee to replace a ruptured cruciate ligament. None of them, however, has reportedly been adequate due to inacceptable plastic deformations after a relatively short period. The functional part of these prostheses is usually made of a single synthetic material with adequate strength properties but not allowing enough elastic elongation as compared to the natural ligament.

Dore *et al.* (1981) developed an original artificial prosthetic ligament capable of large elastic deformation and having a high resistance to breakage. This composite ligament comprises an elastic core having a low modulus of elasticity and opposed ends, a tensionable wrapping of thread having a high resistance to breakage.[16] A further object of their invention is to provide a tension spring, where in the helix angle of the threads wound about the core is selected to achieve a predetermined characteristic of the spring. The design of the composite prosthesis was optimized using a mathematical model of the elastic behavior of a two-material composite prosthesis made of high-strength fibers spirally wound around a soft elastic core.[17] At each end of the core, the fibers are attached to a pulling device. Under a tension load, the fibers exert a pressure on the core, which deforms radially, permitting the elongation of the prosthesis. This allows the achievement of large deformation while both the fibers and the core remain in the elastic domain. The high strength of the spring is provided by the high yield strength of the fibers. The results show the influence of the design variables on the deformation of the prosthesis (see Figure 2).

The developed structures were circular braids, axially reinforced with several core yarns or braided structures. Tensile behavior of these structures was characterized and the effects of number of axial yarns or braids and, the number of yarns used in the axial braids were thoroughly investigated. From the experimental results, it was observed that the braided structures with axial braids could mimic the load-elongation behavior of native ACL. According to the literature,

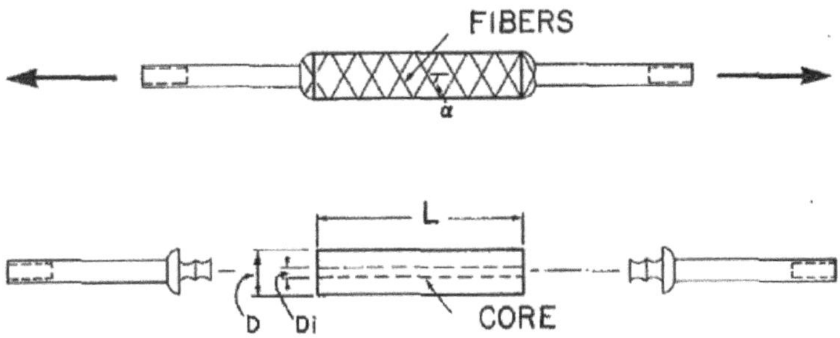

Figure 2. Composite ligament developed by Drouin in 1981 made of high-strength fibers spirally wound around a soft elastic core[17]

natural ACLs possess ultimate tensile load in the range of 739–2300 N, stiffness between 111 and 397 N/mm, toe region strain between 1.5% and 4.8% and failure strain between 19% and 36%.

The average breaking extension and strain at toe region of the braided structures were 30% and 4.3%, respectively, which are in the range of native ACLs. The maximum breaking force and stiffness achieved with seven axial braids, each produced using six yarns were 274 N and 13.5 N/mm, respectively and, both breaking force and stiffness showed linear increase with the number of axial braids as well as number of yarns used in the axial braids. Therefore, it is possible to design an artificial graft using these novel braided structures with mechanical properties similar to that of native ACLs, through adjustment of these structural parameters, as these braided structures have much smaller diameter (0.5 mm) than native ACLs (11 mm).

This prosthesis composed of a fiber mesh sheath wrapped around a silicon rubber cylindrical core (see Figure 3), reproduces satisfactorily the ligament response in tension. However, the prosthesis does not only undergo elongation. Its intra-articular portion, composed of a fiber mesh sheath wrapped around a silicone rubber cylindrical core, reproduces satisfactorily the natural ACL response in tension. The fiber used to develop these structures was polyamide 6.6 having mechanical properties similar to biocompatible fibers such as polyglycolic acid. The idea was to conceive a suitable fibrous structure that can be subsequently developed using biocompatible fibers.

Properties	Values
Linear density (dtex)	160±10
Number of filaments	40
Diameters of filaments (mm)	0.011±0.000
Breaking load (N)	6.7±0.5
Elongation (mm)	160±12
Tenacity (N/tex)	0.39

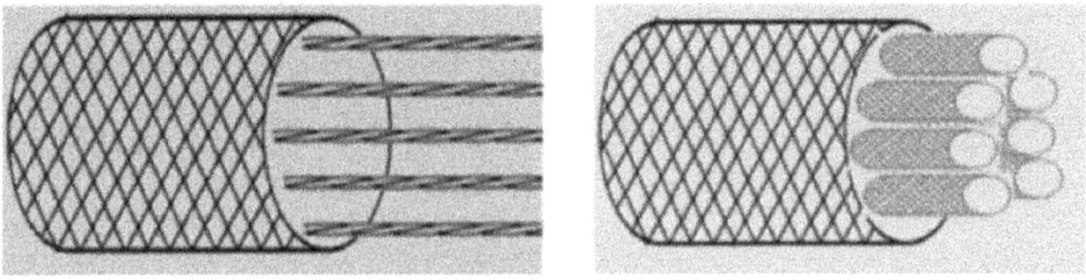

(a) (b)

Figure 3. Properties of polyamide 6.6 fibers (Top) Structure of braided fibers with axial yarns (a) axial braids (b)[18]

Unfortunately, due to the lack of industrial partners, this first biomimetic composite prosthesis able to reproduce biomechanical properties of natural ACL remained a prototype. In 2013, Cruz *et al.* developed a novel braided structure using polyamide 6.6 fibers for application as artificial ACLs. The developed structures were circular braids, axially reinforced with either several core yarns or braided structures.[18]

The advancement in the chemical industry and associated fields, such as biomaterials, provided more suitable materials for medical use. From then on, clinical application of artificial ligaments was initiated. The artificial ligaments are categorized into three distinct groups: (1) prosthetic, (2) augmentation, and (3) scaffold. The prosthesis functions as a permanent implant due to their high mechanical properties. The augmentation device is bioresorbable and it acts as a temporary stent to increase the initial strength of the graft.[19] The scaffold consists of a porous structure that stimulates tissue ingrowth transforming loads to new tissue.[20]

Polytetrafluoroethylene (PTFE), also known as Gore-Tex® ligament, was introduced in 1986 and it was approved in the United

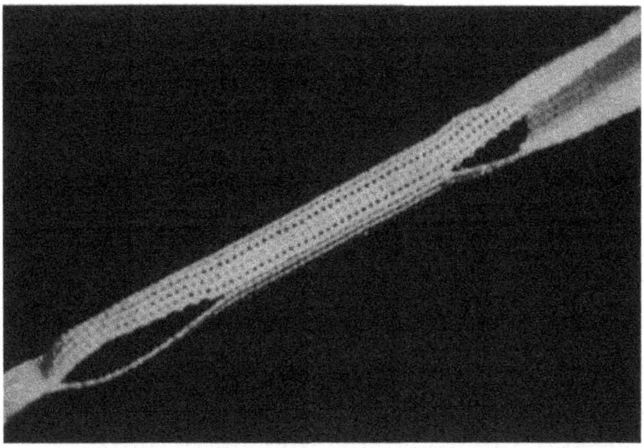

Figure 4. *LK* artificial ligament structure[27]

States of America and used in revision reconstruction autologous grafts. These synthetic ligaments have a very high ultimate tensile strength as well as a good stiffness. They had very encouraging results initially, but later studies showed complications in 76% of the cases: 17% with up to 29% graft failure rate,[21] tunnel osteolysis,[22] and PTFE particles' deposits in lymph nodes distant to the knee.[23] They were eventually withdrawn from the market in 1993.

Polyester, also called Dacron® ligament, was then introduced. Despite initial encouraging results,[24] a very high rupture rate ranging from 29% to 60% was reported in the literature.[25,26] While presenting the long-term outcomes, authors also noted that 83% of the patients had degenerative changes in the knee joint with only 14% of patients having an acceptable stability and functional outcome.[25] This product was later withdrawn from the market in 1994.

The polyethylene terephthalate Leeds-Keio® (LK) ligament was developed in 1982. The LK ligament is a "scaffold" type of prosthesis, as it acts as an inducer for tissue ingrowth. Its porous coating allows the induction of biological tissue and promotes the formation of a neo-ligament on the intra-articular portion (see Figure 4). In a study of 152 patients with a follow-up of more than 4 years, 90.1% had a negative Lachman test and 82.2% had a negative anterior drawer sign; no major complications were noticed.[27] Engström *et al.*;

in a prospective randomized controlled trial comparing LK ligament vs autologous bone–patellar tendon–bone (BPTB) grafts, noticed increased anterior laxity and positive pivot shift test after an average follow-up of 27 months.[28] According to Senni *et al.* (2007), the reported characteristics are the following: a toxicity, biocompatibility, mechanical strength, an easy handling, a low cost/benefit ratio and an ability to induce tissue because it acts as a scaffold.[29] In literature, many authors report further advantages that is the possibility of early returning to high levels of activity,[30] the lack of the donor site morbidity that could be seen following autologous reconstruction, shorter operative times and a reproducible implant design.

Ligament Advanced Reinforcement System (LARS™) made of polyethylene terephthalate (PET) as the structural component had encouraging results (see Figure 5). The LARS™ has been designed to mimic ligamentous anatomy. It is composed of two parts, i.e. intra-articular and intra-osseous part. The intra-osseous part is composed of longitudinal fibers of PET held together with transverse knitted structure. While the intra-articular part has parallel longitudinal fibers of PET twisted perpendicular to each other. These parts should be

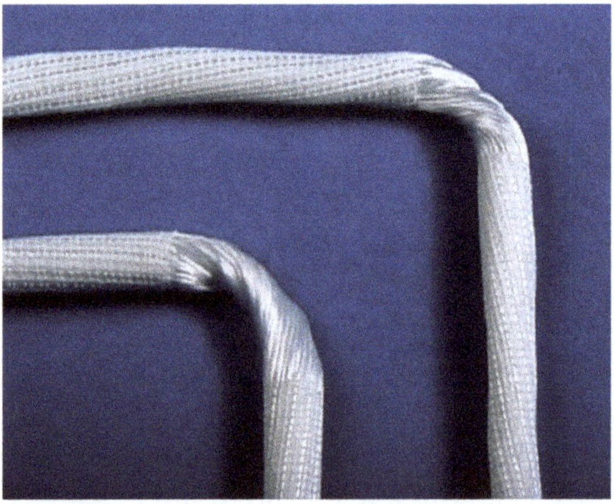

Figure 5. Torsion of the *LARS* ligament mimicking the ACL's properties[37]

aligned perfectly while doing the ACLR to avoid early graft failures. The orientation of the fibers is modified to be side specific, i.e. different for left and right knees thus mimicking the 3D cross-sectional anatomy of intra-articular part of the native ACL. This is supposed to help overcome rotational fatigue of the synthetic ligament. Although this is a far superior structural construct compared to other synthetic substitutes, getting the LARS™ intra-osseous part and intra-articular part exactly in their place during the surgery requires excellent surgical skill. The LARS™ also promotes tissue ingrowth.[31] It allows tissue ingrowth in the intra-articular part. Lavoie *et al.* presented their study of 47 patients with a follow-up of 8–45 months with good results in subjective parameters and satisfying Tegner activity level.[32] The results with LARS™ ligament are promising however long-term results are awaited. Preliminary results for newer-generation devices, specifically the LARS™, show lower reported rates of failure, revision, and sterile effusion/synovitis when compared with older devices.[33]

Several studies considering the outcomes following LARS™ for the ligamentous reconstruction showed good to excellent functional outcomes and good patient satisfaction.[34–38] A few of the papers even rated LARS™ as better than the autograft ACLRs.[39,40] Histopathological studies do support the cellular ingrowth with LARS™ acting as a scaffold.[31]

A study done by Machotka *et al.* in 2010 which was a meta-analysis of the literature published on LARS™ for ACLR from year 2000 to 2010 showed that none of the studies done on LARS™ provided autologous “ligamentous” healing along the synthetic meshwork of LARS™.[41] None of the studies compared return to previous level of function with LARS™ nor with traditional ACLR. This meta-analysis was based on the four studies and stated that LARS™ may not be good for chronic ACL injuries as in such cases quality of remnant of the ACL, i.e. ACL stump is problematic, and LARS™ may not carry good ligamentous ingrowth on fibrotic stump.

Alberto *et al.* published in 2014 a study of few patients with failed reconstruction using PET synthetic grafts.[42] Fourteen of such patients underwent revision surgery performed as two-staged revision. All these patients had histopathological evidence of granulomatous

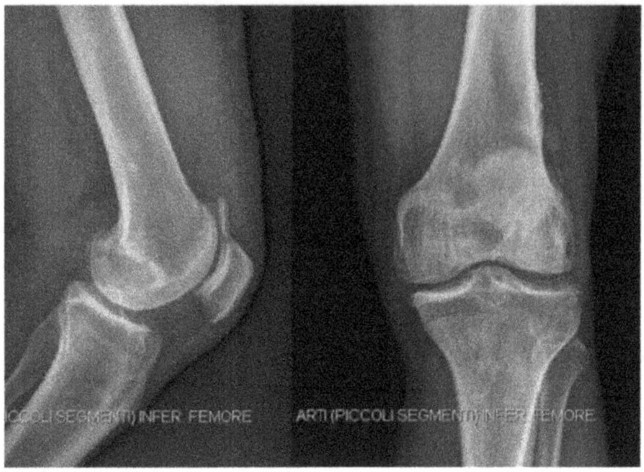

Figure 6. Signs of OA 4 years after revision surgery in a patient that underwent a surgery of reconstruction of the ACL with synthetic graft[42]

reaction due to PET. And even the revision surgeries done with the autografts did not improve functional status of these patients nor stop the progressive osteoarthritis (OA) occurring in these patients (see Figure 6). In another study, the rate of failure of LARS™ in a 19 years outcome study was reported to be 27.5% with 100% patients presenting with degenerative arthritis.[42]

When tested using new battery of tests, which are used to evaluate return to sports status of the patients with ACLR; patient's ability to return to sports related activities was better in patients treated with autograft ACLR than LARS™ ACLR and further evaluation of these patients is being done.[43]

Finally, the results of Tiefenboeck *et al.* (2015) indicate that the LARS™ system should currently not be suggested as a potential graft for primary reconstruction of the ACL. In special cases, however, the LARS™ system can serve as an alternative graft.[44]

3. Biomaterial Aspects

Several prosthetic devices for ACL replacement have been made over the past 30 years using a wide range of materials. The materials which have been considered for these devices include polyester

(Stryker Dacron® ligament prosthesis, Leeds-Keio), polytetrafluoroethylene *PTFE* and *fluoropolymers* (Gore-Tex®), *carbon fibers, polyethylene, nylon and polystyrene*. However, none of these artificial ligaments have demonstrated positive long-term results *in vivo*. Failures of previous devices mostly originate from mechanical failures or from a lack of biocompatibility.

Mechanical failures include (i) rupture caused by wear, by fatigue or by severe loading in the knee and (ii) laxity in the joint after creep of the prosthetic ligament or after loosening of the fixation element in the bone. Biocompatibility issues primarily manifest as immunogenic particulation leading to chronic synovitis. Due to high incidence of such problems, most, if not all the previous artificial ligaments, have been withdrawn from the commercial market. For example, the Food and Drug Administration (FDA) of the United States of America currently approve no such devices for clinical use.

Over the last decades, statistics have been collected that confirm the poor long-term efficacy of existing artificial ligaments. A study of 855 artificial ACL*s* over a 15-year period found that there was 40–78% failure rate.[45] Another report found that around 80% of knees, which had been reconstructed using Dacron® prosthetic ligaments, had developed significant OA symptoms at a 9-year follow up.[45] Similarly, a study of 268 patients revealed that Gore-Tex® ACL prosthesis yielded a failure rate of 42% with case of effusions, rupture and strong loosening.[46] Overall, complication rates for artificial ligament operations are of the order of 40–50%, which is much higher than the rate with autologous and allogenic ligaments.

In October 1986, the FDA approved the Gore-Tex® cruciate ligament prosthesis in ACLR, followed by the 3M Kennedy ligament augmentation devices (LADs) in 1987 and the Stryker Dacron® ligament prosthesis in 1988. Other popular products were the LK ligament and the LARS™. These last two types were adopted in Europe and Asia. However, since the early 1990s, poor outcomes of long-term follow-ups have halted the use of artificial ligaments. A high incidence of complications such as reactive synovitis, instability, loosening, and even rupture of the prostheses was constantly reported.[47]

In Section 4, the causes of these catastrophic failures will be examined. Several types of ligament prostheses, therefore, have been withdrawn from the market due to their long-term drawbacks. The augmentation devices, on the other hand, did not show significant complications in early stages.[48] Scaffolds are the third generation of implants, and their long-term drawbacks have not yet been studied completely. The initial satisfactions of synthetic prostheses are due to their lack of harvest site pathology, availability, accelerated rehabilitation period and significant strength.[49] Moreover, less surgical operation is required, which is more convenient for the patient.

4. Causes of Failures

Since the 1990s, artificial ligaments provide a significant improvement of patients' life quality for a limited period but from a mechanical point of view, no ideal replacement device does exist Failures were attributed to rupture (66%), to synovitis (12%), to elongation (18%), and to mal implantation (10%). Most ruptures were localized at the femoral or at the tibial site of use of synthetic devices in the surgical repair of the knee ligaments. The highest rupture rate was found for Stryker (50%). A foreign-body reaction of the synovial membrane was caused by abrasion particles. The abrasion process is due to the relative motion between the bony canal and the prosthesis. Furthermore, no materials showed yet a complete bone ingrowth in the drill tunnels.

Contact with sharp edges of the bone tunnel causes abrasions, which weaken the implant and create debris that can cause synovitis in the joint. Woven prostheses face the additional problems of axial splitting, low tissue infiltration, low extensibility, and abrasive wear. Eventually, these implants fail due to fragmentation, to stress shielding of new tissue, to fatigue, to creep, and to production of wear debris.[50–52]

Indeed, in the early 1990s Seemann *et al.* observed osteolytic widening of the tibial tunnels during revision surgeries.[22] Failure mode for the pullout tests and the pre-existing partial failure of the studies as a common issue found in clinical situations.[53,54] Fukubayashi *et al.*

performed a 5–11 years follow-up study of Gore-Tex® ACL and they reported that most of the non-ruptured implants resulted in tunnel widening.[55] Muren *et al.* came to the same conclusions more recently in their 13–15 years follow-up study whereby tunnel widening occurred in 15 of their 17 patients.[53]

Poddevin *et al.* (1997) investigated the explanted failed ligaments and made some highly interesting observations.[54] They noticed that most ligaments failed at the bone interface, which induced an acute inflammatory response, a thick disorganized scar tissue surrounded the ligament preventing further tissue infiltration and hence no ligamentization could occur (see Figure 7).

The early failures of the prostheses made of polyester composites, together with many other prototypes, were microscopically analyzed in a retrospective study by Guidoin *et al.* (2000).[56] The authors reported that failure was related to inadequate resistance to abrasion and to torsion forces, together with structural changes of the grafts due to unpredictable tissue infiltration. By interpreting the damaged fiber images from clinically failed and retrieved ACL prostheses, Guidoin *et al.* (2000) confirmed that the predominant cause of synthetic ACL failure was yarn on bone abrasion.[56] Improvements in future ACL prosthesis designs will only be possible by eliminating or by minimizing the effect of this type of abrasive wear.

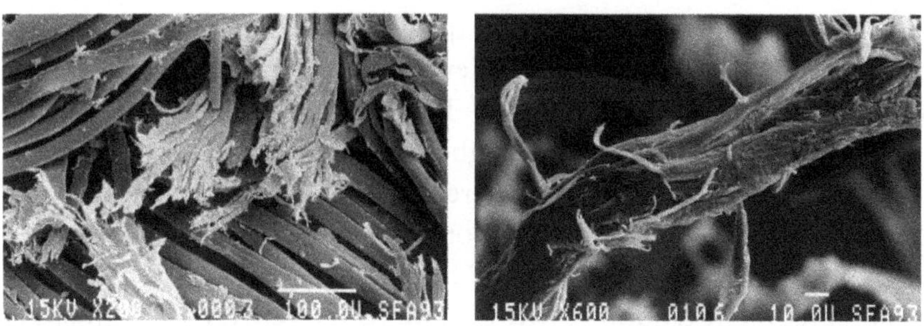

(a) (b)

Figure 7. Scanning electron photomicrograph of PET after 5000 cycles of wear against the bone interface showing crushed fibers and bushy ends. (a) Scanning electron photomicrograph of PET after 500 cycles of wear against the surface. Short peeling is observed at the surface (b)[55]

The reasons for the immense failure of artificial ligaments are multiple such as the biomaterials used in the fabrication of the ligament that were not necessarily adequate for repetitive loading. Another reason, less understood, is related to *in vivo* combined loading imposed to these artificial ligaments.[57] An *in vitro* evaluation of different types of ligament prostheses subjected to combined tension, bending and torsion carried out in laboratories has led to a better understanding of the problems related to ligament prostheses.[16] Usually, the FDA guidelines recommend fatigue tests during traction loading.

Most of these prostheses were soon removed from the market. It is important to mention that some synthetic ligaments, not approved by the FDA, have escaped recall and have survived in Europe and Asia until this day. This is particularly the case with LARS™, Trevira and LK ligaments. These PET ligaments, just like the biological grafts, have similar ultimate tensile strength compared to the human ACL. This resemblance in some mechanical properties led to a lower rate of complications compared to other synthetic implants. The stability and the risk of failure of these grafts for ACLR rely not only on the source and on the mechanical properties of grafts but also on their fixation method. In addition, the biological or the synthetic graft is secured within the bone tunnel in femur and tibia. The attachment site, therefore, plays a significant role in graft performance.

Improvements in the polymer quality and in the fiber's manufacturing process have enabled the development of a better and a safer PET artificial ligament (surch as Trevira, LARS™, etc.). PET is a polyester with a melting point higher than 250°C. It is an inert and a not biodegradable material, where, therefore, cellular attachment is difficult. In order to make it more attractive with respect to cell attachment, to cell proliferation, to collagen regeneration, and to biointegration in tendon repair, Li *et al.* (2013) covered it with layers of chitosan and of hydroxyapatite by a self-assembly technique.[58] It was found that such treatment improves cell attachment and proliferation while reducing the inflammatory response.

Ciobanu *et al.* have developed a radical graft polymerization of polystyrene sodium sulfonate (PolyNASS) onto PET in order to enhance the interaction of the LARS™ ligament with relevant cells,[59] that are, fibroblasts.[7] This method proved very efficient at accelerating fibroblasts adhesion along with achieving enhanced control over the fibroblast morphology and alignment onto the PolyNaSS grafted fibers.[7]

This suggests that the PolyNASS grafting was capable of initiating bone formation, which would later colonize the center of the ligament in a more predictable manner and hence enhance the ligament integration. This is of particular relevance as tunnel osteolysis is generally associated with the use of synthetic ligaments and it is considered as a crucial parameter for ligament biomechanical stability.

Vaquette *et al.* investigated the performance of bioactive grafted PET LARS™ ligaments onto human osteoblasts both *in vitro* and to subsequently evaluated their osseo-integration *in vivo* using an ovine relevant orthopaedic model. Taken together their results provide evidence that PolyNaSS grafting of PET ligaments, improves artificial ligament osseo-integration within the bone tunnels.[60]

Another aspect that is poorly investigated is the simulation of ligament failure and injury. With current commercial software, anatomically realistic 3D models can accurately simulate local strains could be easily enriched in order to predict crack initiation and propagation by the use of extended finite element (FE) methods.[61] However, data available about ligament failure only concern uniaxial tension along the main axis of the ligament and are therefore insufficient for the development of adequate failure criteria to be implemented with extended FE methods.[62]

The reasons for clinical failure after ACLR are numerous but can be broadly separated into three categories: technical, biological, and mechanical failures. It is generally thought that poor tunnel positioning (especially the femoral tunnel) is the most common technical error.

5. The *FDA* Guidelines

Poor device design is the primary reason for a device recall in approximately 17% of cases each year. In most instances, the design fails in one of the two ways. The most common failure occurs when an internal device comes loose in the body. Another common design failure causes the product to leak into a patient. With a defective medical device, lawyer can hold the manufacturer responsible for either failing to instruct doctors on the proper method of installation or for designing the product in such a way that safe installation was impossible.

The FDA published a guidance document for intra-articular prosthetic knee ligament devices in September 1, 1987 and revised the guidance in February 18, 1993. This guidance suggests some important evaluation criteria, test procedures and end points. Since its introduction, several new ligaments have been approved for market bringing the current number of approved ligaments in the US to three. The three approved ligaments are the Gore-Tex® by W.L. Gore and Associates approved on October 10, 1986, the Stryker Dacron® by Meadox Medicals Inc.; approved on December 30, 1988 and the 3M Kennedy *LAD* which was first approved on May 7, 1987 for the Marshall-MacIntosh procedure and then the indication was expanded on December 31, 1992 to include the use of the patellar tendon graft of 10 mm or smaller in patients more than 3 weeks since injury.

It has been determined by the FDA that all intra-articular prosthetic ligament devices are post-amendment significant risk devices. Therefore, an investigational device exemption (IDE) application is required prior to the start of clinical trials and a premarket approval (PMA) application is required prior to marketing these devices. It is the purpose of this guidance document to aid in the preparation of IDEs and PMAs for intra-articular prosthetic knee ligament devices. Specifically, this document is intended to inform the device manufacturer or the investigation sponsor of the preclinical and the clinical testing that should be performed to generate data that will provide reasonable assurance of the safety and of the effectiveness of these devices for their intended use.

Nevertheless, all these FDA approved artificial ligaments were later removed from the market and the American Academy of Orthopedic Surgeons (AAOS) in its Bulletin of October 1995. While a variety of synthetic materials have been used for grafts, these materials have not become particularly popular for a variety of reasons. The inherent mechanical properties of synthetic grafts do not closely resemble those of the normal ligament and these artificial ligaments do not have the capability to repair and to remodel.[63]

The AAOS is careful not to specify which of these mechanical properties were involved. It is known that cruciate ligaments have viscoelastic behavior that is often overlooked. The researchers also demonstrated that these ligaments undergo a combined loading of tension, flexion and torsion; which accelerates the phenomenon of fatigue and wear while tested *in vivo*.

Alternatively, biological grafts (autografts and allografts) are frequently used. Varieties of autografts such as a portion of a bone–patellar tendon–bone complex, the iliotibial tract, the semitendinosus tendon, and the gracilis tendon have been used to replace the ACL. The bone–patellar tendon–bone graft is the most popular and it has been most extensively investigated. In brief, the patellar–tendon–graft complex exhibits approximately 30–50% of the ultimate load of the ACL complex at 1–2 years post-surgery in animal studies. Allografts have been considered for many patients due to the availability of tissue and the potential morbidity associated with autograft procedures.

The ideal graft to use in ACL*R* should have structural and biomechanical properties similar to those of the native ligament, allowing secure fixation and rapid biological incorporation, and it should limit donor site morbidity. However, in general, patellar tendon autografts are preferable for high-performance athletes, and hamstring autografts and allografts have some relative advantages for lower-demand individuals. No current indications exist for synthetic ligaments.

In the face of these failures and for the seek of anything better, clinicians turned to grafts and to allografts in the 2000s. Bioengineers said that "Nature has done things right". The inconstancy of the results with synthetic ligaments pushed the new generations either to take up old concepts of biological grafts or to innovate with bioinspired designs.[64]

This review concerning the failure of artificial ligaments brings the researchers to wonder why artificial ligaments fail and how they can improve the design and the materials selection to solve these problems. Both mechanical and biological studies conducted during the last 40 years by the authors' research group and others have given them a better understanding of the natural ligament. An exhaustive description of the natural ligament was given in the first chapter of this book. Here, the principal features of the natural ligament that have not been addressed by previous existing designs will be pointed out. Based on recent progress, the hope is to come up with a new conceptual design of prosthetic ligaments that both mimics the main functions of the tissue and considers the present problems.

6. Biomimetic ACL Prostheses

The natural world is the source and the subject of nearly all-human knowledge and its beauty is derived from its functionality more than its outer form. Therefore, looking on Nature is the first step that bio-engineers and biomaterial specialists should take for improving their current designs, for solving the inefficiency and the lack of space problems.

The emphasis in the field of orthopedic tissue engineering is on imparting biomimetic functionality to tissue-engineered bone or to soft tissue grafts and enabling their translation to the clinic. A significant challenge in achieving extended graft functionality is engineering the biological fixation of these grafts with each other as well as with the host environment. Biological fixation will require re-establishment of the structure–function relationship inherent at the native soft tissue-to-bone interface on these tissue-engineered grafts. To this end, strategic biomimicry must be incorporated into advanced scaffold design. To facilitate integration between distinct tissue types (e.g., bone with soft tissues such as cartilage, ligament, or tendon), a stratified or multi-phasic scaffold with distinct yet continuous tissue regions is required to pre-engineer the interface between bone and soft tissues. Using the ACL-to-bone interface as a model system, this review outlines the strategies for stratified scaffold design for interface tissue engineering, focusing on identifying the relevant design parameters derived from an understanding of the structure–function relationship inherent at the soft-to-hard tissue interface. The design approach centers on first addressing the challenge of soft tissue-to-bone integration *ex vivo*, and then subsequently focusing on the relatively less difficult task of bone-to-bone integration *in vivo*.

In addition, the authors of this chapter will review stratified scaffold design aimed at exercising spatial control over heterotypic cellular interactions, which are critical for facilitating the formation and maintenance of distinct yet continuous multi-tissue regions. Finally, potential challenges and future directions in this emerging area of advanced scaffold design will be discussed.

The specific biomimetic approach chosen for this research is to imitate the triple helix hierarchal structure of collagen. The triple helix formed by natural collagen molecules gives rise to a special property of ligaments known as the toe region.[26] The toe region refers to a nonlinear structural property that allows a material to stretch a certain distance without a linear increase in material strain. In native ligaments, the toe region is produced by the tendency of collagen fibril helices to form a crimped and wavy macrostructure. Increasing stress causes the collagen bundles to straighten, allowing the ligament to stretch some distance before the collagen fibrils experience any increase in strain.[65] By assembling scaffold material fibers with a triple helix structure, the toe region of the scaffold can more accurately mimic the toe region of the native ligament while maintaining the other factors of biocompatibility previously mentioned.

The ligaments of the knee are among the most complicated structures to simulate and at the same time the most critical in determining the biomechanics of the joint.[17,66]

Several topics concerning the biomechanics of the knee ligaments remain poorly understood. Fluid flow during deformation of the ligaments is one of these. Following the studies of the transient mechanics and the mechanobiology of the intervertebral disk,[53] models including osmotic swelling due to the presence of proteoglycans would allow for a more accurate prediction of their time-dependent response and the overcoming of the incompressibility assumption. However, experimental data about permeability for the ligamentous tissue is still lacking.[67]

Based on the studies on natural ligaments, which relates structural, physiological, biomechanical and surgical conditions to be respected in the development of ligament prosthesis, the design criteria for the development of a new generation of ACL ligament prosthesis have been earlier established.[68] In collaboration with orthopedic surgeons using PET artificial ligaments (Dr. Laboureau in France and Dr. Krudwig in Germany), Hagemeister *et al.* have been among the first to suggest a biomimetic approach for improving the ACL artificial prosthesis.[69,70]

The design of LARS™ ligament prosthesis was initially based on the surgeon's intuition (see Figure 5). In fact, Dr. Laboureau had noticed that the intra-articular fibers of the natural ligaments were arranged in a helical pattern, as Yahia had shown in his thesis of 1984.[71] They have supposed that this self-organization would reduce the fatigue and the wear of cruciate ligaments during physiological twisting movements (screw home). This hypothesis was validated by performing fatigue tests on different commercial ligaments, including LARS™ ligaments, using cruciate ligament fatigue/wear testing system TTF600 developed at Polytechnique Montreal by Drouin *et al.* (1991).[72]

This machine was designed to subject the ligaments to simultaneous tension, bending and torsion in order to better reproduce the *in vivo* loading conditions and the environment conditions. Six devices can be tested simultaneously in a liquid environment at 37°C. Computer monitored the loading conditions and the behavior of the prosthesis.

Unfortunately, most companies producing artificial ligaments have not followed these concepts,[73] nor by the FDA, which has not updated its guidelines for cruciate ligament fatigue tests to date. The latter being know through the catastrophic failure of most synthetic ligaments in North America and their withdrawal from the market.

In 2015, Brulez *et al.* from LARS™ company patented a biodegradable and "biointegrable" artificial ligament which makes it possible to take away all the apprehensions and the uncertainties due to their previous non-degradable synthetic support.[74] It consists of polycaprolactone (PCL) fibers, inspired by and similar to the native tissue, which is biodegradable while being sterilizable. It can optionally be seeded in order to facilitate the formation of functional tissues with controlled cell and tissue activity, having the required mechanical properties. The prosthesis may slowly be resorbable in order to be gradually replaced with a functional tissue identical to that of the native ligament.

6.1. *Nitinol ACL*

Nickel–titanium (NiTi) alloys are used in a variety of medical devices, due to its combination of mechanical properties that include super-elasticity, shape memory and corrosion resistance.[75]

Yahia *et al.* have been the first to propose the use of Nitinol wires in ACLR.[76] Their strategy was to take advantage on the mechanical compatibility of Nitinol with soft tissue to reproduce the mechanical behavior of the natural ligament; i.e. super-elasticity, hysteresis, and biocompatibility. This is impossible with other conventional materials. A new orientation in the design of the ligament prosthesis need to be taken. A solution would be to use super-elastic springs or helical structures. In fact, these structures are able to undergo large macroscopic deformation while the microscopic strain remains small.

The excellent biocompatibility, very high corrosion resistance, and excellent cytocompatibility of Nitinol has made these unique applications possible.[75] Nitinol is an alloy of nickel and titanium chemically joined with a strong intermetallic bond and in which these two elements are mostly present in the same percentages. Of course, the necessary regulatory approvals must still be received for each new application. For a more thorough review of the biocompatibility of Nitinol, please consult the references below.[75] The FDA regulation of NiTi remains a challenge, particularly for musculoskeletal applications.[77]

In 2013, Bogdan *et al.* performed a study of the behavior of an artificial ACL made from Nitinol using a FE analysis (see Figure 8).[78] Considering the human ACLR aspects, the proposed artificial ACL was inserted into the *FE* model of the knee joint. Results showed that the values of the stress are below the transformation plateau of

(a)

(b)

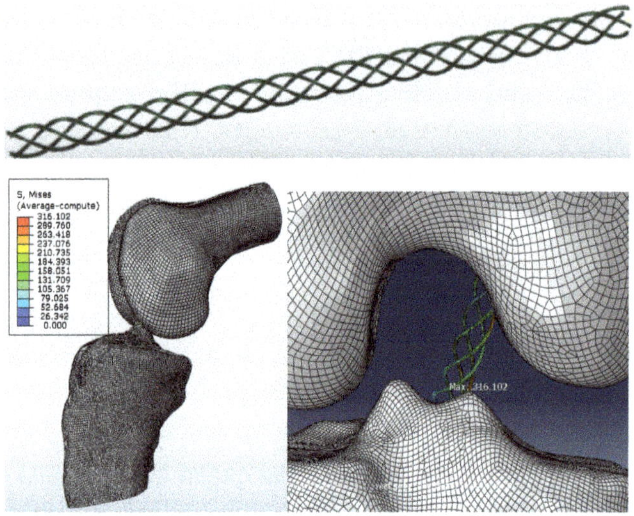

Figure 8. Model of the synthetic ACL made from Nitinol (a) Stress distribution at a 60 degrees flexion (b)[78]

Nitinol's martensitic phase and the material can recover all the strain (see Figure 8).

Super-elastic Nitinol alloys are becoming integral to the design of a variety of medical products. The considerable elasticity of these alloys is the most important advantage afforded by this material but by no means the only advantage. The nickel in Nitinol is chemically joined to the titanium with a strong intermetallic bond, so the risk of reaction, even in patients with nickel sensitivity, is extremely low.[79,80] Despite all these structural properties, there is insufficient evidence showing that these alloys could be used in reconstruction of a natural ligament. In one patient, early implant failure occurred when he was running smoothly without any landing, stopping, or cutting maneuver mechanism and without a strong valgus or a rotary force to his knee. They blamed non-anatomic placement of the graft and low elasticity and strength of the graft material for early fatigue behavior. In addition, probable metallic irritation cannot be neglected for synovial joints such as the knee joint. The researchers found multiple free-floating intra-articular metallic particles. Metal hypersensitivity and impaired renal function should be considered during decision making when choosing the graft type. Nevertheless, current evidence is not enough to suggest a metallic graft as an option for an ideal allograft. Above all, this is the second growing in popularity of similar synthetic grafts in the past 20 years. Such grafts should not be able to be adapted to daily practice so easily. The researchers believe that using grafts of similar structure should be avoided because of their lack of biocompatibility. It is a fact that they are doomed to early mechanical failure. Further research is necessary to standardize the processes involved in ACLR including the graft choice and the graft fixation methods.

6.2. *Knee-T-Nol ACL Prosthesis*

A promising new ligament implant from Israel is now entering the market, kicking months of recovery time off any current treatment. Inspired by stents, the device is developed by Israeli company Tavor. The Knee-T-Nol implant is made from a metal and titanium alloy, Nitinol, and looks a little like a dart. NiTi alloys, or Nitinol, is different from conventional titanium alloys.

Idan *et al.* conceived a new design for ligament or for tendon prosthesis made from two or more of cables braided into a helical structure, where each cable is made from two or more strands.[81] The strands may be made from an alloy exhibiting pseudo-elastic properties at body temperature and may be twisted into a helical structure in the cable. Each cable of the prosthesis comprises two or more strands that are twisted together (see Figure 9). The strands may be made from a pseudo-elastic alloy (also known as a "super-elastic alloy") such as an implantable Nitinol conforming to the ASTM Standard 2063. As shown below, strands made from a super-elastic alloy endow the prosthesis with mechanical properties particularly suitable to replace a torn ligament or a tendon.

The prosthesis tends to have a relatively low resistance to bending and to twisting movements as compared to the tensile resistance of the prosthesis, in comparison to a regular braid of solid wires of the same diameter. This allows implanting the prosthesis as a replacement

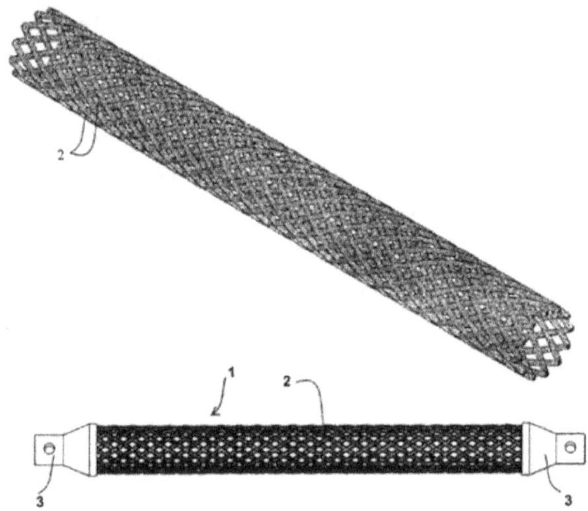

Figure 9. Structure of the prosthesis for replacement of the ACL[81]

for intra-articular ligaments or for tendons, which undergo extensive twisting and bending as compared to extra-articular ligaments or tendons.

The invention thus provides a ligament or a tendon prosthesis comprising two or more of cables braided into a helical structure, each cable comprising two or more strands. The prosthesis may further comprise an attachment device at one or both ends configured to allow an end of the prosthesis to be attached to bone (see Figure 9). The prosthesis may have a hollow circular cross-section.

Each cable may have a helical shape in the prosthesis, and may have, for example, a radius of 2–8 mm. The prosthesis may have a number of cables in a range from 24 to 96, and the cables may be connected at points of contact between the cables in the braided structure.

The strands of the prosthesis may be made, for example, of an alloy exhibiting pseudo-elastic properties at body temperature. The strands may be twisted together. The number of strands in a cable may be in a range from 3 to 19. The strands may be made from a pseudo-elastic alloy such as Nitinol. Each strand in a cable may have a helical shape having a radius, for example, of 0.2–0.6 mm. The helical shape of a strand may have a ratio of radius to pitch that is smaller than a ratio of radius to pitch of cables having a helical shape in the prosthesis.

The prosthesis may have a nonlinear force–elongation relationship. In an embodiment of the invention, the prosthesis comprises 48 cables, each cable being 0.5 mm thick and comprising 19 strands, 0.1 mm thick, made of Nitinol with an austenitic final temperature of 25°C. The prosthesis may have a 3-mm elongation in a toe region, a 2.4-mm elongation in the pseudo-elastic region, and an ultimate tensile load of 750 N.

When implanted laparoscopically through three small incisions, the flexible metallic tubing works to anchor the knee to its upper and lower bones, while providing strength, support and ligament-like freedom of movement almost immediately. The braided, super-elastic Nitinol strands are spring-like, much like a natural tendon.

Idan Tobis started a clinical study in 2015. This study is designed to evaluate the safety and the efficacy of implanting the Tavor ACL prosthesis in patients with a ruptured ACL by improvement of healing kinetics as well as major adverse treatment events. It is designed to test the hypothesis that there is a difference in healing kinetics of ACL deficient knees treated by ACLR using autografts and those in which such procedure was performed with the Tavor prosthesis.

The Tavor implant reportedly failed in two people, and occasional fractures in Nitinol wire were found in these cases.[82] This device is now in place in 14 patients in Israel. It offers great promise for athletes who have everything to lose.

With a *Conformité Européenne* (CE) Mark approval for Europe, the procedure and the implant are currently only available in Turkey's clinics that accept foreign patients. To break into the US market, due to stringent FDA requirements, it will take a significant investment of about $10 million, a 200-patients clinical trial, and 3 years of use in the operating room.

In summary, artificial biomimetic ligaments provide alternatives for both autograft and allograft which have a risk of donor site morbidity and risks of possible disease transmission, whereas artificial ones can be widely available with a long shelf life and simple storage and inventory arrangements.

As well as availability, convenience, lack of disease transmission risk and cost, the other advantage of synthetic ligament reconstruction is the potential for dramatically accelerated rehabilitation with return to sport significantly earlier than for autograft or for allograft. This is because biological grafts require prolonged period (probably at least 1 year) for incorporation of the graft tissue into the host bone.

7. Alternatives: Biologic Grafts

As it was mentioned previously, following the failures of the first generation of synthetic ligaments, North American orthopedists have turned to autograft or to allograft transplants for ACLR. Other strategies have emerged since the 2000s, such as the improvement of the healing process (Chapter 1), biomimetic prostheses (Chapter 11) or ligament engineering.[64] In other words, this "ligament disaster" has led clinicians and bioengineers to realize that nature has done things too well. As a result, clinicians have returned to the old practice of transplants, and bioengineers to new biological and bioinspired approaches.

Tissue engineering is still in its infancy to restore, maintain and improve ACL functions. Fibrous scaffolds composed of natural or synthetic polymers were cultured via ligament cells to reproduce the performance of native ACL. Some of these biodegradable scaffolds have been implanted into animal models and they have shown promising regeneration of ACL. Their clinical evaluation, however, has not been assessed for these engineered ligaments. Long-term development in this field may resolve the issue of ACL by complete regeneration of this tissue. Therefore, in the following sections, techniques for closer use in the clinical environment will be presented.

In 2015 and 2017, two excellent overviews of different approaches using tendon and ligament grafts and augmentation (of auto-, allo-, and xenobiotic origin) were published.[83,84] Xenografts, ligaments from other animals, and allografts from cadaveric human tissue are possibilities that overcome the need to autologous tissues and avoid the risk of donor-site morbidity. However, their use poses several issues including risks of disease transmission, graft rejection and inflammation. Moreover, in the case of allografts, the supply is so small that the market demand can never be met from this source. Autograft tissues extracted from the patellar tendon, the quadriceps tendon–patellar bone or the hamstring tendons are currently the most common sources of grafts for ACLR. Yet, this therapy relies on the extraction of healthy tissue which implies risks of donor-site morbidity, an initial low strength, a high probability of rupture at the initial stages and a long and painful recovery period.

The typical treatment of tendon or ligament injuries involves the use of tissue allografts or autografts to allow patients to return rapidly to ordinary activities of daily living. However, evidence suggests that these procedures do not substantially convalesce long-term patient outcomes.[85–87]

All the different types of grafts used in everyday practice for the reconstruction of a ruptured ACL have a place in this complex field of surgery. There are good data to support all of them. The most commonly used grafts in ACLR are the hamstring tendon and the patellar tendon. Hamstring and bone–patellar tendon–bone autografts are described to allow approximately 50% of patients to return to their pre-injury sporting activity level. There is no clear "best" graft to use.[88] Despite the vast amount of research, a great deal of debate still surrounds graft choice during ACLR and the effect of graft choice on subsequent graft failure. However, there are some clear advantages with respect to the different grafts. The factors considered by the surgeon include donor-site morbidity, reported rates of graft failure, familiarity with the graft, surgical time, associated complications, ability to restore the patient's activity to pre-injury level, and cost-effectiveness.

The ideal graft for ACLR should reproduce the histological and the biomechanical characteristics of the native ligament, incorporate fully and quickly within bone tunnels, have no risk of rejection nor disease transmission, have minimal donor site morbidity, be of sufficient length and diameter, and be cost-effective, as well as readily available.[89] The ultimate physical and mechanical properties of implanted graft should approximate or exceed the native ACL.

7.1. *Autograft*

Autologous grafts remain the most popular method for ACLR and are considered as "gold standard" because of the high rate of success (85–90%) of their long-term clinical outcomes.[90–92]

In this method, the injured ligament is substituted with a tendon of the patient. Patella tendon, hamstring tendons (e.g. semitendinosus and gracilis), and quadriceps tendons are commonly used as an alternative tissue.[92]

7.1.1. *Bone-patellar tendon-bone (BPTB) grafts*

BPTB grafts allow for bone-to-bone healing within the tunnels, seen to have favorable time-zero biomechanical strength and have good-to-excellent clinical outcomes on long-term follow-up.[89] Histologic studies have shown that osteonecrosis occurs at the graft tunnel interface, followed by creeping substitution and rapid incorporation into surrounding host bone. Dense fibrous tissue surrounds the bone block at 3 weeks with complete incorporation of the grafted bone to the host bone by 6 weeks.[89]

The ultimate tensile load, the stiffness and the cross-sectional area of the BPTB are comparable with the intact ACL. Thus, the BPTB autograft has the intrinsic properties that allow immediate active rehabilitation, and these favorable biomechanical properties combined with bone to bone healing and rigid, aperture fixation with interference screws account for the graft's excellent initial and continued long-term performance.

Literature has described many disadvantages of patellar tendon autograft. First, the length of the BPTB graft is fixed and is vulnerable to graft tunnel mismatch when tunnel length is not adjusted accordingly. Second, patella fracture is another disadvantage that is associated, following ACLR using BPTB autograft.

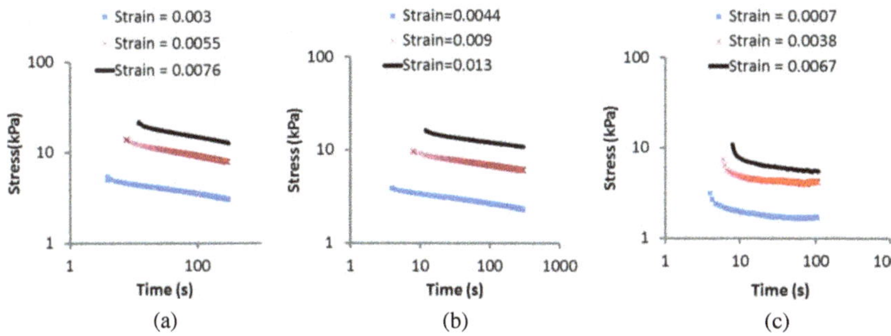

Figure 10. Stress relaxation as a function of initial strain for ACL (a), BLB in adult sheep (b) and adult patellar tendon (c)[90]

However, the patellar tendon has been shown to differ in viscoelastic properties, as the initial stiffness and the strain to failure rate are dissimilar, leading to an increasing failure incidence (see Figure 10).[90,93]

It significantly promotes bone-to-bone healing, initial fixation securing and returning to pre-injury activities.[94] Donor site morbidity including anterior knee pain, kneeling pain, patellar fracture, higher graft failure rates, and patellofemoral pain are its main complications.[95]

7.1.2. *Hamstring tendon*

Hamstring tendon (HT) is another alternative in autogeneic grafts. Their mechanical properties include ultimate tensile yield strength, stiffness, and stress relaxation curve mimicking the native ACL.[96] The widening of femoral tunnel and the weakness of the hamstring muscles after the operation are considered as their potential adverse effect.[97] ACLR is favorable due to the higher rate of satisfaction and a lower degree of OA in HT grafts.

7.1.3. *Semitendinosus tendon*

Semitendinosus tendon (STT) seems to be an ideal autograft for ACLRs.[98–100] Goradia *et al.* showed that an STT autograft can be transformed into a histologically very similar tendon as the ACL, after 1 year.[98,99] For that purpose, this group performed an ACLR in one of the hind limbs of eleven sheep and used a doubled STT autograft, which was attached to the femur with an endoscopic button and to the tibia with sutures tied around a screw. After the surgery, histological analysis revealed a successful adaptation of the tendon structure compared to the natural ACL. The conclusion was that the STT autograft led to good results compared to the usually used patellar tendon autograft.[98,99] However, during the first-year post-operation, the biomechanical properties of STT autograft in a sheep model were lower than those of native ACL.[83] Kondo *et al.* (2012) found that after 52 weeks post-operation, the maximum load of the femur–graft–tibia complex was significantly lower than the femur–ACL–tibia complex.[100]

7.1.4. *Complications associated to autografts*

These autografts pretend to be "gold standard" because they give the illusion to be made of biologic human tissues and therefore have more opportunities to be completely integrated by the patient's organism. However, with some investigation, it is possible to recognize some drawbacks. The necessity of harvesting tissue from the patient adds further damage to an already damaged knee with destruction of the proprioceptive neuroreceptors. Nevertheless, with synthetic ligaments, there are 0% of these complications because no harvesting is required. Regarding HT, several studies showed that their removal can cause a diminution of the rotational control and consequently decrease the protection of the new ligament during rotational stresses. During the first few weeks following the implantation, the graft resistance decreases reaching only 30% of the initial one and after 9 years the final resistance is only 50%. This explains why the return to physical activities including sports must be reported within seven to eight months.

Nevertheless, several studies give a rate of good results near to 80% but some to 60%. Therefore, the so-called biologic autografts can be defined as "gold standard". In any case, it is necessary to find other possible grafts, avoiding "robbing Peter to pay Paul" by harvesting, respecting the proprioceptivity and vascularization and cutting no bridges in case of further failures.

There are many reports of the morbidity and complication associated with BTPB grafts. Complications include patella tendon rupture, patella/tibial fracture, quadriceps weakness, loss of full extension, anterior knee pain and difficulty kneeling.[88]

Autograft failure is found in ACLR due to harvesting not enough graft material, inaccurate bone tunnel orientation, and low tension in the BPTB autograft.[101]

7.2. *Allograft*

The allografts are able to eliminate completely the donor site morbidity. The use of allografts shortens the operation period and it reduces the size of incisions.[102] Further advantages of allograft include no size limitation appropriate for revision surgery, and lower incidence of postoperative arthrofibrosis and knee stiffness.[103] That is the reason, why there has been steadily increasing demand of the allograft.

Allograft causes an immunogenic response of the host to the graft and thus delay graft incorporation when compared to the autograft. A histological study has shown poor vascularization in the center portion of the graft at an autopsy 2 years after reconstruction.[104]

In 2010, Foster *et al.* conducted a systematic review and analyzed the graft sources affecting the functional outcomes in ACLR.[105] Out of 31 studies, there were only four studies on the functional outcome after allograft used in ACLR. There was no difference in the outcome for allografts compared to autografts in patients with up to 6 years of follow-up.

The most applicable allograft materials include patellar ligament, and Achilles tendon.[106] Other tissues such as anterior or posterior tibialis and peroneus longus have also been used for allograft ACLR.[107]

The 5-year follow-up on the ACLR revealed that the allograft leads to less pain and to better short-term function compared to autograft.[108] In a recent systematic review comparing long-term outcomes after ACLR with either autograft BPTB or autograft HT, no significant differences in manual/instrumented laxity and in graft failures between graft types were suggested. An increase in long-term anterior knee pain, kneeling pain, and higher rates of OA were noted with BPTB graft use.[109]

The main drawback of these grafts is the significant risk of disease transmission that can be minimized by sterilization of graft prior to reconstruction.[84] Moreover, an allograft may lead to immune rejection, delayed incorporation,[110] and bone tunnel enlargement,[111] that enhances the rate of failure. Besides, the remodeling activity of allograft tissue is slower compared to autograft due to the lower cellularity and to the absence of allograft's revascularization.[110] The mechanical properties of allografts for ligament are lower than autografts in terms of knee laxity, of stress to failure, and of postoperative traumatic rupture rate.[112,113]

Sterilized or fresh frozen allografts after aseptic harvesting have the same advantages as synthetic ligaments in terms of no harvesting, therefore no complications on the donor side. In addition, allografts are more available than autografts but less than the synthetics by lack of donors. However, the fibroblastic ingrowth is slower than with autografts.

Even considering the above doubts and the quality of the results, the major problem with this system is the real risk of transmitting bacterial infections (*Clostridium* spore infection for example) or viral infections (such as hepatitis, HIV and so on). Despite rigorous precaution when harvesting the graft in a sterile theatre and during the conditioning, the risk of contamination, even if bounded, remains. Firstly, because there is a window period between the moment of the contaminated donor and death, making the infection non-detectable and secondly, human error is always possible.

7.3. *Xenograft*

Current techniques to reconstruct ruptured ACLs utilize either autologous tissue or allograft (cadaver) tissue. Both treatments have well-documented shortcomings (i.e. autologous tissue exposes patients to increased morbidity and allograft tissue use is limited by global availability and quality). There are currently no effective artificial materials or xenograft tissue substitutes widely available.

Xenogeneic tissues are derived from other animal species and provide a source of material for engineering mechanically functional tissue grafts, such as heart valves, tendons, ligaments, and cartilage. Xenogeneic tissues, however, contain molecules, known as antigens, which invoke an immune reaction following implantation into a patient. Therefore, it is necessary to remove the antigens from a xenogeneic tissue to prevent immune rejection of the graft. Antigen removal can be accomplished by treating a tissue with solutions and/or with physical processes that disrupt cells and that solubilize, degrade, or mask antigens. However, processes used for cell and antigen removal from tissues often have deleterious effects on the extracellular matrix of the tissue, rendering the tissue unsuitable for implantation due to poor mechanical properties. Thus, the goal of an antigen removal process should be to reduce the antigen content of a xenogeneic tissue while preserving its mechanical functionality.[114]

Replacement of torn ligament with animal tissue, xenograft, has been attempted in less than 10% of ACLR.[115] The xenograft tissue is rigorously treated prior to implantation to reduce the immunologic side effects. Decellularization, enzymatic cleavage, glutaraldehyde cross-linking and terminal sterilization by irradiation are the optimized treatments for xenograft reconstruction.[116] These therapeutic techniques have the same advantages and disadvantages of allograft reconstruction. Immunological rejection and diseases transmission, however, are the serious drawbacks of xenograft replacement.[117]

Since young healthy human tissue is always in short supply, Dr. Stone initiated a program in 1996 to solve the rejection problem when animal tissues are transplanted into humans. Animal tissues are plentiful, young strong and healthy and can be sterilized. Dr. Uri Galili had identified the cause of rejection when live animal organs were transplanted into people as a specific carbohydrate called the Gal epitope.[115]

A novel method was developed for processing porcine tendon and other ligament implants that enables *in situ* remodeling into autologous ligaments in humans.[118] The method allows for gradual remodeling of porcine tendon into autologous human ACL while maintaining the biomechanical integrity. The method was first evaluated in a preclinical model of monkeys and subsequently in patients. The method overcomes detrimental effects of the natural anti-Gal antibody and harnesses anti-non-Gal antibodies for the remodeling process. This ligamentization process lasts around 2 years and the biomechanical integrity of the graft is maintained throughout the whole period. These studies are the first, and so far, the only, to demonstrate remodeling of porcine tendon implants into permanently functional autologous ACL in humans. Porcine BPTB served as a model in reconstruction of ruptured ACL. The porcine tendons were processed for removal of Gal epitopes by recombinant a-galactosidase, followed by partial cross-linking with glutaraldehyde. Studies in rhesus monkeys demonstrated that implantation of such processed tendons, for replacement of respected ACL, resulted in gradual ligamentization of the implant into autologous ACL. Subsequent studies in humans demonstrated a similar process of remodeling of the tendon implant into autologous ACL within a period of about 2 years, while the biomechanical integrity is maintained.

After successful primate testing, a human clinical trial, of BPTB ACL replacement was designed and carried out at The Stone Clinic initiated in 2003 demonstrating the ligament could be successfully and safely implanted and that it would be a sustained treatment in patients. The FDA accorded the success of this human clinical trial and a wide US clinical trial was accorded up to 10 sites for 326 patients. This trial is ongoing. In the meantime, a European clinical trial comparing xenograft tissue to allograft tissue was initiated and it was successfully completed. Recently the Z-Lig (a pig bone patellar tendon bone), invented by Kevin R. Stone, and subsequently developed by Apeiron Biologics, was cleared for marketing and distribution in the European Union and other markets which recognize the CE Mark.

The Z-Lig™ ACLR Device is an engineered porcine tendon that has been "humanized" to allow the tissue to be turned into an off-the-shelf scaffold device that can be used by surgeons to replace a ruptured ACL in the knee. In being granted Europe's CE Mark, the Z-Lig is the only non-human biologic device for revision and multi-ligament ACLR to be approved anywhere in the world.

8. Concluding Remarks

Synthetic grafts have been developed over the years and are currently on their "third generation" but have encountered considerable problems in the past. None of the first FDA approved artificial ligaments have demonstrated positive long-term results *in vivo*. Failures of these first-generation devices mostly originate from mechanical failures or from a lack of biocompatibility. Eventually, these implants failed due to fragmentation, to stress shielding of new tissue, to fatigue, to creep, and to production of wear debris. Most of these prostheses were soon after removed from the market.

It is important to mention that some synthetic ligaments, not approved by the FDA, have escaped recall and have survived in Europe and Asia until this day. This is particularly the case with LARS™, Trevira and LK ligaments, which are currently the most widely accepted synthetics; however, their use remains somewhat controversial.

On the other hand, both mechanical and biological studies conducted during the last 30 years provide a better understanding of the natural ligament. For example, the triple helix formed by natural collagen molecules as well as the helical arrangement of fibers and fascicles gave rise to a special property of ligaments known as the toe region. These findings lead to the development of biomimetic design of ligaments (2nd generation) such as LARS™ and Nitinol ACL. The helical arrangement of fibers was found to reduce the fatigue and the wear of cruciate ligaments during physiological twisting movements. A promising new ligament implant, developed by the Israeli company Tavor, is now entering the market. The Knee-T-Nol implant that is made from a nickel and titanium alloy, Nitinol, and it looks a little like a dart. With a CE Mark approval for Europe, the procedure and the Tavor implant are currently only available in Turkey in clinics that accept foreign patients.

Synthetic grafts are slowly regaining popularity as these show good general results with no donor site morbidity and the ability to perform multi-ligament reconstructions without compromising the patella or the hamstrings. They offer an off the shelf solution which shortens operative time and renders the surgical procedure somewhat less complex, and no graft harvest is required. However, the surgery is technically different and should ideally be performed on a different timescale form conventional ACL surgery.

Regarding the biological grafts, there is no ideal graft for ACLR without any complications. The ideal graft for ACLR should reproduce the histological and the biomechanical characteristics of the native ligament, incorporate fully and quickly within bone tunnels, have no risk of rejection or disease transmission, have minimal donor site morbidity, be of sufficient length and diameter, and be cost-effective, as well as readily available. Substitution of torn ACL with biological graft (i.e. autogenic or allogenic) is nonetheless currently the most successful technique in ACLR. The success rates of autogenous grafts are more than 80% in long-term clinical studies. The donor site morbidity and the feasibility of disease transmission, however, are the main drawbacks of biological grafts. Moreover, most of the patients do not return to pre-injury level of activity, due to structural differences between the graft and the native ACL.

A novel method was developed for processing porcine tendon and other ligament implants that enables *in situ* remodeling into autologous ligaments in humans. The Z-Lig xenograft (a pig bone patellar tendon bone), invented by Kevin R. Stone, and subsequently developed by Apeiron Biologics, was cleared for marketing and distribution in the European Union and other markets which recognize the CE Mark. A wide US clinical trial accorded by the FDA is ongoing.

Further studies are necessary to standardize the processes involved in ACLR including the graft choice, the graft fixation methods, and the rehabilitation protocol

Acknowledgments

The author would like to acknowledge the financial support from the Natural Sciences and Engineering Research Council of Canada (NSERC).

References

1. Shelton, W. R.; Fagan, B. C. *J. Am. Acad. Orthop. Surg.* **2011**, *19*(5), 259–264.
2. Leiter, J. R.; Gourlay, R.; McRae, S.; de Korompay, N.; MacDonald, P. B. *Knee Surg. Sports Traumatol Arthrosc.* **2014**, *22*(5), 1061–1069.
3. Bach, J. S.; Cherkaoui, M.; Corté, L.; Cantournet, S.; Ku, D. N. *J. Med Dev.* **2012**, *6*(4), 045004–045009.
4. Goldblatt, J. P.; Fitzsimmons, S. E.; Balk, E.; Richmond, J.C. *Arthroscopy* **2005**, *21*(7), 791–803.
5. Colombet, P.; Allard, M.; Bousquet, V.; Delavigne, C. *The History of ACL Surgery.* Orthopedic Mastery, No. 87, **1999**.
6. Altman, G. H.; Horan, R. L.; Lu, H. H.; Moreau, J.; Martin, I.; Richmond, J. C.; Kaplan, D. L. *Biomaterials* **2002**, *23*, 4131–4141.
7. Pavon-Djavid, G.; Gamble, L. J.; Ciobanu, M.; Gueguen, V.; Castner, D.G.; Migonney, V. *Biomacromolecules* **2007**, *8*, 3317–3325.
8. Benson, B. J. *J Biomed Mater Res.* **1972**, *5*(6), 41–47.
9. Forster, I. W.; Ralis, Z. A.; McKibbin, B.; Jenkins, D. H. R. *Clin. Ortho. Rel. Res.* **1978**, 131, 299–307.
10. Jenkins, D. H. R. *J Bone Joint Surg. Brit.* **1978**, *60*(4), 520–522.
11. Jenkins, D. H. R.; Forster, I. W.; McKibbin, B.; Ralis, Z. A. *J. Bone Joint Surg. Brit.* **1977**, *59*(1), 53–57.
12. Tandogan, R. N.; Taşer, Ö.; Kayaalp, A.; Taşkiran, E.; Pinar, H.; Alparslan, B.; Alturfan, A. *Knee Surg. Sports Traumatol., Arthro.* **2004**, *12*(4), 262–270.
13. Jenkins, D. H. R.; McKibbin, B. *J. Bone Joint Surg. Brit.* **1980**, *62*(4), 497–499.
14. Rushton, N.; Dandy, D. J.; Naylor, C. P. E. *J. Bone Joint Surg. Brit.* **1983**, *65*(3), 308–309.
15. Insall, J.; Joseph, D. M.; Aglietti, P.; Campbell, Jr. R. D. *J. Bone Joint Surg. Am.* **1981**, *63*(4), 560–569.
16. Doré, R.; Drouin, G. Deformable high energy storage tension spring. U.S. PATENT, NO 4,301,551, 1981.
17. Drouin, G.; Doré, R.; Thiry, P.S.; Jean-Francois, C. *J. Biomech. Eng.* **1980**, *102*(3), 194–198.
18. Cruz, J.; Rana, S.; Fangueiro, R.; Guedes, R. *Fibers and Polymers.* **2014**, *15*(1), 181–186.

19. Mascarenhas, R.; MacDonald, P.B. *McGill J. Med.* **2008**, *11*(1), 29–37.
20. Nishimoto, H.; Kokubu, T.; Inui, A.; Mifune, Y.; Nishida, K.; Fujioka, H.; Yokota, K.; Hiwa, C.; Kurosaka, M. *Int. Orthop.* **2012**, *36*(11), 2379–2386.
21. Sledge, S. L.; Steadman, J. R.; Silliman, J. F.; Peloza, J.; Flistone, H. A. *Am. J. Knee Surg.* **1992**, *5*, 65–70.
22. Seemann, M. D.; Steadman, J. R. *Am J Knee Surg.* **1993**, *6*, 31–38.
23. Wilson, W. J.; Lesis, F.; Scranton, P. E. *J. Bone Joint Surg. Am.* 1990, 72A: 742–748.
24. Lukianov, A. V.; Richmond, J. C.; Barrett, G. R.; Gillquist, J. *Am. J. Sports Med.* **1989**, *17*, 380–385.
25. Gillquist, J.; Odensten, M. *Am. J. Sports Med.* **1993**, *21*, 358–366.
26. Barrett, G.R.; Line, L.L. Jr.; Shelton, W.R.; Manning, J.O.; Phelps, R. *Am. J. Sports Med.* **1993**, *21*, 367–373.
27. Matsumoto, H.; Fujikawa, K. *Keio J Med.* **2001**, *50*, 161–166.
28. Engström, B.; Wredmark, T.; Westblad, P. *Clin. Orthop. Relat. Res.* **1993**, *295*, 190–197.
29. Senni, C. *et al.* (2007). Additional advantages of using artificial ligaments in orthopaedic surgery. *Keio J. Med.* **2007**, *56*(2), 66–67.
30. Nau, T.; Lavoie, P.; Duval, N. *J. Bone Joint Surg. Br.* **2002**, *84*, 356–360.
31. Trieb, K.; Blahovec, H.; Brand, G.; Sabeti, M.; Dominkus, M.; Kotz, R. *Eur Surg Res.* **2004**, *36*(3), 148–151.
32. Lavoie, P. Fletcher, J.; Duval, N. *The Knee* **2000**, *7*, 157–163.
33. Batty, L.M.; Norsworthy, C.J.; Lash, N.J.; Wasiak, J.; Richmond, A.K.; Feller, J.A. *Arthroscopy* **2015**, *31*(5), 957–968.
34. Ventura, A.; Terzaghi, C.; Legnani, C.; Borgo, E.; Albisetti, W. *The Knee* **2010**, *17*, 108–113.
35. Huang, J.M.; Wang, Q.; Shen, F.; Wang, Z.M.; Kang, Y.F. (2010). Cruciate ligament reconstruction using LARS artificial ligament under arthroscopy: 81 cases report. *Chin. Med. J.* **2010**, *132*(2), 160–164.
36. Chen, J.; Gu, A.; Jiang, H.; Zhang, W.; Yu, X. *Arch Northup Trauma Surg.* **2015**, *135*, 95–102.
37. Gao, K.; Chen, S.; Wang, L.; Zhang, W.; Kang, Y.; Dong, Q.; Zhou, H.; Li, L. *Arthro.: The J. Arthro. Rel. Surg.* **2010**, *26*(4), 515–523.

38. Papadopoulos, G. *et al.* Long-term results. In: *The Treatment of* ACL*CL Ruptures Using The LARS — Artificial Ligament.* (A.L.S., Salzburg, **2005**).
39. Fan, Q.; Fan, J. *Chin J Rep Reconstruc. Surg.* **2008**, (6), 676–679.
40. Liu, Z. T.; Zhang, X. L.; Jiang, Y.; Zeng, B. F. *Int. Ortho.* (*SICOT*) **2010**, *34*, 45–49.
41. Machotka, Z.; Scarborough, I.; Duncan, W.; Kumar, S.; Perraton, L. Sports Med Arthroscopy, Rehab, Therapy and technology, 2: 29.
42. Ventura, A.; Legnani, C.; Terzaghi, C.; Borgo, E.; Albisetti, W. *Eur. J. Orth. Surg. Traumatol.* **2014**, *24*, 93–98.
43. Cerulli, G. *et al.* (2007). *S.I.O.T* **2007**, *33*(3suppl. 1), 8238–8242.
44. Tiefenboeck, T. M.; Thurmaier, E.; Tiefenboeck, M. M.; Ostermann, R. C.; Joestl, J.; Winnisch, M.; Schurz, M.; Hajdu, S.; Hofbauer, M. *Knee* **2015**, *22*(6), 565–568.
45. Fu, F. H.; Bennett, C. H.; Ma, C. B.; Menetrey, J.; Lattermann, C. *Am. J. Sports Med.* **2000**, *28*, 124–130.
46. George, M. S.; Dunn, W. R.; Spindler, K. P. *Am. J. Sports Med.* **2006**, *34*(12), 2026–2037.
47. Miller, M. D.; Peters, C. L.; Allen, B. *J. Arthroplasty* **2006**, *21*(5), 765–770.
48. Muren, O.; Dahlstedt, L.; Dalén, N. *Arch Orthop. Trauma Surg.* **2003**, *123*(4), 144–147.
49. Legnani, C. Ventura, A.; Terzaghi, C.; Borgo, E.; Albisetti, W. *Int Orthop.* **2010**, *34*(4), 465–471.
50. Smith B. A.; Livesay, G. A.; Woo, S.L. *Clin. Sports Med.* **1993**, *12*, 637–670.
51. Woo, S. L. Y.; An, K. N.; Arnoczky, S. P.; Wayne, J. S.; Fithian, D. C.; Myers, B. S. Anatomy, biology, and biomechanics of tendon, ligament and meniscus. In: Simon, S. R. (ed.), *Orthopaedic Basic Science.* (AAOS, **1994**), pp. 45–87.
52. Laurencin, C. T.; Ambrosio, A. M. A.; Borden, M. D.; Cooper, J. A. Tissue engineering: Orthopedic applications. In: Yarmush, M. L.; Diller, K. R.; Toner, M. (eds.), *Annual Review of Biomedical Engineering.* (Palo Alto, CA: Annual Reviews, **1999**), pp. 19–46.
53. Fukubayashi, T.; Ikeda, K. *J. Long Term Eff. Med. Implants* **2000**, *10*, 267–277.

54. Muren, O.; Dahlstedt, L.; Brosjö, E.; Dahlborn, M.; Dalén, N. *Acta Orthop.* **2005**, *76*, 270–274.
55. Poddevin, N.; King, M. W.; Guidoin, R. G. *J. Biomed. Mater. Res. Winter* **1997**, *38*(4), 370–381.
56. Guidoin, M. F.; Marois, Y.; Bejui, J.; Poddevin, N.; King, M. W.; Guidoin, R. *Biomat.* **2000**, *21*, 2461–2474.
57. Gely, P.; Drouin, G.; Thiry, P. S.; Tremblay, G. R. *J. Biomech. Eng.* **1984**, *106*(4), 285–294.
58. Li, H. *et al. J. Biomater. Sci. Polym.* **2013**, *24*, 431–446.
59. Ciobanu, M.; Siove, A.; Gueguen, V.; Gamble, L. J.; Castner, D. G.; Migonney, V. *Biomacromolecules* **2006**, *7*, 755–760.
60. Vaquette, C.; Viateau, V.; Guérard, S.; Anagnosto, F.; Manassero, M.; Castner, D. G.; Migonney, V. *Biomaterials* **2013**, *34*(29), 7048–7063.
61. Moës, N.; Dolbow, J.; Belytschko, T. *Int. J. Numer. Meth. Eng.* **1999**, *46*, 131–150.
62. Weiss, J. A.; Gardiner, J. C.; Ellis, B. J.; Lujan, T. J.; and Phatak, N. S. *Med. Eng. Phys.* **2005**, *27*, 845–861.
63. Soslowsky, L. J.; Goldstein, S. A. Many unknowns in ACL repair. AAOS Bulletin, **1995**.
64. Yahia, L. H. *Ligaments and Ligamentoplasties.* (Berlin, Heidelberg: Springer Berlin Heidelberg, 1997).
65. Goh, J. C.; Ouyang, H. W.; Teoh, S. H.; Chan, C. K.; Lee, E. H. (*Tissue Eng.* **2003**, *9*(1), 31–44.
66. Thiry, P. S.; Tabbal, M.; Drouin, G.; Laurin, C. A. (1981). A large deformation composite model for quasi-cylindrical ligamentous structure. Mechanics of structural media. In: *Proceedings of International Symposium on the Mechanical Behavior of Structured Media*, Ottawa, Canada, Part A, **1981**, pp. 209–217.
67. Schroeder, Y.; Wilson, W.; Huyghe, J. M.; Baaijens, F. P. *Eur. Spine J.* **2006**, *15*(Suppl. 3), S361–S371.
68. Yahia, L. H.; Hagemeister, N.; Drouin, G.; Sati, M.; Rivard, C. H. *Biomimetics* **1994**, *2*(4), 309–330.
69. Hagemeister, N.; Duval, N.; Yahia, L. H.; Krudwig, W.; Witzel, U.; de Guise, J. A. *Knee* **2002**, *9*(4), 291–299.
70. Hagemeister, N.; Long, R.; Yahia, L. H.; Duval, N.; Krudwig, W.; Witzel, U.; de Guise, J. A. *J. Biomed. Mater. Eng.* **2002**, *12*(1), 47–57.

71. Yahia, L. H. *Étude de la nature composite des ligaments croisés du genou. Thèse de PhD sous la direction de PS Thiry*, Polytechnique Montréal, **1984**.
72. Drouin, G.; Masson, M.; Yahia, L.H. *Biomed. Mater. Eng.* **1991**, *1*(3), 159–165.
73. Yahia, L. H.; Hagemeister, N.; Drouin, G.; Rivard, C. H.; Newman, N. Evaluation of cruciate ligament prostheses — Critique of current concepts and procedures. In: Yahia (ed.), *Ligaments and Ligamentoplasties.* (Springer, **1997**), pp. 1–16.
74. Brulez, B.; Migonney, V.; Guilard, R. Publication number: WO2015/075397 Al; 28 mai, **2015**.
75. Yahia, L. H. *Shape Memory Implants* (Springer, **2000**).
76. Hagemeister, N.; Yahia, L. H.; Lours, T. *J. Phys. IV France* **1995**, *05*, C2-403–C2-408.
77. Yahia, L. H.; Rayes, F.; Warrak, A. O. *Shape Memory Alloys for Biomedical Applications* (Woodhead Publishing, **2009**), pp. 306–326.
78. Bogdan, L.; Faur, N.; Parente, M.; Pătraşcu, J. M. *E-Health Bioeng. Conf. (EHB)*, **2013**.
79. Mantovani D. (2000). Shape memory alloys: Properties and biomedical applications. *JOM.* **2000**, *52*, 36–44.
80. Pfeifer, R.; Müller, C. W.; Hurschler, C.; Kaierle, S.; Wesling, V.; Haferkamp, H. *Procedia CIRP* **2013**, *5*, 253–258.
81. Idan Tobis. Ligament and tendon prosthesis made from cables of filaments US 20130131803 A1. PCT/IL2011/00067. 13 mai, **2013**.
82. Bilal, Ö.; Kınaş, M.; Güney, A.; Doğar, F. *Orthop. J. Sports Med.* **2014**, *2*(11) (3 Suppl).
83. Buschmann, J.; Bürgisser, G. M. *Biomechanics of tendons and Ligaments. Tissue Reconstruction and Regeneration.* (WP, Elsevier, **2017**).
84. Negahi Shirazi A.; Chrzanowski W.; Khademhosseini A.; Dehghani F. Anterior cruciate ligament: structure, injuries and regenerative treatments. In: Bertassoni L.; Coelho P. (eds.), *Engineering Mineralized and Load Bearing Tissues. Advances in Experimental Medicine and Biology*, vol. 881. (Springer, Cham., **2015**).
85. Breidenbach, A. P.; Dyment, N. A.; Lu, Y.; Rao, M.; Shearn, J. T.; Rowe, D. W.; Kadler, K. E.; Butler, D. L. *Tissue Eng. Part A.* **2014**, *21*(3–4), 438–450.

86. Lohmander, L. S.; Ostenberg, A.; Englund, M.; Roos, H. *Arthritis Rheum.* **2004**, 50: 3145–3152.
87. Streich, N. A.; Zimmermann, D.; Bode, G.; Schmitt, H. *Int. Orthop.* **2011**, *35*, 607–613.
88. Shaerf, D. A.; Pastides, P. S.; Sarraf, K. M.; Willis-Owen, C.A. *World J. Orthop.* **2014**, *5*, 23–29.
89. Ranjan, R.; Asif, N. *Saudi J. Sports Med.* **2016**, *16*, 7–14.
90. Ma, J.; Smietana, M. J.; Tatiana, Y.; Kostrominova, T. Y.; Wojtys, E. M.; Larkin, L. M.; Arruda, E. M. *Tissue Eng. Part A.* **2012**, *18*(1–2), 103–116.
91. Leong, N. L.; Petrigliano, F. A.; McAllister, D. R. *J. Biomed. Mater. Res.* **2014**, *102*(5), 1614–1624.
92. Haut Donahue, T. L.; Howell, S. M.; Hull, M. L.; Gregersen, C. *Arthroscopy* **2002**, *18*(6), 589–597.
93. Danto, M. I.; Woo, S. L. Y. *J. Orthop. Surg.* **1993**, *11*, 58–67.
94. Forster, M. C.; Forster, I. W. *Knee* **2005**, *12*(3), 225–230.
95. Laboute, E.; Savalli, L.; Puig, P.; Trouve, P.; Sabot, G.; Monnier, G.; Dubroca, B. *Ann. Phys. Rehabil Med.* **2010**, *53*(10), 598–614.
96. Bogunovic, L.; Yang, J. S.; Wright, R. W. *Oper. Techniq. Sports Med.* **2013**, *21*, 64–71.
97. Struewer, J. Ziring, E.; Frangen, T. M.; Efe, T.; Meissner, S.; Buecking, B.; Bliemel, C.; Ishaque, B. *Int. Orthop.* **2013**, *37*(2), 271–277.
98. Goradia, V. K.; Rochat, M. C.; Grana, W. A.; Rohrer, M. D.; Prasad, H.S. *Am. J. Knee Surg.* **2000**, *13*, 143–151.
99. Goradia, V. K.; Rochat, M. C.; Kida, M.; Grana, W. A. *Am J Sports Med.* **2000**, *28*, 40–46.
100. Kondo, E.; Yasuda, K.; Katsura, T.; Hayashi, R.; Kotani, Y.; Toyama, H. *Am. J. Sports Med.* **2012**, *40*, 315–324.
101. Vališ, P.; Sklenský, J.; Repko, M.; Rouchal, M.; Novák, J.; Otaševič, T. *Acta Chir. Orthop. Traumatol. Cech.* **2014**, *81*(6), 371–379.
102. Caborn, D. N. M.; Selby, J. B. *Arthroscopy* **2002**, *18*(1), 102–105.
103. Amendola, A.; Stolley, M. P. *Clin. Sports Med.* **2009**, *28*(2), 215–222.
104. Malinin, T. I.; Levitt, R. L.; Bashore, C.; Temple, H. T.; Mnaymneh, W. *Arthroscopy.* **2002**, *18*, 163–170.
105. Foster, T. E.; Wolfe, B. L.; Ryan, S.; Silvestri, L.; Kaye, E. K. *Am. J. Sports Med.* **2010**, *38*, 189–199.

106. Sherman, O. H.; Banffy, M. B. (2004). Anterior cruciate ligament reconstruction: which graft is best? *Arthroscopy* **2004**, *20*(9), 974–980.
107. Pearsall, A. W. 4th, Hollis, J. M.; Russell, G. V. Jr.; Scheer, Z. *Arthroscopy* **2003**, *19*(10), 1091–1096.
108. Poehling, G. G.; Curl, W. W.; Lee, C. A.; Ginn, T. A.; Rushing, J. T.; Naughton, M. J.; Holden, M. B.; Martin, D. F.; Smith, B. P. *Arthroscopy* **2005**, *21*(7), 774–785.
109. Poehling-Monaghan, K. L.; Salem, H.; Ross, K. E.; Secrist, E.; Ciccotti, M. C.; Tjoumakaris, F.; Ciccotti, M. G.; Freedman, K. B. *Orthop. J. Sports Med.* **2017**, *5*(6), 1–9.
110. Jackson, D. W.; Grood, E. S.; Goldstein, J. D.; Rosen, M. A.; Kurzweil, P. R.; Cummings, J. F.; Simon, T. M. *Am. J. Sports Med.* **1993**, *21*(2), 176–185.
111. Fahey, M.; Indelicato, P. A.; Frank, C. B. *Am. J. Sports Med.* **1994**, *22*(3), 410–414.
112. Nagda, S. H.; Altobelli, G. G.; Bowdry, K. A.; Brewster, C. E.; Lombardo, S. *J. Clin. Orthop. Relat. Res.* **2010**, *468*(5), 1418–1422.
113. Scheffler, S. U. Schmidt, T.; Gangéy, I.; Dustmann, M.; Unterhauser, F.; Weiler, *Arthroscopy* **2008**, *24*(4), 448–458.
114. Cissell, D. D.; Hu, J. C.; Griffiths, L. G.; Athanasiou, K. A. *J. Biomech.* **2014**, *47*(9), 1987–1996.
115. Marx, R. G.; Jones, E. C.; Angel, M.; Wickiewicz, T. L.; Warren, R. F. *Arthroscopy* **2003**, *19*(7), 762–770.
116. Stone, K. R.; Walgenbach, A. W.; Turek, T. J.; Somers, D. L.; Wicomb, W.; Galili, U. *Arthroscopy* 2007, 23(4), 411–419.
117. Ekwueme, E. C.; Kwansa, A. L.; Sharif, K.; El-Amin, S. F.; Freeman, J. W. *Recent Pat. Biomed. Eng.* **2011**, *4*(3), 196–204.
118. Stone, K. R.; Walgenbach, A. W.; Galili, U. *Tissue Eng.: Part B* **2017**, *23*(4), 412–419.

https://doi.org/10.1142/9789811204630_0004

Chapter 4

Animal Models for Anterior Cruciate Ligament Reconstruction: Using *Ex Vivo* and *In Vivo* Models

Bertrand Lussier

DMV MSc Diplomate ACVS, Professor of Surgery,
Department of Clinical Sciences, Associate Member,
GREPAQ (Research Group in Animal Pharmacology of Quebec),
Faculty of Veterinary Medicine, Associate Researcher,
Osteoarthritis Research Unit, Hospital Research Centre (CRCHUM),
Université de Montréal
bertrand.lussier@umontreal.ca

Abbreviations

ACL	Anterior cruciate ligament
BMP-2	Bone morphogenetic protein 2
CPC	Calcium phosphate cement
HA	Hydroxyapatite
IACUC	Institutional Animal Care and Use Committee
IHH	Indian hedgehog signaling molecule
LARS	Ligament advanced reinforcement system
MSC	Mesenchymal stem cells
OA	Osteoarthritis
PDGF-B	Platelet-derived growth factor subunit B
PLLA	Poly(L-lactid) acid
UHMWPE	Ultra high molecular weight polyethylene
VEGF	Vascular endothelial growth factor

1. Introduction

Biomedical research is a vast domain that covers a plethora of disorders, from disease processes to therapeutic solutions. Numerous techniques are also available: from computer models to *in vivo* studies, not forgetting *ex vivo* or cadaveric models. The rupture of the anterior cruciate ligament (ACL) is a serious knee injury that affects a wide range of patients. The rupture of the ACL causes joint instability, which leads to pain, decreased function and predisposes to osteoarthritis (OA).[1]

There are several aspects of surgically correcting this disease that can be evaluated, and by several means. There are diverse aspects of surgically correcting this disease that can be evaluated, and by various methods. The use of computer models in orthopedic research has limited use: these predictive models cannot represent the complex integrative interactions of live beings. Evaluating biological systems requires using biological systems. The complex phenomenon of healing can only be reproduced and studied using animal models.

When studying healing, several key facts are essential to take into account, validating the use of *in vivo* models. *In vitro* studies are useful when evaluating specific aspects of healing or integration. They provide essential preliminary results that lead to pursuing with *in vivo* proof of concept studies. Using devices, implants or grafts must take into account their biofunctionality: how does the cellular environment react to the presence of such devices, implants or grafts? Furthermore, for regulatory agencies, two points are of utmost importance: the safety/biocompatibilty of an implant and its efficacy. Safe/biocompatible implant must be: non-toxic, non-thrombogenic, non-carcinogenic, non-antigenic, and non-mutagenic. In addition, any breakdown products or any products eluding from them must be safe/biocompatible.

Moreover, even if small animal models are adequate for safety and biofunctionality, only larger models such as dogs, sheep/goats and pigs can mimic the local healing/integrating capacities under physiologic loads.[2] According to the available literature, amongst the large animal models, the sheep/goat might be the one having the most resemblance with Humans.[2–4] Its use is frequent when evaluating orthopedic implants in spine surgery.[5] The quest for the perfect model in all domains of biomedical research is universal. As it does not exist, the best we can do is try to get consensus through a work group. This has been proposed for animal models in fracture research.[6] A consensus seems hard to reach with ACL models.[4]

This chapter will try to help researchers identify potential models to investigate further one or several aspects of their field of expertise. Hence, animal models play an important role in the endeavor for medical advances in the evaluation of ACL reconstruction, may it be in the pathobiology or in the evaluation of new techniques or devices.

2. Ethical Consideration

The responsible use of animals in research is a universal duty. Animal welfare is a topic that is well recognized and is of utmost importance. Most countries regulate the conduct of biomedical research using animal models. Furthermore, peer reviewed journals will not accept to revise manuscripts if the research protocol has not been approved by an Institutional Animal Care and Use Committee (IACUC). The role of this committee is to facilitate the investigative work and to ensure that the latter is conducted in accordance with the highest standards of animal ethics and care.

We, as researchers, must thrive to use animals responsibly in our investigative work and comply with the guidelines, rules and regulations of our respective ethics' organizations and regulatory agencies. All researchers, from medical to non-medical disciplines, must observe this compliance.

Ethics committees will evaluate the submitted protocols taking into account the following:

- Scientific merit of the project.
- The category of invasiveness of the procedure.
- If the model has been validated or reported.
- The number of animals:
  - Should have enough to have statistically sound analyses;
  - Should take into account attrition in groups:
    - Outliers, deaths, euthanasia.
- The anesthetic, analgesic and surgical protocol and post-op care;
- The respect of the 3Rs principles by Russell and Burch[7–9]:
  - **Replacement:** Refers to methods which avoid or replace the use of animals.
  - **Reduction:** Refers to strategies to decrease the numbers of animals used, without compromising the validity of the results.
  - **Refinement:** Refers to modifications of husbandry or experimental procedures which lead to minimizing pain and distress, thus decreasing morbidity and mortality. Also aims at enhancing animal welfare.
- The establishment of critical points and end-points.

It is important to inform the IACUC of all of these aspects when submitting your demand, making sure that committee's members have all the pertinent data to approve, approve conditionally or refuse the protocol. Once approved, the research protocol must be observed and the use and care of animals realized with strict adherence to the protocol. If deemed necessary, modifications can be brought to the protocol, but these must be approved, in advance, by the IACUC.

The use of animals in research is a privilege and is under the responsibility of each researcher. All efforts should be directed to benefit from their use for the comprehension and advancement of medical conditions for our benefit.

3. Hints to Select the Most Appropriate Model

The use of animals in research is a privilege and is under the responsibility of each researcher. All efforts should be directed to benefit from their use for the comprehension and advancement of medical conditions for our benefit. Researchers, who develop, validate and use different animal models are frequently asked which is the best model for this or that condition. As a veterinary surgeon and an investigator, the author of the chapter, Dr. Bertrand Lussier, always asks himself, which model is most appropriate for each individual project? The answer is, in most instances: he doesn't not know, but he will identify the desired primary outcome, search the literature and come back with a well-thought-out proposal.

Dr. Lussier is sharing in this chapter, hints to help you decide for your specific project, which is the most appropriate model. These questions can guide you in orienting your decision in choosing the most appropriate model for your study.

- Is this problematic found as a naturally occurring disease in animals?
  - This is the most important question!
  - The answer is no for rupture of the ACL. Even if dogs are afflicted by naturally/spontaneous rupture of their ACL, the underlying pathological process leading to rupture is totally different. Moreover, the surgical treatment for ACL rupture is also completely different: intra-articular repairs are not used because they fail due to enzymatic degradation and weakening of the grafts.

- Which question or problematic do you specifically want to answer?
  - As a rule of thumb, the "big" question is, "Is this technique or device efficient or better than this other one?" This is a bad question because it is too vague. It needs to be refined. The real question should be, "Which specific question do we want to answer?"
  - As examples:
    - In ACL replacement, do we want to evaluate the mechanical resistance of a fixation device at time of insertion or do we want to evaluate the biological integration of this method of fixation?
    - In ACL replacement, how are the device and the graft integrated through time?
- Which method or outcome measure (or measures) do you want to use?
  - Do we need histopathological evaluation alone or combined with mechanical resistance assessment? If so, we cannot use the same samples.
  - Do we need to run cytokine profiles of synovial fluid samples? If so, we need a certain volume of fluid to perform the analyses. We need then to choose large animal models (like rabbits or larger).
- Has this question or problematic been investigated in the past, and if so, which model was used?
  - Using validated or at least published models should be preferred.
  - Why reinvent the wheel?
- Did this model proven efficacious in conducting such studies?
  - Carefully read the limitations of the previously published studies to understand the potential use of this model.
- Does this model have a translational value?
  - Can we extrapolate your results to the clinical situation[10–12]?
  - If we measure the pullout strength of a 2 mm in diameter interferential screws in rabbits, can we extrapolate the results to Humans?
- Is this model technically feasible in your hands?

  - Do we have in our facilities all the resources necessary to conduct the study? Do we have the equipment, the personnel, the expertise and the funding?
- Did you consider the 3Rs?
  - **Replacement:** Did we look at all the different models and must we use an *in vivo* model?
  - **Reduction:** And if so, is it the most reproducible, and necessitating the least number of animals? Did we determine via the literature or a pilot project, the minimum number of animals necessary to establish statistical significance and adequate power?
  - **Refinement:** Is it the model that causes the least distress? Moreover, can we adapt the protocol to decrease distress, pain and complications?
- Is the use of this model publically accepted in your country? Is another model better accepted?
  - There are national and/or cultural differences for which animal models are chosen upon. These must be taken into consideration.
- Which animal model is readily available in your country?
  - Making sure that the chosen model is available or we might end up not being able to have sufficient numbers…
- Which model has less zoonotic risks for the investigative team and animal facility personnel?
  - It is important to know that some diseases are transmissible from animals to humans (and vice-versa). These are called zoonoses.
  - They comprise viruses, bacteria, fungi and protozoa. In general, viruses are more species' specific.
  - Is this zoonotic disease highly morbid for humans, or are the complications of contracting such a disease severe?
  - Is the risk of transmission high and is the infection easily prevented?
  - Can we make sure that the animals are free of this disease before they enter our research facility?
- Which model can be consistently reproduced in your setting?

  - This point is of utmost importance.
  - The use of a model that cannot be reproduced consistently will create greater variability in the results thus necessitating a greater number of subjects. This goes against the 3R principles.
- Which model is easier to handle?
  - If we want to evaluate the influence of exercise on our model, choosing one that can spontaneously exercise in our facility is preferred to one that necessitates reinforcement.
  - It is easy to walk and trot a dog VS walking or trotting a pig or a sheep.
  - It is easier to examine and manipulate rats or mice than monkeys.
- How much will this model cost to use?
  - Finally, it often comes down to financial resources.
  - Efforts should be directed to obtain the most valid results in sufficient numbers to determine or not statistical significance, not losing perspective of animal welfare and care.

These are all important questions that an investigator must ask in order to guide his decisions in regards to the necessity of using animal models and to which might be the most appropriate one to use.

4. *Ex Vivo* Models

In this section, the term *ex vivo* must be taken in its broad significance, which means outside of a living organism. Using this broad definition, once explanted, it is not necessarily perfused and reimplanted in a living organism. In its strict definition, *ex vivo* relates to a biological part, which is taken out of a living organism, kept alive and reimplanted.

As a more practical guide for investigators, instead of a long enumeration of studies and models, find Table 1 in which *ex vivo* models have been used for different types of evaluation. This is of course a non-exhausted list. These few *ex vivo* studies cover several topics and use several large animal models. Some *ex vivo* studies using human

Table 1. *Ex vivo* models in the evaluation of ACL repair techniques and devices. A non-exhaustive list

Evaluated outcome	Title	*Ex vivo* animal model	Objective of study
Fixation strength • Femur	Femoral fixation strength following soft-tissue posterolateral corner reconstruction using fibular-based technique: Biomechanical analysis of four techniques in normal and low-density synthetic bone[13]	Synthetic bone and **bovine** tendon	To evaluate 4 methods of fixation for posterior corner reconstruction
Fixation strength • Femur	A biomechanical comparison of ACL suspensory fixation devices in a porcine cadaver model[14]	**Porcine**	To evaluate 4 methods of femoral suspension systems of ACL
Fixation strength • Tibia	A comparison of the fixation strengths provided by different intraosseous tendon lengths during ACL reconstruction: a biomechanical study in a porcine tibial model[15]	**Porcine**	To evaluate tendon length (2 cm vs 4 cm) on tibial fixation strength
Fixation strength • Tibia	*In situ* comparison of varying composite tibial tunnel interference screws used for ACL soft tissue graft fixation[16]	**Porcine**	To evaluate 4 methods of fixation using interferential screws on tibial fixation strength
Fixation strength • Allografts	Mechanical strength of four allograft fixation techniques for ruptured cranial cruciate ligament repair in dogs[17]	**Canine**	To evaluate 4 methods of ACL replacement with allografts in a controlled study
Fixation strength • *LARS* (ligament advanced reinforcement system)	Mechanical evaluation of a ligament fixation system for ACL reconstruction at the tibia in a canine cadaver model[18]	**Canine**	To evaluate the initial mechanical stability of two techniques with an interference screw on the tibial side of an ACL repair with the *LARS* ligament
Fixation strength • Femur	Mechanical stability of the femoral fixation for single- and double-bundle ACL reconstruction in an *in vitro* experimental model[19]	**Porcine**	To evaluate the influence of a single vs a double bundle ACL on femoral fixation strength

(*Continued*)

Table 1. (*Continued*)

Evaluated outcome	Title	*Ex vivo* animal model	Objective of study
Fixation strength • Mesh augmentation	Improvement of primary stability in ACL reconstruction by mesh augmentation of an established method of free tendon graft fixation. A biomechanical study on a porcine model[20]	**Porcine** • 4 different techniques	To evaluate the initial primary stability of a mesh augmented hamstring graft
Kinematics and strength 3 tunnels with double bundle	Biomechanical comparison of three anatomic ACL reconstructions in a porcine model[21]	**Porcine**	To evaluate the knee kinematics and strength in ACL reconstruction with 2 femoral/single tibial vs single femoral/double tibial tunnels
Kinematics	A biomechanical study of two distinct methods of ACL rupture, and a novel surgical reconstruction technique, in a small animal model of posttraumatic OA[22]	**Rat**	To evaluate the effect of knee stabilization using rat tail tendon after surgical or biomechanical injury of the ACL
Kinematics	Primary and coupled motions in the intact and the ACL-deficient knee: an ***in vitro*** study in the goat model[23]	**Goat** ACL transection	To evaluate the effects of ACL transection on kinematics of the goat knee joint
Tunnel position • Femur	Femoral tunnel positioning using an anteromedial technique for ACL reconstruction: A radiographic study with a cadaveric model[24]	**Human**	To evaluate the accuracy of femoral tunnel placement using anteromedial arthroscopy portal
Fixation strength • Femur	Comparison of initial mechanical properties of 4 hamstring graft femoral fixation systems using non-permanent hardware for ACL reconstruction: an ***in vitro*** animal study[25]	**Porcine**	To evaluate the initial mechanical properties of 4 hamstring fixation systems
Tunnel position • Femur	Cadaveric knee observation study for describing anatomic femoral tunnel placement for two-bundle ACL reconstruction[26]	**Human**	To describe anatomic landmarks for double bundle ACL replacement

Tunnel position • Femur	Effect of tunnel position for anatomic single-bundle ACL reconstruction on knee biomechanics in a porcine model[27]	**Porcine**	To evaluate the effect of 5 tunnel positions on knee biomechanics
Allograft types	What is the best candidate allograft for ACL reconstruction? An *in vitro* mechanical and histologic study in a canine model[28]	**Canine**	To evaluate the mechanical (friction) and histological properties of several allografts.
Alternative model	White-tailed deer as an *ex vivo* knee model: Joint morphometry and ACL rupture strength[29]	**White-tailed deer**	To evaluate the validity of using white-tailed deer for *ex vivo* ACL rupture and repair studies
Fixation strength	Biomechanical comparison of four coupled fixation systems for ACL reconstruction with bone socket or full-tunnel on the tibial side[30]	**Porcine** knee and **bovine** tendons	To evaluate the biomechanical properties of 4 coupled fixation devices used in ACL reconstruction
Fixation strength	*In vitro* biomechanical testing of ACL reconstruction: traditional vs physiologically relevant load analysis[31]	**Bovine**	To evaluate the biomechanical characteristics of the cross-pin and button type fixation devices under practical rehabilitation loads
Fixation strength • Tibia • Various tunnel size	Influence of the diameters of tendon graft and bone tunnel in hamstring ACL reconstruction. A bovine model[32]	**Bovine** (calf)	To evaluate whether pull out forces and failure modes were influenced by changing tendon and bone tunnel diameters
Fixation strength ACL reinforcement	Intra-articular reinforcement of a partially torn ACL using newly developed *UHMWPE* biomaterial in combination with Hexalon ACL/*PCL* screws: *ex vivo* mechanical testing of an animal knee model[33]	**Porcine** knee	To evaluate the use of *UHMWPE* biomaterial reinforcement of partial ACL tears
Anterior tibial translation model	A potential animal model for creating a controlled and reversible ACL insufficiency[34]	**Ovine** Knee	To validate the use of a device to reproduce and evaluate anterior tibial translation

Table 2. *In vivo* models in the evaluation of ACL repair techniques and devices. A non-exhaustive list

Evaluated outcome	Title	*In vivo* animal model	Objective of study
Validation of ACL reconstruction model	ACL surgery in the rabbit[35]	**Rabbit** • extensor digitorum longus tendon • sutured to periosteum	To evaluate the feasibility and outcome of ACL replacement in rabbits
Validation of ACL reconstruction model	ACL reconstruction with semitendinosus tendon autograft without detachment of its tibial insertion: a histologic study in a rabbit model[36]	**Rabbit** • semitendinosus autograft • undetached from tibia	To evaluate the feasibility and viability of this type of graft in rabbits
Validation of ACL reconstruction model	A canine hybrid double-bundle model for study of arthroscopic ACL reconstruction[37]	**Dog** • digital extensor tendon • preserving posterolateral band	To evaluate the feasibility and outcome of ACL replacement in dogs
Validation of ACL reconstruction model	Mechanical strength of four allograft fixation techniques for ruptured cranial cruciate ligament repair in dogs[38]	**Dog** • 4 techniques	To evaluate the feasibility and outcomes of 4 ACL replacement techniques in dogs
Validation of ACL reconstruction model	Early joint tissue changes are highly correlated with a set of inflammatory and degradative synovial biomarkers after ACL autograft and its sham surgery in an ovine model[39]	**Ovine** • ACL autograft	To evaluate the feasibility and outcome of ACL autograft replacement in sheep and its influence on synovial biomarkers
Validation of ACL reconstruction model	Changes of early post-traumatic OA in an ovine model of simulated ACL reconstruction are associated with transient acute post-injury synovial inflammation and tissue catabolism[40]	**Ovine** • ACL autograft	To evaluate, over 20 weeks, the outcome of ACL autograft replacement in sheep and its effect on synovial biomarkers

Validation of ovine model	The mature sheep as an animal model for bio-enhanced ACL repair and reconstruction[41]	**Ovine** • Bioenhanced ACL repair	To validate the ovine model to study bio-enhanced healing of ACL tears
Validation of ovine model	OA develops in the operated joint of an ovine model following ACL reconstruction with immediate anatomic reattachment of the native ACL[42]	**Ovine** • Post traumatic OA	To evaluate the development of OA even after immediate stabilization of knee joint
Validation of ovine model	An animal model to study ACL reconstruction during growth[43]	**Ovine** • Immature (4 months)	To evaluate healing of ACL reconstruction in immature patients
Validation of porcine model	Investigating the effects of anterior tibial translation on anterior knee force in the porcine model: is the porcine knee ACL dependent? [44]	**Porcine**	*Ex vivo* study To prove that the knee is ACL dependent in pigs which supports is use in *in vivo* studies for ACL reconstruction strategies.
Validation of ACL reconstruction model	Use of a bioactive scaffold to stimulate ACL healing also minimizes posttraumatic OA after surgery[45]	**Porcine** • Bioenhanced graft	To evaluate the biomechanical properties and joint structural effects of a bioactive scaffold in ACL repair
Efficacy of ACL reconstruction • Interferential screws	High-purity magnesium interference screws promote fibrocartilaginous entheses regeneration in the ACL reconstruction rabbit model via accumulation of *BMP-2* and *VEGF*[46]	**Rabbit** • Semitendinosus tendon • Interference screws	To evaluate the efficacy of high-purity magnesium interference screws in the ligamentization process of tendon grafts
Efficacy of ACL reconstruction • Bioenhanced ACL repair	Effects of suture choice on biomechanics and physeal status after bioenhanced ACL repair in skeletally immature patients: a large-animal study[47]	**Pig** • Immature	To evaluate the effects of absorbable or non-absorbable sutures in bioenhanced ACL repair on suture tunnel and growth plate healing and biomechanical outcomes

(*Continued*)

Table 2. (*Continued*)

Evaluated outcome	**Title**	***In vivo* animal model**	**Objective of study**
Efficacy of ACL reconstruction • Blood derived mesenchymal stem cells (*MSC*) ACL	Efficacy and safety of human umbilical cord blood-derived *MSC* in ACL reconstruction of a rabbit model: New strategy to enhance tendon graft healing[48]	**Rabbit** • Hamstring • Sutured to periosteum	To evaluate the safety and efficacy of human umbilical cord *MSC* enhanced ACL reconstruction
Efficacy of ACL reconstruction • Novel silk-collagen scaffold	ACL reconstruction in a rabbit model using silk-collagen scaffold and comparison with autograft[49]	**Rabbit** • Sutured around screws in femur and tibia	To evaluate a novel silk-collagen scaffold for ACL reconstruction
Efficacy of ACL reconstruction • Bioenhanced ACL repair using *MSC* with whole blood	Addition of autologous mesenchymal stem cells to whole blood for bioenhanced ACL repair has no benefit in the porcine model[50]	**Porcine** • Immature	To evaluate the biomechanical efficacy of adding *MSC* to whole blood in bioenhanced ACL repair
Efficacy of ACL reconstruction • 3D bioartificial graft	Generation of stem cell-based bioartificial ACL grafts for effective ACL rupture repair[51]	**Porcine** • Immature	To evaluate the efficacy of combined stem cell technology with a non-absorbable biomaterial for the reconstruction of the ruptured ACL.
Efficacy of ACL reconstruction • Graft tensioning	Effect of graft tensioning on mechanical restoration in a rat model of ACL reconstruction using free tendon graft[52]	**Rat** • Flexor digitorum longus tendon • Sutured to periosteum	To evaluate the effect of graft tensionning on healing following ACL reconstruction
Efficacy of ACL reconstruction • Tripeptide copper complex	Tripeptide-copper complex GHK-Cu (II) transiently improved healing outcome in a rat model of ACL reconstruction[53]	**Rat** • Flexor digitorum longus tendon • Sutured to periosteum	To evaluate the efficacy of a tripeptide copper complex could improve graft healing following ACL reconstruction

Healing of ACL reconstruction • Effect of low-magnitude motion	Effect of short-duration low-magnitude cyclic loading vs immobilization on tendon–bone healing after ACL reconstruction in a rat model[54]	**Rat** • Flexor digitorum longus tendon • Sutured to periosteum and fascia	To evaluate the effect of low magnitude motion vs immobilization on tendon–bone interface
Healing of ACL reconstruction • *IHH* signaling	Indian hedgehog signaling and the role of graft tension in tendon-to-bone healing: Evaluation in a rat ACL reconstruction model[55]	**Rat** • Flexor digitorum longus tendon • Sutured through transverse bone tunnels	To evaluate the effect of *IHH* signaling on healing through pretensioning graft
Healing of ACL reconstruction • Ligament augmentation	Therapeutic advantage in selective ligament augmentation for partial tears of the ACL: Results in an animal model[56]	**Rat** • Partial ACL tear/ augmentation • ACL repair	To evaluate the outcome of augmentation in partial ACL tears
Healing of ACL reconstruction • Longitudinal gaps	Effects of gaps induced into the ACL tendon graft on tendon–bone healing in a rodent ACL reconstruction model[57]	**Rat** • Flexor digitorum longus • Created longitudinal gaps within tendon	To evaluate the effect of gaps for cell invasion in this ACL reconstruction
Healing of ACL reconstruction • Tissue engineering	Allograft integration in a rabbit transgenic model for ACL reconstruction[58]	**Rabbit** • Extensor digitorum longus tendon • Sutured to periosteum	To better understand the tendinous allograft integration, ligamentization and repopulation processes.
Healing of ACL reconstruction • Strontium enriched calcium phosphate	Use of a strontium–enriched calcium phosphate cement in accelerating the healing of soft-tissue tendon graft within the bone tunnel in a rabbit model of ACL reconstruction[59]	**Rabbit** • Achilles tendon • Suspension system around screws in femur and tibia	To evaluate the effect of enriched graft on healing

(*Continued*)

Table 2. (*Continued*)

Evaluated outcome	Title	*In vivo* animal model	Objective of study
Healing of ACL reconstruction • Influence of low dose radiation in autograft vs allograft	Bony incorporation of soft tissue ACL grafts in an animal model: autograft vs allograft with low-dose gamma irradiation[60]	**Rabbit** • Semitendinosus tendon graft • Sutured to collateral ligaments	To evaluate the effect of low dose sterilization of tendon grafts on ACL healing
Healing of ACL reconstruction • Influence of low dose radiation on allograft with seeding of cells	ACL reconstruction in a rabbit model using irradiated Achilles allograft seeded with mesenchymal stem cells or *PDGF-B* gene-transfected mesenchymal stem cells[61]	**Rabbit** • Achilles tendon allograft • Seeded with *MSC* or *PDGF-B* gene transfected *MSC*	To evaluate the effect of irradiated allograft treatment with *MSC* or gene-transfected *MSC*
Healing of ACL reconstruction	*In vivo* bone tunnel evaluation of nanoparticle-grafts using an ACL reconstruction rabbit model[62]	**Rabbit** • Acellular human gracilis tendons with gold nanoparticles	To evaluate the remodeling outcomes of these grafts.
Efficacy of ACL reconstruction • Tissue engineered grafts	Fresh vs frozen engineered bone–ligament–bone grafts for sheep ACL repair[63]	**Ovine**	To evaluate the efficacy of freezing tissue-engineered constructs as a method of preservation before use for ACL reconstruction
Efficacy of ACL reconstruction • Bioenhanced ACL repair	Biomechanical outcomes after bioenhanced ACL repair and ACL reconstruction are equal in a porcine model[64]	**Porcine**	To evaluate the biomechanical outcomes of bioenhanced vs control ACL repair
Efficacy of ACL reconstruction • Suture types	Effects of suture choice on biomechanics and physeal status after bioenhanced ACL repair in skeletally immature patients: a large-animal study[65]	**Porcine**	To evaluate the effect of absorbable or non-absorbable suture in bioenhanced ACL repair

Efficacy of ACL reconstruction • Attachment type	Bone-to-bone fixation enhances functional healing of the porcine ACL using a collagen–platelet composite[66]	**Porcine**	To evaluate if bony stabilization between the tibia and femur improves the structural properties of an "enhanced" ACL repair using a collagen–platelet composite
Efficacy of ACL reconstruction • Attachment type	Suspensory vs interference screw fixation for arthroscopic ACL reconstruction in a translational large-animal model[67]	**Canine**	To evaluate the healing of suspensory vs interference screws
Healing of ACL reconstruction	Temporal changes in cellular repopulation and collagen fibril remodeling and regeneration after allograft ACL reconstruction: An experimental study using Kusabira–Orange transgenic pigs[68]	**Porcine**	To evaluate the ability to track the distribution and differentiation of recipient cells using genetically engineered transgenic animals
Healing of ACL reconstruction • Bioenhanced scaffold	Electron beam sterilization does not have a detrimental effect on the ability of extracellular matrix scaffolds to support *in vivo* ligament healing[69]	**Porcine**	To evaluate a method of sterilization of extracellular matrix without significantly impairing *in vivo* function
Healing of ACL reconstruction • Bioenhanced scaffold	ACL regeneration using mesenchymal stem cells and silk scaffold in large animal model[70]	**Porcine**	To evaluate the implantation of *MSC*-seeded silk scaffold to regenerate the ACL in a porcine model.
Healing of ACL reconstruction	Tendon-to-bone healing of a semitendinosus tendon autograft used for ACL reconstruction in a sheep model[71]	**Ovine** • Double semitendinosus graft	To evaluate the osteointegration of double tendon graft
Healing of ACL reconstruction	Does fibrin clot really enhance graft healing after double-bundle ACL reconstruction in a caprine model? [72]	**Caprine** • Double bundle • Partial achilles tendon	To evaluate the influence of a fibrin clot on the optimizing healing

(*Continued*)

Table 2. (*Continued*)

Evaluated outcome	Title	*In vivo* animal model	Objective of study
Healing of ACL reconstruction • Using *HA/PLLA* screws	Polymer-hydroxyapatite composite vs polymer interference screws in ACL reconstruction in a large animal model[73]	**Ovine** • Bone patellar tendon graft	To evaluate the influence of *HA/PLLA* vs *PLLA* screws on healing
Healing of ACL reconstruction • Influence of Gender on biomechanical outcomes	Sex influences the biomechanical outcomes of ACL reconstruction in a preclinical large animal model[74]	**Porcine** • Females vs males	To evaluate the outcomes of ACL reconstructions on female vs males Yucatan minipigs
Healing of ACL reconstruction • Influence of age on healing	The effect of skeletal maturity on functional healing of the ACL[75]	**Porcine** • Juvenile vs adolescent vs adult	To evaluate the effect of age on healing of ACL reconstructions in Yucatan minipigs
Healing of ACL reconstruction • *LARS*	Biological and biomechanical evaluation of the ligament advanced reinforcement system (*LARS* AC) in a sheep model of ACL replacement: A 3-month and 12-month study[76]	**Ovine** • *LARS* and interference screws	To evaluate tissue ingrowth within the *LARS*
Healing of ACL reconstruction • Collagen-platelet composite graft	The use of platelets to affect functional healing of an ACL autograft in a caprine ACL reconstruction model[77]	**Caprine** • Patellar bone-tendon bone	To evaluate the use of *CPC* graft on post-operative laxity
Healing of ACL reconstruction • Augmented repair of remnant ACL tear	Biomechanical and biological findings between acute ACL reconstruction with and without an augmented remnant repair: A comparative ***in vivo*** animal study[78]	**Rabbit** Semitendinosus autograft	To evaluate the outcome of ACL remnant repair

cadavers are also included. The following Table 1 will permit the investigator to find and develop research protocols based on previously published articles. These studies will act as a springboard to launch new ideas for research in this field.

5. *In Vivo* Models

Once again, like in the previous section, as a more practical guide for investigators, Table 2 is presented below in which *in vivo* models have been used for different types of evaluation. This is of course a non-exhausted list.

6. Conclusion

The selection of an animal model is not a simple task. The perfect animal model does not exist; it is a question of selecting the most appropriate model for your project. Choosing an animal model can be facilitated by identifying precise objectives and questions to be answered by the investigative work. Then, here are a few hints: first, identify if an animal model is necessary?; Second, can *ex vivo* (cadaveric) models be used? If not, refer to Table 2 to verify in the literature what other models have been used previously which had similar objectives and were evaluating similar outcomes. Dr. Bertrand Lussier hopes this will facilitate your endeavor.

References

1. Frobell, R. B.; Roos, E. M.; Roos, H. P.; Ranstam, J.; Lohmander, L. S. *N. Engl. J. Med.* **2010**, *363*(4), 331–342.
2. Wancket, L. M. *Vet Pathol.* **2015**, *52*(5), 842–850.
3. Proffen, B. L.; McElfresh, M.; Fleming, B. C.; Murray, M. M. *Knee* **2012**, *19*(4), 493–499.
4. Madry, H.; Ochi, M.; Cucchiarini, M.; Pape, D.; Seil, R. *J. Exp. Orthop.* **2015**, *2*(1), 9.
5. Allen, M. J.; Turner, A. S.; Sairyo, K.; Ferrara, L. *SAS J.* **2008**, *2*(4), 195–200.

6. Auer, J. A.; Goodship, A.; Arnoczky, S.; Pearce, S.; Price, J.; Claes, L.; von Rechenberg, B.; Hofmann-Amtenbrinck, M.; Schneider, E.; Muller-Terpitz, R.; Thiele, F.; Rippe, K. P.; Grainger, D. W. *BMC Musculoskelet Disord.* **2007**, 8, 72.
7. Russell, W.; Burch, R. *The Principles of Humane Experimental Technique.* (London, UK" Universities Federation for Animal Welfare, **1959**).
8. Fenwick, N.; Griffin, G.; Gauthier, C. *Can. Vet. J.* **2009**, *50*(5), 523–530.
9. CCAC. Three Rs Microsite: About the Three Rs. Retrieved August 31, **2017**.
10. Sah, R. L.; Ratcliffe, A. *Tissue Eng. Part B Rev.* **2010**, *16*(1), 1–3.
11. Vavken, P.; Murray, M. M. *Tissue Eng. Part B Rev.* **2010**, *16*(1), 5–11.
12. Hast, M. W.; Zuskov, A.; Soslowsky. L. J. *Bone Joint Res.* **2014**, *3*(6), 193–202.
13. Gallo, R. A. *et al. Knee* **2015**, *22*(6), 591–596.
14. Rylander, L. *et al. Clin. Biomech.* (*Bristol, Avon*) **2014**, *29*(2), 230–234.
15. Bohn, M. B. *et al. Scand. J. Med. Sci. Sports* **2013**,. *23*(3), 263–270.
16. Yang, D. L. *et al. Clin. Orthop. Surg.* **2014**, *6*(2), 173–179.
17. Nyland, J. *et al. Knee* **2015**, *22*(6), 554–558.
18. Biskup, J. J. *et al. Am. J. Vet. Res.* **2015**, *76*(5), 411–419.
19. Debandi, A. *et al. Knee Surg. Sports Traumatol. Arthrosc.* **2011**, *19*(5), 728–735.
20. Dong, Y. L. *et al. Technol. Health Care.* **2016**.
21. Espejo-Baena, A. *et al. Arthroscopy* **2006**, *22*(4), 433–40.
22. Mochizuki, T. *et al. Arthroscopy* **2006**, *22*(4), 356–361.
23. Kato, Y. *et al. Knee Surg. Sports Traumatol Arthrosc.* **2010**, *18*(1), 2–10.
24. Qu, J. *et al. J. Biomech.* **2015**, *48*(10), 1811–1816.
25. Zaino, N. L. *et al. Ann. Biomed. Eng.* **2017**, *45*(4), 1093–1100.
26. Mochizuki, T.; Muneta, T.; Nagase, T.; Shirasawa, S.; Akita, K.; Sekiya, I. *Arthroscopy* **2006**, *22*(4), 356–361.
27. Trump, M. *et al. Knee* **2011**, *18*(3), 193–201.
28. Bachy, M. *et al. J. Orthop Surg. Res.* **2013**, *8*, 27.
29. Papachristou, G. *et al. Knee Surg. Sports Traumatol. Arthrosc.* **2007**, *15*(10), 1175–1180.
30. Cook, J. L. *et al. J. Orthop. Res.* **2015**, *33*(8), 1171–1179.

31. Biskup, J. J. *et al. Am. J. Vet. Res.* **2015**, *76*(5), 411–419.
32. Heard, B. J. *et al. J. Orthop. Res.* **2011**, *29*(8), 1185–1192.
33. Heard, B. J. *et al. Osteoarthritis Cartilage* **2013**, *21*(12), 1942–1949.
34. Proffen, B. *et al.* The mature sheep as an animal model for bio-enhanced anterior cruciate ligament repair and reconstruction. In: M. R (ed.), *The Knee: Current Concepts in Kinematics, Injury Types, and Treatment Options.* (Nova Science Publishers: New York, 2012), pp. 117–129.
35. O'Brien, E. J. *et al. J. Orthop. Res.* **2013**, *31*(1), 35–43.
36. Meller, R. *et al. Technol. Health Care* **2009**, *17*(5-6), 403–410.
37. Boguszewski, D. V. *et al. J. Orthop. Res.* **2011**, *29*(5), 641–646.
38. Murray, M. M.; Fleming, B. C. *Am. J. Sports Med.* **2013**, *41*(8), 1762–1770.
39. Cheng, P. *et al. Biomaterials* **2016**, *81*, 14–26.
40. Vavken, P. *et al. Arthroscopy* **2013**, *29*(1), 122–132.
41. Jang, K. *et al. Arthroscopy* **2015**, *31*(8), 1530–1539.
42. Bi, F. *et al. PLoS One* **2015**, *10*(5), e0125900.
43. Proffen, B. L. *et al. Am J. Sports Med.* **2015**, *43*(2), 320–330.
44. Kouroupis, D. *et al. Stem Cell Res.* **2016**, *17*(2), 448–457.
45. Fu, S. C. *et al. Knee Surg. Sports Traumatol. Arthrosc.* **2013**, *21*(5), 1226–1233.
46. Fu, S. C. *et al. J. Orthop. Res.* **2015**, *33*(7), 1024–1033.
47. Brophy, R. H. *et al. J. Bone Joint Surg. Am.* **2011**, *93*(4), 381–393.
48. Carbone, A. *et al. J. Orthop. Res.* **2016**, *34*(4), 641–649.
49. Mifune, Y. *et al.* Therapeutic advantage in selective ligament augmentation for partial tears of the anterior cruciate ligament: results in an animal model. *Am. J. Sports Med.* 2013. 41(2), 365-73.
50. Lovric, V. *et al. Muscles Ligaments Tendons J.* **2011**, *1*(3), 91–99.
51. Bachy, M. *et al. Orthop Traumatol Surg. Res.* **2016**, *102*(2), 189–195.
52. Kuang, G. M. *et al. Bone Joint J.* **2013**, *95-B*(7), 923–928.
53. Bhatia, S. *et al. Am. J. Sports Med.* **2012**, *40*(8), 1789–1798.
54. Li, F.; Jia, H.; Yu, C. *Knee Surg. Sports Traumatol Arthrosc.* **2007**, *15*(10), 1219–1227.
55. Grant, S. A. *et al. J. Biomed. Mater. Res. A* **2017**, *105*(4), 1071–1082.
56. Mahalingam, V. D. *et al. Tissue Eng. Part C Meth.* **2015**, *21*(6), 548–556.
57. Vavken, P. *et al. Arthroscopy* **2012**, *28*(5), 672–680.

58. Murray, M. M. *et al. Arthroscopy* **2010**, *26*(9 Suppl), S49–57.
59. Smith, P. A. *et al. Arthroscopy* **2016**, *32*(6), 1086–1097.
60. Takeuchi, H. *et al. Am. J. Sports Med.* **2016**, *44*(9), 2375–2383.
61. Proffen, B. L. *et al. J. Orthop. Res.* **2015**, *33*(7), 1015–1023.
62. Fan, H. *et al. Biomaterials* **2009**, *30*(28), 4967–4977.
63. Goradia, V. K. *et al. Am. J. Knee Surg.* **2000**, *13*(3), 143–151.
64. Hensler, D. *et al. Knee Surg. Sports Traumatol Arthrosc.* **2015**, *23*(3), 669–679.
65. Hunt, J. A.; Callaghan, J. T. *Knee Surg. Sports Traumatol Arthrosc.* **2008**, 16(7), 655660.
66. Kiapour, A. M. *et al. Am. J. Sports Med.* **2015**, *43*(7), 1623–1631.
67. Murray, M. M. *et al. J. Bone Joint Surg. Am.* **2010**, *92*(11), 2039–2049.
68. Viateau, V. *et al. Arthroscopy* **2013**, *29*(6), 1079–1088.
69. Spindler, K. P. *et al. J. Orthop. Res.* **2009**, *27*(5), 631–638.
70. Song, G. Y. *et al. Arthroscopy* **2016**, *32*(2), 307–319.
71. Goradia, V. K. *et al. Am. J. Knee Surg.* **2000**, *13*(3), 143–151.
72. Hensler, D. *et al. Knee Surg. Sports Traumatol Arthrosc.* **2015**, *23*(3), 669–679.
73. Hunt, J. A.; Callaghan, J. T. *Knee Surg. Sports Traumatol Arthrosc.* **2008**, *16*(7), 655–660.
74. Kiapour, A. M. *et al.* S *Am. J. Sports Med.* **2015**, *43*(7), 1623–1631.
75. Murray, M. M. *et al. J. Bone Joint Surg. Am.* **2010**, *92*(11), 2039–2049.
76. Viateau, V. *et al. Arthroscopy* **2013**, *29*(6), 1079–1088.
77. Spindler, K. P. *et al.* T *J. Orthop. Res.* **2009**, *27*(5), 631–638.
78. Song, G. Y. *et al. Arthroscopy* **2016**, *32*(2), 307–319.

https://doi.org/10.1142/9789811204630_0005

Chapter 5

The Fibrocartilaginous Ligament Enthesis

Johnathan L. Sevick[*], David A. Hart[*,†], and Nigel G. Shrive[*,‡,§]

[*]*McCaig Institute for Bone and Joint Health,*
University of Calgary, Calgary, Alberta, Canada
[†]*Department of Surgery, Cumming School of Medicine,*
University of Calgary, Calgary, Alberta, Canada
[‡]*Department of Civil Engineering, Schulich School of Engineering,*
University of Calgary, Calgary, Alberta, Canada
[§]*ngshrive@ucalgary.ca*

Abbreviations

ACL	Anterior cruciate ligament
AFM	Atomic force microscopy
BLB	Bone–ligament–bone
BMP-2	Bone morphogenetic protein-2
BPB	Bone–patellar ligament–bone
β-TCP	β-tricalcium phosphate
CFC	Calcified fibrocartilage
DIC	Digital image correlation
EMD	Enamel matrix derivative
FE	Finite element
FTIR	Fourier transform infrared
HA	Hydroxyapatite
MCL	Medial collateral ligament
MSCs	Mesenchymal stem cells
PCL	Polycaprolactone
PEGDA	Polyethylene glycol diacrylate
PGA	Propylene glycol alginate
PLA	Poly-lactide acid
QLV	Quasi-linear viscoelastic
RBX	Recombined bone xenograft
rt-PCR	Real-time polymerase chain reaction
Runx2	Runt-related transcription factor 2
SAM	Scanning acoustic microscopy
SEM	Scanning electron microscope
SHG	Second harmonic generation
Smad8ca	Constitutively active Smad8

TGF	Transforming growth factor
TPEF	Two-photon excitation fluorescence
UFC	Uncalcified fibrocartilage

1. Introduction

A complex, well-adapted transitional region of tissue called the enthesis typifies the attachment of tendon and ligament to bone.[1] The enthesis serves to transfer mechanical loads between soft and hard tissue, a considerable challenge from an engineering standpoint. In healthy subjects the enthesis performs this function well; however, in degenerative disease, injury or post-surgical intervention, the reformed enthesis does not provide the same level of function.[2,3] For clinicians, scientists and the patients they serve, this has remained a persistent source of frustration, and has spawned significant academic and clinical investment into the understanding of entheses, and their functioning and repair.

Two types of entheses are recognized in the literature,[4] differentiated primarily by their histological structure. These are fibrous and fibrocartilaginous. Fibrous entheses occur at the junction of metaphyses, where little relative rotation occurs between ligament/tendon and bone. Examples include the tibial attachment of the medial collateral ligament (MCL) and the clavicular attachment of the deltoid. Fibrocartilaginous entheses, on the other hand, occur near epiphyses and apophyses, often continuous with articular cartilage, and where relative motion between ligament/tendon and bone is significant. Examples include the attachment of the anterior cruciate ligament (ACL) to the femur/tibia and supraspinatus tendon to the humerus. Due to their relevance in injury and frequency in the body, fibrocartilaginous entheses have received the bulk of investigative attention, and will also be a focus in this chapter.

The most common examples (rightly) used to justify research interest in the enthesis are rotator cuff repair and ACL reconstruction. In the shoulder, the supraspinatus tendon attaches to the humeral head via a fibrocartilaginous enthesis. Many tears of this tendon and degenerative processes occur near the enthesis,[5] hence, this tendon often requires surgical reattachment post-injury. Unfortunately, healing of reattachments progresses via a scar-mediated process without regeneration of the original structure and composition of the enthesis.[3,6] The result is too often a re-injured rotator cuff (20–94% of cases[7,8]), and continuing pain and lack of function for patients. ACL reconstruction differs from rotator cuff repair in that grafted tissue is used and attached in a different configuration than the native ACL (i.e. through bone tunnels). Thus, the healing graft–bone interface generally does not resemble the native enthesis and is a frequent point of early weakness, resulting in graft failure.[9–11] As such, strategies to improve healing for both rotator cuff repair and ACL reconstruction are numerous and ongoing.

In this chapter, a thorough but non-exhaustive review of understanding of the fibrocartilaginous enthesis is presented. This will include the topics of enthesis development, structure and composition, and mechanics. Additionally, re-attachment strategies centered on ACL reconstruction will be briefly touched on. The authors intend that readers will be able to develop their own basic understanding of the enthesis to act as a springboard for ideas with the potential to overcome the challenges of soft tissue reattachment.

2. The Native Enthesis Structure, Composition and Function

The defining feature of entheses is gradation; gradation in structure and composition and thereby mechanical properties. Structural and compositional features of entheses have been well-documented, as will become evident. Additionally, the developmental processes and mechanical cues that generate these gradations have begun to be elucidated.

2.1. *Comparison of Fibrocartilaginous Entheses*

The different environments of fibrocartilaginous entheses (e.g. location in the body, biological conditions and mechanical stimulation) are likely to account for the differences seen between them. Benjamin *et al.*[12] detailed the histological appearance of numerous tendon entheses throughout the body, noting that, although differences within entheses (e.g. varying proportions of fibrocartilage and fibrous regions) and between entheses (e.g. fibrocartilage quantity) exist, many features of the physical attachment are common throughout, particularly the presence of tissue zonation. Benjamin and McGonagle[13] advocate the concept of an "enthesis organ" that encompasses not only the physical attachment but also the surrounding tissues and their interactions (e.g. the fat pad and retrocalcaneal bursa of the Achille's tendon), which likely differs between entheses. In an allometric study of the characteristics of the supraspinatus enthesis of different animal species, Deymier-Black *et al.*[14] showed that humeral head diameter increased geometrically with animal mass and that the area of enthesis attachment increased nearly isometrically with muscle cross sectional area, whereas interfacial roughness and mineral gradient width (discussed later) did not vary with muscle load. This is interesting because the increasing attachment area with increasing load combine to produce similar stresses at the interface regardless of animal size. This may account for the minimal changes in interfacial roughness and mineral gradient observed, since cells at the enthesis would experience similar mechanical environments.[14] It further supports the conclusion that, while every enthesis is unique, they share many of the same characteristics.

Although tendon and ligament entheses share overarching similarities in structure and are frequently referenced in the same conversation[15] (including in the discussion that follows), it is still worth recalling that every enthesis is operating in and influenced by a unique environment.

2.2. *Structure and Composition*

A great deal of literature exists describing what the fibrocartilaginous enthesis is made of and what it looks like. Fibrocartilaginous entheses typically occur at epiphyses and apophyses[4] where the attaching ligament undergoes large angular or rotational changes during movement.[16] As the ligament approaches bone, the enthesis exhibits an increase in cross-sectional area relative to the ligament mid-substance, further amplified by scalloping of the interface between the two tissues.[16] Where an enthesis begins and stops is not easy to identify, as the transitional tissues are contiguous with those that they connect; however, entire entheses are small (e.g. in the range of 380 μm to 1 mm[17,18]). Four broadly identified material zones have been used traditionally to describe the material transition at fibrocartilaginous entheses. From ligament to bone they are: ligament, UFC, CFC, and bone (e.g. Figure 1). Although exhibiting such a tissue transition, fibrocartilaginous entheses still consist of one part that is primarily fibrous and another that is primarily fibrocartilaginous.[4]

The ligamentous portion of the enthesis consists of densely packed, longitudinally organized fibers (primarily type I collagen with some type III collagen and elastin).[20,21] Cells in this location are no different from those in the ligament proper (i.e. elongated fibroblasts).[20]

The UFC region comprises the proteoglycan aggrecan and types I, II and III collagen[16,20,22]; the proteoglycans attract water into the tissue matrix and are typically present where the enthesis sustains compression.[16] Cells in this region are classified as fibrochondrocytes due to their rounded shape and the matrix they produce.[23] UFC differentiates itself from ligament by an apparent loss of cell-cell interaction as indicated by the loss of gap junctions, rounding and enlargement of cells.[23] Cells often appear in longitudinal rows/columns, similar to the organization of fibroblasts in ligament proper.[12] Ligament/tendon fibers unravel across a portion of the enthesis, indicated by decreasing fiber diameter.[2] Additionally, the parallelism of fibers lessens as they advance through the enthesis, splaying out at angles from the main fiber direction in the ligament/tendon.[2,24]

In the CFC region, fibers and matrix become mineralized. The region consists primarily of type II collagen but also contains type I and type X.[25–28] Fibrochondrocytes again comprise this portion of the enthesis, albeit in fewer numbers than in the UFC, a possible result of the deposition of calcium salts resulting in cell death.[16] In a study of rat Achilles tendon, pyknotic cell nuclei were observed in CFC,[29]

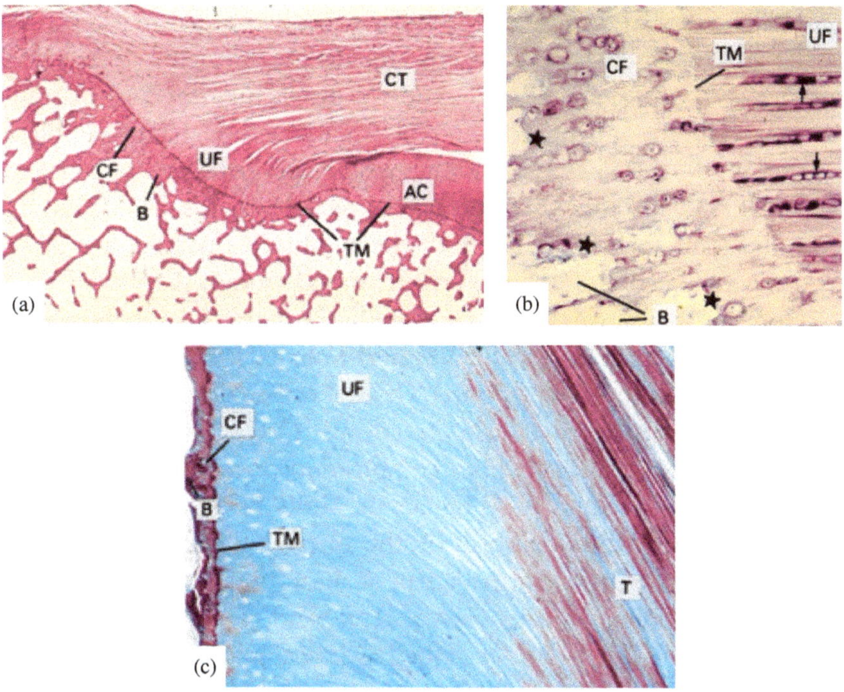

Figure 1. (a) Human supraspinatus tendon showing the four zones of a fibrocartilaginous insertion (H&E x8): dense fibrous connective tissue (CT), uncalcified fibrocartilage (UF), calcified fibrocartilage (CF) and bone (B). A visible tidemark (TM) separates the UF and CF; (b) Increasingly magnified view of the supraspinatus enthesis: asterisks indicate irregularly shaped junction with bone; (c) Insertion of rat quadriceps tendon into the patella (Toluidine blue x180) showing angular change of collagen fibers; Taken from Ref. [19], published with permission of Wiley

suggesting that apoptotic/necrotic cells occupy this zone. However, conflicting evidence suggests living cells also occupy this zone. In the calcified zone of articular cartilage, mineralization has been shown to stop short of cell boundaries, and is instead occupied by proteoglycans,[30] suggesting these cells are living. Whether the CFC is more or less calcified than bone is inconclusive.[4,20] The true union of ligament to bone is made at a highly irregular/undulating interface between CFC and bone.[4,31] Both the mature UFC and CFC regions are generally considered avascular.[4] Similarly, no functional nerve supply exists within the enthesis itself, though neural elements (e.g. nerve endings, receptors) have been reported to be present.[32,33] Instead, microvasculature and neuroregulatory elements are mainly supplied by surrounding tissues (e.g. joint capsule, periosteum).[32] Collagen content has been shown to decrease across both regions transitioning from ligament to bone, with fibrils becoming less parallel and their arrangement becoming increasingly random through the CFC.[34]

Bone at a fibrocartilaginous enthesis is characterized by a thin subchondral bone plate, small amounts of compact bone followed by more substantial trabecular bone.[4] The trabeculae demonstrate alignment with the principal tensile direction.[35] Osteoclasts, osteoblasts, and osteocytes act to maintain a composition of type I collagen and carbonated apatite mineral.[25] Ligament fibrils have been shown to both intertwine with bone fibrils (in the anteromedial band of the pig ACL) as well as to be embedded in shallow bone sockets with no intertwining evident (in the posterolateral band of the pig ACL).[36] In the rabbit patella, fibers are described as interdigitating with lamellar bone structures but not truly joining with bone fibers.[37] Thus, the precise configuration and integration of enthesis collagenous structures with bony collagenous structures is not entirely clear.

A basophilic line termed the tidemark is apparent histologically at the prescribed boundary between UFC and CFC, generally thought to demarcate the soft/hard tissue boundary.[4] Collagen fibers are continuous across the tidemark, and typically oriented nearly perpendicularly to it.[4,12,29] While no obvious cause of a tidemark could be identified in a scanning electron microscope (SEM) study of the rabbit patellar tendon enthesis,[37] a SEM study of human articular cartilage described the tidemark as a band of fibrils oriented perpendicularly to UFC/CFC fibrils,[38] highlighting the uncertainty of its origin. Traditionally, based on knowledge of a similar line in articular cartilage, the line is thought to represent a mineralization front, or the point at which the tissue ceases to be mineralized.[4] In fact, where entheses are adjacent to articular cartilage, their tidemark is continuous with that of the cartilage.[12] However, subsequent evidence points to a gradation in mineralization near the tidemark which has motivated the notion that its histologically abrupt-appearance is an artifact of staining (i.e. that the stain only gains noticeable visibility at a threshold concentration of mineral).[39] For example, a linear increase in mineral content has been shown to occur over 120 μm in the rat supraspinatus using Raman spectroscopy,[40] and over 20 μm in the mouse supraspinatus using micro-computed tomography.[41] Different methodologies provide alternative results though, such as an abrupt/step-wise increase in mineralization at the tidemark of the bovine ACL using Fourier transform infrared (FTIR) spectroscopic imaging.[34] Results from multiphoton imaging studies provide some evidence contrasting the idea that the tidemark is an artifact of the histological process. In these studies, a fluorescent boundary between two-photon excitation (TPE) signal (autofluorescence) and second harmonic generation (SHG) signal exists that shares similarities to the histologically identified tidemark, including the shape of cell lacunae, and the relative smoothness of the boundary, suggesting that it could be the same feature (Figure 2).[42–44] If this is the case, it would be intriguing based on the fact that these multiphoton signals are not known to be caused or affected by mineralization. In a study by Mansfield and Winlove[44] decalcified samples of the boundary displayed the same characteristics on multiphoton images as those that remained calcified. These authors suggested that the origin of the boundary could be increased collagen cross-linking, or cellular debris. In spite of the above discussion, such a boundary could equally still be an artifact of multiphoton imaging. In brief, there is a definitive gradation in mineralization near, or across the tidemark; however, whether the tidemark is visible as a result of this mineralization or some other structural/composition aspect is still to be determined.

A last, intriguing finding in relation to the potential tidemark seen in multiphoton studies is the possible presence of elastin. Likely due to the difficulties entailed in staining elastin for light microscopy,[45] its relatively low content as measured by immunohistochemistry at the enthesis,[2] and for being refractory to a majority of electron microscopy stains,[45] elastin has not been a popular topic of enthesis research. In multiphoton imaging however, elastin produces a strong, characteristic TPE signal in tissues that include cartilage, intervertebral disc,

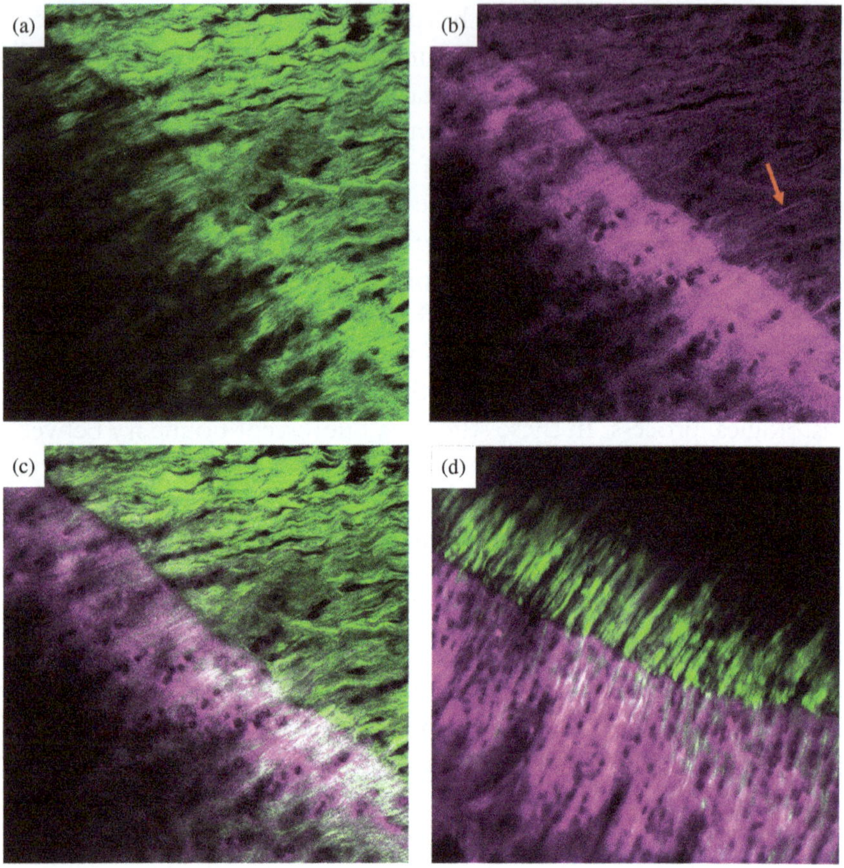

Figure 2. Static image (single slice) of MCL femoral enthesis; SHG channel (a); TPEF channel, arrow indicating example of a highly fluorescent fiber (b); combined channels (c); combined channels (d); FOV = 425 μm × 425 μm (A–C); FOV = 318 μm × 318 μm (D); Taken from Ref. [42], published with permission of Wiley

adipose, chordae tendinae, dermis and ligament.[45–48] Similarly characteristic signals can be seen at the fibrocartilaginous enthesis in Figure 3, and thus, may be resultant from elastin.[42] Still, further investigation of elastin's possible presence and role at the enthesis may be merited.

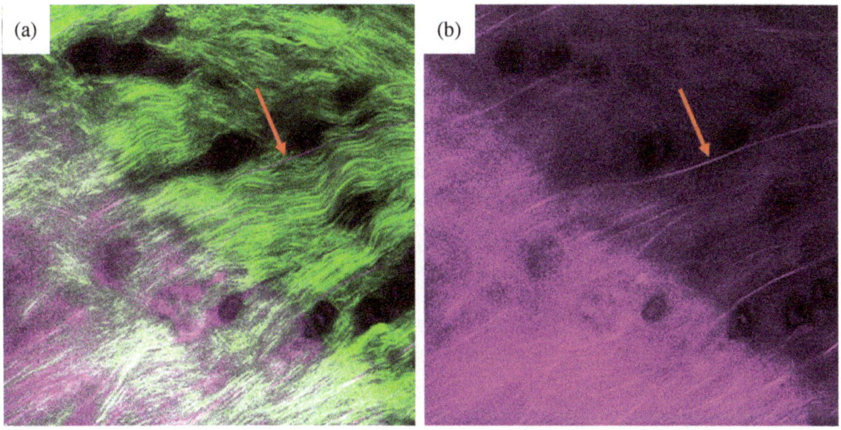

Figure 3. Static image (single slice) of MCL femoral enthesis; Combined channels (a); TPEF channel, arrow indicating example of a highly fluorescent fiber (b); FOV = 145 μm × 145 μm; Taken from Ref. [42], published with permission of Wiley

2.3. *Development*

Pioneering studies of enthesis development relied upon postnatal histology and immunohistochemistry, offering insight into the compositional progression of the enthesis after birth. These studies, and the bulk of the body of work on entheses, draw on animal models such as the mouse, rat and rabbit. At birth in a rat model, the femoral enthesis of the MCL attaches to the femur via perichondrium.[49] Soon thereafter, zones of ligament, fibrocartilage, proliferative epiphyseal cartilage, calcified cartilage and trabecular bone can be identified.[49] With further maturation, the epiphyseal cartilage calcifies and is replaced by bone while the fibrocartilaginous zone remains.[49] Gao *et al.*[50] observed labelling of type I collagen in ligament and type II collagen in adjacent cartilage at the femoral enthesis with no overlap between the two. At the onset of endochondral ossification, as cartilage was eroded on the bony side of the enthesis it was promptly replaced by fibrocartilage (as evidenced by type II collagen labeling) developing on the ligamentous side of the enthesis. This type II labeling (in a region of ligament where previously there had not been detectable collagen II) and the lack of type I/type II overlap initially, was used to make the suggestion of ligament metaplasia (i.e. resident ligament cells becoming fibrochondrocytes and producing type II collagen). Nawata *et al.*[51] reported findings similar to those of Gao *et al.*[49] providing further evidence of this phenomenon. Analogous patterns of collagen gene expression to those mentioned above were shown in the developing mouse supraspinatus enthesis by Galatz *et al.*[52] This group additionally identified a mineralized fibrocartilage zone consisting of hypertrophic chondrocytes embedded in matrix stained positively for type X collagen.[52] The fibrocartilaginous enthesis thus develops (postnatally) from a direct attachment to the perichondrium to the traditionally described zonal tissue attachment as evidenced by the changing expression of key matrix components.

The cellular signaling patterns that guide these changes are coming into clearer focus, predicated on the idea that understanding the signals necessitated in development will open the door to biological strategies for repair and regeneration. Owing to their regulatory functions in chondrogenesis and ligamentogenesis/tenogenesis respectively, SRY-box containing gene 9 (Sox9), and scleraxis (Scx) have been probed at the developing fibrocartilaginous enthesis. A progenitor population of cells positive for both transcription factors was shown to be present at several tendon/ligament attachment sites in mouse embryos, capable of chondrocyte, tenocyte or ligamentocyte differentiation.[53,54] What specific aspects of development Scx controls at the enthesis are still unclear; however, Killian and Thomopoulos[55] have demonstrated that a loss of Scx impairs mineral deposition and collagen organization. Scx and Sox9 expression therefore, help define a population of cells from which the enthesis originates, as well as play a part in the ensuing enthesis development.

Thereafter, early cell differentiation at the enthesis is thought to be driven by bone morphogenetic protein 4 (BMP4), while transforming growth factor beta (TGFβ) signaling drives cell specification.[53] TGFβ expression, in particular, is relevant to regenerative healing. A switch in expression in skin from TGFβ-3 to TGFβ-1 in fetal development was concomitant with a loss in regenerative capacity.[56] Such a shift has been shown to occur prenatally at the enthesis as well,[52] marking these growth factor genes as potential candidates for regenerative strategies. Later developmental events, particularly mineralization and fibrocartilage formation, are likely guided by Indian hedgehog (Ihh) coupled to parathyroid hormone-related peptide (PTHrP) signalling. For instance, Shwartz *et al.*[57] detected a distinct population of Hh-responsive cells at the developing enthesis as measured by positive Gli1 expression, the progeny of which eventually populate the entire enthesis. They were also able to show that a reduction in Ihh signaling led to decreases in the mineralization of fibrocartilage. It follows that, in a subsequent study, a portion of this cell population was found to mature into fibrochondrocytes, while retaining some Gli1 positive cells.[58] The regenerative implications of the Gli1 positive cell population came to light in the same study: before enthesis maturation, Gli1 positive cells regenerated native enthesis structure after injury, whereas mature cells did not. Moreover, while Gli1 expression was elevated in mature entheses after injury, it was to a much lower degree than in immature entheses. This combined body of work suggests that the metaplasia previously hypothesized is likely partially correct in that cells on the ligamentous side of the enthesis are responsible for enthesis development. However, these progenitor cells are unique from those of the ligament and differentiate under the influence of several signalling molecules to form the enthesis. Furthermore, many of these cell signalling pathways offer promising targets for regenerative therapeutics.

Mechanical stimulation is known to play an important role in many developing tissues, and studies have shown the same to be true for the fibrocartilaginous enthesis. Mature fibrocartilaginous entheses were demonstrated to occur only postnatally,[52] supporting that mechanical cues (of much greater significance after birth) are necessary for enthesis development and maturation. Indeed, paralysis of mouse shoulders at birth resulted in delayed and impaired fibrocartilage development, decreased mineralization of bone at the enthesis, and collagen fiber disorganization at maturity.[59] With that said, the entheses of paralyzed shoulders had an appearance similar (including some formation of fibrocartilage) to controls early on,[59] indicating that in the initial postnatal period biological cues may be driving development. Whether these entheses could recover a normal structure after paralysis is not clear, although, as Benjamin and Ralphs[15] point out in their discussion of papers by Ploetz[60] and Pauwels,[61] tendon has been shown to develop fibrocartilage-like tissue (where previously there was none) when subjected to compression. Such compression could likely be categorized as repeated in nature, given that Ploetz[60] translocated tendon insertions. In mature animals, a response to load was implied by the changing shape of the tidemark with unloading resulting from ligament transection in a model by Matyas.[33] Despite the progress evidenced herein, delineating the contributions of biomechanical cues during development, and their effects later on (i.e. at maturity) could still use research attention.

2.4. *Enthesis Mechanics*

Though the small size of entheses makes their observation under loaded conditions exceedingly difficult, several groups have had some measure of success doing so, thus facilitating study of their mechanical behavior. Analytical and finite element (FE) models have been used variously as well to assess aspects of enthesis mechanics, or a suspected relationship between a biological parameter and mechanical behavior. Several main themes constitute how an enthesis behaves mechanically and these are discussed here.

To begin with, the interface of CFC and bone makes a visibly undulating, interdigitated line that has been proposed to increase tissue "toughness". While this area of the enthesis has generated relatively less interest, Hu *et al.*[31] tested this theory using an analytical approach. Their findings indicate that increasing the interface roughness and stochasticity of interdigitations may act to increase insertional toughness, but it represents a trade-off in ultimate strength.

That fiber orientation of soft tissues directionally influences mechanical properties has been well established in the literature. Quantification of this parameter and its correlation with mechanical properties at the enthesis has thus received due attention. To this point, in an FE model by Matyas *et al.*,[62] whose geometry derived from a real histological slice, principal tensile stresses corresponded nearly exactly to the main collagen fiber direction at the fibrocartilaginous enthesis. Meanwhile, in regions of compressive stress, noted to be along the inner curvature of the enthesis, cell roundness was more pronounced, and the tissue phenotype resembled fibrocartilage. Analyses such as this can be used to hint at the prevailing stresses at an enthesis by visual inspection, and demonstrate the effect of load on tissue phenotype/organization. Additional examination of fiber orientation was performed with the help of FE models representing the physiological fiber orientations of the rat supraspinatus enthesis developed in work by Thomopoulos *et al.*[63] As could be expected, the fiber orientation was shown to dictate material properties in the tendon and enthesis. The FE model was further used to show that physiological fiber orientation likely serves to lessen the stress in the outward splay of this enthesis. These studies[62,63] verify that overall collagen fiber orientation at the enthesis is designed to transfer load efficiently and in correspondence with its direction.

A large divide in mechanical properties occurs over a very short distance at the enthesis, easily appreciated by considering the substances, ligament/tendon and bone, that they connect. Dividing the rat supraspinatus tendon enthesis into two sections, bony and tendinous, for example, and fitting quasilinear viscoelastic (QLV) properties to each section began to quantitatively elucidate just how much tissue mechanical properties change over an enthesis.[2] Principally, the authors of this study found that, at least in tension, the tendinous end of the enthesis was mechanically superior to its bony end. Sano *et al.*[64] found that the transition to the CFC region was depicted by an abrupt/sharp change in acoustic properties (i.e. sound speed), a pseudo measure of elastic modulus, while elastographic imaging mapping strain and deformation at the ACL enthesis under tension, suggested a stiffness gradation over the enthesis (i.e. increasing towards bone).[65] To investigate compressive properties, Moffat *et al.*[66] performed microcompression tests of the enthesis, demonstrating substantially greater compressive mechanical properties in the CFC region compared to the UFC region, and that the UFC region experiences greater strain than the CFC region.

Such large changes in mechanical behavior have spawned several well-formed opinions of contributing factors, chief among them, mineralization. For ligament/tendon to connect to bone, it stands to reason that in some form or another a transition in mineralization occurs. As previously indicated, Genin *et al.*[39] showed that the transition to CFC from UFC can be described as a gradient, albeit a gradient over a very short distance. In the rat supraspinatus enthesis, their experimental model, the mineral content increased linearly over 120 μm. Although occurring over a short distance, this gradation is thought to alleviate adequately the stress concentrations that would otherwise occur at an attachment of two dissimilar materials.

Moreover, this group developed several FE models of individually mineralized collagen fibers. The models suggested that substantial fiber stiffening does not occur until after a minimum mineral content, or percolation threshold is reached. At this point, a continuous network of mineralization encompasses a fiber. Combined with increasing fiber disorganization across the enthesis (shown to vastly decrease stiffness in the absence of mineral for small angular changes), the theorized percolation threshold supports a previously identified region between tendon and bone that is less stiff than either tissue.[2,39,67] At first glance such a region may seem counterintuitive; however, researchers have gathered targeted evidence to support its existence. For example, atomic force microscopy (AFM) of tendon-to-bone beams of the mouse supraspinatus was employed to estimate elastic modulus, resiliency and toughness along the beam length.[68] A highly compliant region bordering the beginning of the mineral gradient was revealed with local image correlation. These authors echoed the idea of prior studies that the region acts as an energy absorber. Mineral content on its own, though, did not explain the changing material properties, suggesting that other parameters (such as increasing collagen disorganization) contribute as well. An optimization algorithm designed to minimize peak stresses was run on numerical models of the rotator cuff by Liu *et al.*,[69] allowing material properties to vary between tendon and bone. By doing so, the algorithm produced a gradation wherein the elastic moduli between tendon and bone decreased below that of either tissue individually, providing an additional functional explanation for the compliance observed experimentally. Confocal microscopy combined with micromechanical testing permitted Rossetti *et al.*[24] to quantify the heterogeneous mechanical response at the porcine Achilles tendon enthesis comprehensively. A characteristic longitudinal (i.e. parallel to loading axis and primary fiber direction) deformation pattern was observed between the bone and tendon, manifesting as an abrupt increase under load application (indicative of a region of greater compliance than either bone or tendon, in accordance with the work just described). What is additionally notable is that here the authors showed the compliant region to coincide with a region where fiber diameters decreased dramatically, fiber crimping becomes absent, and fibers begin to splay out. In other words, the arrangement of the fibers becomes increasingly disorganized, contributing to the enthesis' compliance. Accordingly, the manner in which mineralization and fiber organization change across the enthesis and the locations and length over which they do so, are largely thought to control how mechanical properties transition between tissues. Interestingly, these changes cultivate a region of greater compliance than either ligament/tendon and bone that seems to be of mechanical benefit at the enthesis.

A second deformation pattern was also noted by Rossetti *et al.*[24] characterized by a much smoother (i.e. not abrupt) transition from bone to tendon. Upon further examination, these investigators determined that, depending on the angle of load application to tendon, a portion of the enthesis could sustain either of the characteristic smooth or abrupt deformation patterns, highlighting a potential load-sharing mechanism dependent on the direction of load application. Both the concept of a percolation threshold and load-sharing were supported in a study by Sevick *et al.*[42] Under load, simultaneous multiphoton image capturing showed qualitatively rapid angular fibril change at a fibrocartilaginous enthesis (Figure 4). The length over which this angle change occurred was in the range over which mineralization has been shown to increase at the enthesis,[39] particularly if one considers that significant rotation would be restricted once a percolation threshold is reached (i.e. rotation would be localized to where

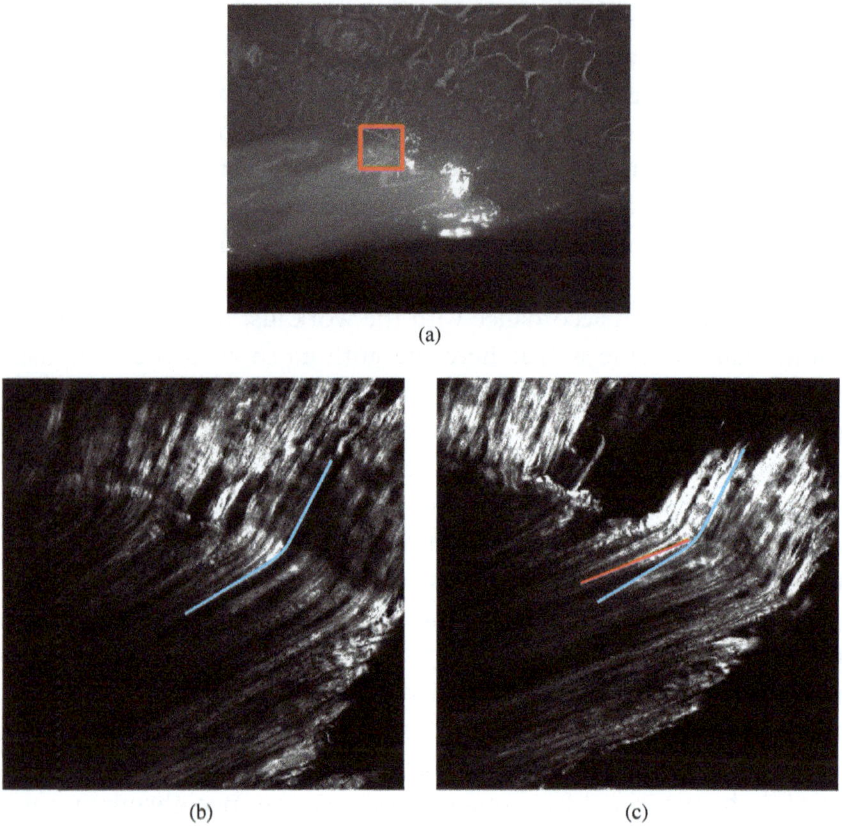

Figure 4. A typical MCL response to load; approximate location imaged by multiphoton microscope indicated by box (509 μm × 509 μm) (a); "Unloaded" SHG image. Line approximates path of a fibril (overall elongation = 9.02 μm, approximate load = 0.605 N) (b); "Loaded" SHG image. Additional line shown next to original approximates the change in fibril orientation due to load (overall elongation = 997 μm, approximate load = 13.5 N) (c); FOV = 509 μm × 509 μm; Taken from Ref. [42], published with permission of Wiley

fibers lose substantial stiffness as a result of decreasing mineralization). In some samples this behavior was not observed, with little uncrimping or reorientation of fibrils under load, thus signifying that a different region of the enthesis may be sharing the load.

The original impetus for this work, however, was to examine fibril embedment. Drawing from engineering examples of fiber reinforced composites[70] and reinforced concrete[71] that establish the concept of a minimum required length of fiber/rebar to develop shear stresses sufficient to avoid failure (embedment length), the authors endeavored to understand how enthesis fibrils accomplish this over such a seemingly short distance. Several ideas resulted from this work that include cable saddle action, pulley action and high fibril density leading to a high interfacial surface area.[42] Additional investigation on this topic, however, would be required to confirm these speculations. Nonetheless, the study outlines a novel method of combined mechanical and imaging testing that could be used or altered in future research.

2.5. *Summary*

Review of the literature pertaining to the composition, structure and function/mechanics of the enthesis reveals several overarching concepts. Namely, the fibrocartilaginous enthesis (regardless of its location in a human or animal) represents a transition over a very short distance in morphology, organic composition, inorganic composition (mineral content), and fiber/fibril orientation. The combination of these variables is thought to dictate the effectiveness of the material transition from relatively pliable ligament to relatively stiff bone. This body of research has underscored numerous components of the enthesis that will likely need to be recapitulated in any ideal ligament/tendon reconstruction or repair. Despite this, questions remain regarding enthesis composition and mechanics, the relationship between the two, and how best to restore them after injury.

3. Effectiveness of Attachment Strategies

In the clinical setting, the relevance of native enthesis composition, structure and function is realized at the attachment sites of graft tissue. Studies investigating the effectiveness of such an attachment, in the sphere of ligaments, are largely focused on one of the most prevalent knee surgeries — ACL reconstructions. Injury to the ACL, be it at either enthesis or at mid-substance, typically requires, in some form or another, the attachment of a ligamentous or tendinous autograft or allograft. Of these, hamstring and bone–patellar ligament–bone (BPB) grafts are the most common.[72]

One of the major issues plaguing the ultimate effectiveness of grafted tissue in ACL reconstruction is its ability to integrate with bone in the femoral and tibial bone tunnels early in the healing process.[3,73] Rodeo *et al.*,[74] in a pioneering study of graft integration in the bone tunnel of dogs found that pull-out failure predominated failure modes early after surgery. They further described in detail gradual collagen fiber continuity from graft to bone through an interface zone between the tissues; however, fibrocartilage-like tissue was not reported. BPB grafts have demonstrated improved healing (better bony integration, and superior mechanical properties) compared to hamstring grafts.[75,76] A potential reason for the better integration is that a BPB graft already possesses fibrocartilaginous entheses at both of its ends, entheses of the same type present at both ends of the ACL. These entheses thus permit a bone-to-bone connection in the bone tunnels, whereas hamstring grafts do not. However, donor site morbidity,[77] osteoarthritis,[78] and the chronic joint pain[77] associated with BPB grafts have pushed surgeons towards the use of hamstring grafts.[75,76] Both grafts can result in bone tunnel widening, a potentially deleterious effect.[79,80] A sampling of the myriad strategies used to affix these and similar grafts mechanically, attempts to improve the attachment healing/integration, as well as to replicate the native enthesis entirely are discussed herein. A focus is given to the recapitulation of fibrocartilage.

3.1. *Mechanical Re-attachment Strategies*

Interference screws have been described as the standard to fix soft tissue grafts in bone tunnels,[81] but suffer from poor integration,[82] in addition to stress shielding as a result of the relatively stiff non-biodegradable materials such as titanium,[83] and acidic breakdown of biodegradable polymers.[84] As an alternative, biodegradable magnesium interference screws have peaked the interest of researchers for their ability to promote osseointegration by mineralization of fibrous tissue.[82] When grafts were fixed by either titanium or magnesium screws there were no differences in the mechanical properties of the graft system with the grafts failing by mid-substance ruptures.[82] Magnesium screws provided the added benefit of a lack of bone tunnel widening when they degraded. Use of biodegradable screws and anatomic fixation in a separate study in the reconstruction of sheep ACLs demonstrated that after early weakness near the graft fixation, the interference screw fixation performed adequately under normal loads in the long term.[85] The same group demonstrated histologically the development of fibrocartilage between graft and bone in the ACL bone tunnel using this system.[86] Their results corroborate those of a study in the rabbit, which also suggested that anatomic fixation by interference screws promotes fibrocartilage development.[86] Yamakado *et al.*[87] re-attached the extensor digitorum longus tendon through an extra-articular bone tunnel drilled perpendicularly through the tibia, and confirmed an influence of mechanical stress on osseointegration. In regions of tensile stress, characteristics more similar to those of a fibrous insertion developed, while in regions of compressive stress characteristics more similar to those of a fibrocartilaginous insertion developed.

Thus, although development of fibrous-like insertions are common at the attachment of graft and bone, and these have been shown in some cases to be points of weakness (particularly early in the healing process), the literature demonstrates that, in general, functional outcomes for mechanical fixation of soft-tissue grafts using anatomic fit interference screws are achievable in the long term, and may promote fibrocartilaginous-like insertions under the right circumstances. Differences between the native ligament enthesis and the grafted attachment may provide some mechanical clues as to the different observed results in interface healing. For instance, whereas the native ACL enthesis only extends as far as bone, grafted tissues extend much further (i.e. along the length of bone tunnels). The loading geometries of grafted tissue have therefore changed: the sides of the tissue graft make contact with the sides of the bone tunnel and presumably transfer load from one to the other via shear with little relative rotation, potentially preferencing the development of a fibrous type connection in studies using non-interference fit fixation. Constraining load to be transferred over only a small portion of the grafted tissue, such as at the entrance to the bone tunnel of an interference fit reconstruction, presents a different geometry and loading condition that might explain the development of fibrocartilaginous-like insertions. With that said, the biological environment is also very likely different, especially compared to when the enthesis is initially developing.

3.2. *Biological Augmentation Strategies*

Biological efforts to enhance the healing of grafts at the graft-bone interface as a means of improving early performance of the graft system, wherein the weakest link of the system can reside, have been wide-ranging. These efforts are demarcated from those discussed in the following section by the fact that engineered scaffolds have not been used.

Periosteum has been recognized for is resident populations of multipotent mesodermal, chondroprogenitor and osteoprogenitor cells — all components that could potentially contribute to the recapitulation of a fibrocartilaginous enthesis under the right conditions. In a rabbit model of ACL reconstruction, periosteum wrapped hamstring grafts were shown to rapidly stimulate cartilage and bone formation around the graft, resulting in a fibrocartilaginous-like interface that mechanically outperformed controls.[88] Bone morphogenetic protein-2 (BMP-2) has been recognized for some time to promote osseointegration in bone tunnels.[89] Hence, the same research group experimented with injectable polyethylene glycol diacrylate (PEGDA) hydrogels seeded with periosteal progenitor cells, incorporating bone morphogenetic protein-2 (BMP-2) which proved to further enhance the development of fibrocartilage at the interface of graft and bone.[88] Recombined bone xenograft (RBX) sutured to graft ends in a rabbit model of ACL reconstruction exhibited an abundance of chondrocyte-like cells (fibrocartilage-like), bone formation and the appearance of a neo-enthesis structure.[90] Likewise, a fibrocartilaginous zone between a hamstring graft and bone in a rabbit model of ACL reconstruction was reasonably produced by coating grafts in a fibrin glue carrying mesenchymal stem cells (MSCs).[91] Hashimoto *et al.*,[92] were able to generate ectopic ossicles by injecting recombinant human (rh) BMP-2 into the flexor digitorum communis tendon of rabbits, and subsequently dissect and reattach the ossicle (with intact tendon) to the tibia via a bone tunnel. Histomorphometry indicated the presence of a fibrocartilaginous type enthesis, while mechanical testing demonstrated a higher load to failure than controls. In a subsequent study, this group reconstructed the rabbit ACL with a rhBMP-2 induced ossicle–tendon–ossicle construct, again showing characteristics similar to the native insertion, and superior mechanical properties compared to controls.[93] Ma *et al.*[94] have been successful in developing ligament enthesis tissue gradations with a similar bone–ligament–bone (BLB) construct. In their study, bone and ligament constructs were engineered separately *in vitro* from BMSCs, before being co-cultured to create the BLB constructs for MCL replacement in rats. While a viable ligament enthesis developed *in vivo*, a fibrocartilaginous region, as present at the native enthesis, was not observed. In a follow-up study, sheep ACLs were replaced with a similarly developed BLB construct.[95] Although structurally inferior to the native ACL after 6 months, constructs did achieve physiologically relevant biomechanical properties. Aspects of both fibrous and fibrocartilaginous enthesis development were observed histologically. Gene delivery via MSCs was investigated by Shahab-Osterloh *et al.*[96] in an ectopic mouse implantation model. Spontaneous development of a fibrocartilaginous-like insertion was achieved by making a viral modification to murine MSC-like cells that included constitutively active Smad8 (Smad8ca) and BMP-2 seeded on a collagen sponge. Together, these studies indicate that osseoinductive factors such as BMP are promising elements in a formula for recapitulating fibrocartilage, but that an optimal route of administration and dose is still to be determined.

Inorganic calcium phosphate (brushite) cement, in a manner similar to hydroxyapatite (HA), is capable of promoting osseointegration, and was therefore chosen as a candidate to improve bone tunnel healing in the study of Wen *et al.*[97] Moreover, whereas HA is relatively insoluble under physiological conditions, brushite is relatively soluble, making it (possibly) a preferable osseoconductive candidate. Placing brushite cement between a hamstring graft and the bone tunnel in rabbit ACL reconstruction yielded the development of a fibrocartilaginous-like integration, as well as superior structural characteristics (e.g. ultimate strength, stiffness) relative to control reconstructions.

In lieu of a bone tunnel, Kanazawa *et al.*[98] created a tibial pit (arguably more closely replicating the native enthesis geometry) and implanted bone marrow-derived MSCs in a carrier comprised of a collagen sponge and fibrin sealant between the semitendinosus graft and bone. Although no significant differences in the number of attachments developing fibrocartilage could be deduced between the MSC treated and control groups, the treatment group developed more fibrocartilage overall. In particular, the posterior regions at the base of the ACL developed fibrocartilage, suggesting that, as discussed previously, mechanical cues can influence cell differentiation.

As evidenced, the biological (i.e. without discussion of mechanical fixation or inclusion of tissue-engineered scaffolds) strategies for attachment improvement are varied. Alterations in the healing process have been produced, often beneficially, with the use of (for instance) periosteum, growth factors, stem cells, gene therapy, and brushite cement. However, all of these strategies are in their infancy, and will require further evaluation and experimentation to be fully characterized, and before they can be proven practical and worthwhile pursuing in larger animals, then humans. Moreover, closer attention to the factors influencing the native development of fibrocartilaginous entheses and more consensus on what constitutes true re-development of the native structure could help guide more focused regenerative/augmentative attempts.

3.3. *Tissue Engineering Strategies*

Before the advent of tissue engineering strategies to replace or augment ligament healing, prosthetic ligaments attained some popular usage. Despite achieving satisfactory knee stability, pain persisted in 70% of patients postoperatively,[99] likely as a result of the gradual breakdown of synthetic products and the body's reaction to foreign materials.[100] Research has subsequently turned to a host of sophisticated attempts at tissue engineering the ligament and its enthesis. A subset of these are presented here, although several in-depth articles have been published on the topic.[72,101]

Different combinations of cells, growth factors, and scaffolds have been used at graft ends in attempts to improve graft integration in bone tunnels. As described by Smith *et al.*,[101] a majority of tissue-engineered attempts at the enthesis can be stratified by those that use a single cell type with a gradation of biological factors and those with multiple cell types seeded on a graded scaffold. As an example of the first case, He *et al.*[102] co-cultured MSCs between bone and ligament cells on hybrid silk scaffolds with sections adapted to each cell type. Their hypothesis that fibrocartilage would develop between bone and ligament regions was confirmed by real-time polymerase chain reaction (rt-PCR) results, immunohistochemistry, and SEM, illustrating the importance of cell–cell interaction in regeneration. Interestingly, calcium deposition at the UFC/CFC interface exhibited a possible mineralization gradient. In a separate study, this group developed a multiphasic scaffold without cell seeding to mimic the native fibrocartilaginous transition.[103] Ligament was fabricated from poly-lactic acid (PLA) microfibers, and bone from microchanneled β-tricalcium phosphate (β-TCP) and a polycaprolactone (PCL) anchor. Varying the amounts of PLGA and β-TCP created intervening UFC and CFC scaffold sections, although the actual ability of such a manufactured scaffold to generate a fibrocartilaginous enthesis *in vivo* has not been determined.

As an example of the second prevalent strategy outlined by Smith *et al.*,[101] cell-seeding on a triphasic scaffold (polyglactin mesh sheets for ligament, PLGA microspheres for fibrocartilage, and PLGA/bioactive glass composite microspheres for bone) was performed by Spalazzi *et al.*[104] The scaffold's heterogeneity and co-culturing of fibroblasts and osteoblasts produced distinct, maintainable (in the short term) cellular distributions and extracellular matrix compositions *in vitro*. Details on the fabrication of such a scaffold were explained in a separate paper.[105] *In vivo* application of the seeded triphasic scaffold was established by implantation in a subcutaneous pouch on the posterior dorsum of athymic rats.[106] Despite the absence of mechanical load, a fibrocartilage-like region developed by 8 weeks post-implantation. A linear calcium phosphate content gradation was successfully implemented on an electrospun PLGA nanofiber scaffold by immersion in simulated body fluid.[107] Seeding of mouse pre-osteoblast cells onto the scaffold illustrated that the mineral gradient influenced cell characteristics (morphology, adhesion, proliferation). Moreover, a dependence in mechanical behavior (stiffness) was shown to relate to the engineered mineral gradient. A strategy like this is a potentially promising step towards replicating the native mineralization gradient at fibrocartilaginous entheses. Phillips *et al.*[108] created a graded tissue interface with a single cell type seeded on a scaffold by first establishing a spatial distribution of a retrovirus encoding runt-related transcription factor 2 (Runx2) along its length. Osteoblastic differentiation of fibroblasts, and accompanying mineralization followed a graded distribution as a result; however, an intervening fibrocartilaginous zone did not develop.

In an effort to grade both cell types and biological factors, Kim *et al.*[109] created human collagen scaffolds, varying chondroitin sulfate crosslinking and artificial calcification and seeding with different cell types (fibroblasts, chondrocytes, osteoblasts). *In vitro* testing showed that the scaffold preferentially supported proliferation of cell types naturally found in the corresponding region of the gradation (including chondrocytes in a fibrocartilaginous region).

Mechanical action has additionally been incorporated into scaffold design, either *in vitro* or *in vivo*. The inherent contraction of PLGA nanofiber scaffolds was taken advantage of by Spalazzi *et al.*[110] on the premise that this contraction could be used to compress a tendon graft, and thereby stimulate fibrocartilage generation. Indeed, scaffold compression increased the expression of fibrocartilage related markers (e.g. aggrecan, type II collagen, and TGF-β3). To test whether fibrocartilage could develop under periodic hydrostatic tension, Thomopoulos *et al.*[111] constructed a 3D-mesenchymal stromal cell seeded collagen matrix looped around two bars and subjected it to either static or cyclic tension. Cell morphology, alignment, gene expression and extra cellular matrix production were shown to vary between tensile and compressive regions. The fibrous portion (tensile) of fibrocartilage could be generated by mechanical stimulation alone. However, the cartilaginous portion (compressive) of fibrocartilage required the application of TGF-β3, demonstrating a reliance on both biological and mechanical cues. Cyclic loading, specifically, was required to stimulate fibrochondrocyte-like development.

As one can see, the field of tissue engineering the fibrocartilaginous enthesis is complex. Numerous variables (e.g. materials, their geometries and scales, cell sources/types, cell culture time/conditions, *in vivo/in vitro* growth, mechanical loading, biological factors, and so on), in numerous combinations have resulted in a diverse array of somewhat successful recapitulations of the native enthesis. Research elucidating which paths are potentially more productive to pursue over others is on-going and should help to pin down the impacts of different variables in a more systematic way. Furthermore, such research should also provide tangible comparison between tissue-engineered constructs and native entheses, comparisons that could be additionally informative.

Additionally, a few constraints on the feasibility of most tissue-engineering strategies are worth considering. Some of these include isolation and proliferation of multiple cell types from multiple host locations, being both costly, potentially painful, and overly time consuming. There is a lack of understanding of the precise stress environment (static vs cyclic, and if cyclic, stress amplitude, frequency, bursts of cycles vs continuous stimulation and effect of mean stress being some of the variables that need to be understood) to which cells at the enthesis are subject through development and maturity, and what effect this stress environment has on cellular behavior; and, along the same lines, what constitutes an adequate tissue-engineered replacement (i.e. what minimum biomechanical and biological standards need to be met in order for outcomes to surpass those of available reparative techniques).[101]

4. Conclusion and Future Directions

As exemplified earlier, a great deal of sophisticated research has generated a comprehensive understanding of the fibrocartilaginous enthesis in terms of its development, structure and composition, and its function/mechanics. Nevertheless, certain obstacles, such as the small size of these complex entheses and the difficulties entailed in viewing them as load is applied, have only just begun to be overcome. Additionally, investigation may be warranted of the cause/significance of the tidemark, the presence or absence of elastin at the enthesis, the way in which enthesis collagen fibrils intertwine (or not) with bone, and the precise influence of mechanical cues on development and healing. Continuing to uncover the basic science of entheses remains a crucial step towards their eventual recapitulation at a surgical attachment site.

From a tissue engineering perspective, the mechanical (stress environment) and biochemical environment experienced by cells along the native enthesis, and subsequently the engineered enthesis, needs better definition. While many tissue-engineered strategies have been tried, comparison of their relative success is difficult. Efforts to standardize what elements of the native enthesis are crucial to recapitulate (e.g. fiber density, mineralization content and gradient length and so on) and how to measure them could facilitate such comparisons. Eventually, engineering for specific activities such as volleyball or soccer may be achievable.

Although imperfect, autografts and allografts have proven to be capable of returning stability to an injured joint in many cases. Problems like graft pull-out are generally avoided in the long term, whereas problems of bone tunnel widening, and graft laxity persist. While such problems continue, there is a need for strategies to improve outcomes. These may be methods of mechanical fixation of, or biological additives to, graft tissue, or entirely tissue-engineered replacements. In every case, a wide variety of ideas have been tested, many showing improved histological and mechanical results (typically as compared to controls). However, in many cases it is unclear to what degree any of these strategies are analogous to the native enthesis. This may be important or not, depending upon one's measurement of success. For instance, if return to function is considered the only measure of successful ligament reconstruction, then recapitulation of the native enthesis may not be necessary. Expecting that a tendon graft in a bone tunnel needs to develop a fibrocartilaginous interface to be functional may not be a necessity when the different materials and geometries of the attachment are considered. That said, any ideal ligament replacement would perfectly mimic the structure that preceded it and remains a goal worthy of pursuit.

Acknowledgments

The authors thank the following funding sources for their support: Canadian Institutes of Health Research (formerly Medical Research Council of Canada), The Arthritis Society of Canada, Alberta Innovates Health Solutions (formerly Alberta Heritage Foundation for Medical Research), Natural Sciences and Engineering Research Council of Canada (NSERC), NSERC Undergraduate Student Research Award, NSERC Collaborative Research and Training Experience Program, McCaig Institute for Bone and Joint Health Professorship, Province of Alberta, and University of Calgary Biomedical Engineering Graduate Program. Additionally, the authors are grateful for the help of personnel at the McCaig Institute of the University of Calgary, particularly Dr. Neil Duncan, Dr. John Matyas, and Dr. Roman Krawetz for use of their equipment.

References

1. Benjamin, M.; McGonagle, D. Scand. *J. Med. Sci. Sport.* **2009**, *19*(4), 520–527.
2. Thomopoulos, S.; Williams, G. R.; Gimbel, J. A.; Favata, M.; Soslowsky, L. J. *J. Orthop. Res.* **2003**, *21*(3), 413–419.
3. Lazarides, A. L.; Eward, W. C.; Green, K.; Cardona, D. M.; Brigman, B. E.; Taylor, D. C. *Am. J. Sports Med.* **2015**, *43*(8), 1935–1940.
4. Benjamin, M.; Kumai, T.; Milz, S.; Boszczyk, B. M.; Boszczyk, A. A.; Ralphs, J. R. *Comp. Biochem. Physiol. A. Mol. Integr. Physiol.* **2002**, *133* (4), 931–945.

5. Derwin, K. A.; Galatz, L. M.; Ratcliffe, A.; Thomopoulos, S. *J. Bone Jt. Surg.* **2018**.
6. Thomopoulos, S.; Williams, G. R.; Soslowsky, L. J. *J. Biomech. Eng.* **2003**, *125*(1), 106.
7. Galatz, L. M.; Ball, C. M.; Teefey, S. A.; Middleton, W. D.; Yamaguchi, K. *J. Bone Joint Surg. Am.* **2004**, *86-A*(2), 219–224.
8. Yamaguchi, K.; Ditsios, K.; Middleton, W. D.; Hildebolt, C. F.; Galatz, L. M.; Teefey, S. A. *J. Bone Joint Surg. Am.* **2006**, *88*(8), 1699–1704.
9. George, M. S.; Dunn, W. R.; Spindler, K. P. *Am. J. Sports Med.* **2006**, *34*(12), 2026–2037.
10. Noyes, F. R.; Barber-Westin, S. D. *J. Bone Joint Surg. Am.* **2001**, *83-A*(8), 1131–1143.
11. Magnussen, R. A.; Taylor, D. C.; Toth, A. P.; Garrett, W. E. *Sport. Med. Arthrosc. Rehabil. Ther. Technol.* **2012**, *4*(1), 22.
12. Benjamin, M.; Evans, E. J.; Copp, L. *J. Anat.* **1986**, *149*, 89–100.
13. Benjamin, M.; McGonagle, D. *J. Anat.* **2001**, *199*(5), 503–526.
14. Deymier-Black, A. C.; Pasteris, J. D.; Genin, G. M.; Thomopoulos, S. *J. Biomech. Eng.* **2015**, *137*(11), 111005.
15. Benjamin, M.; Ralphs, J. R. *J. Anat.* 1998, 193, 481–494.
16. Benjamin, M.; Toumi, H.; Ralphs, J. R.; Bydder, G.; Best, T. M.; Milz, S. *J. Anat.* **2006**, *208*(4), 471–490.
17. Wang, I. N. E.; Mitroo, S.; Chen, F. H.; Lu, H. H.; Doty, S. B. *J. Orthop. Res.* **2006**, *24*(8), 1745–1755.
18. Gao, J.; Messner, K. *J. Anat.* **1996**, *188*(Pt 2), 367–373.
19. Benjamin, M.; Ralphs, J. R. *J. Anat.* **1998**, *193*(Pt 4), 481–494.
20. Apostolakos, J.; Durant, T. J.; Dwyer, C. R.; Russell, R. P.; Weinreb, J. H.; Alaee, F.; Beitzel, K.; McCarthy, M. B.; Cote, M. P.; Mazzocca, A. D. *Muscles. Ligaments Tendons J.* **2014**, *4*(3), 333–342.
21. Kumagai, J.; Sarkar, K.; Uhthoff, H. K.; Okawara, Y.; Ooshima, A. *J. Anat.* **1994**, *185*(Pt 2), 279–284.
22. Waggett, A. D.; Ralphs, J. R.; Kwan, A. P. L.; Woodnutt, D.; Benjamin, M. *Matrix Biol.* **1998**, *16*(8), 457–470.
23. Ralphs, J. R.; Benjamin, M.; Waggett, a D.; Russell, D. C.; Messner, K.; Gao, J. *J. Anat.* **1998**, *193*(Pt 2), 215–222.

24. Rossetti, L.; Kuntz, L. A.; Kunold, E.; Schock, J.; Grabmayr, H.; Sieber, S. A.; Burgkart, R.; Bausch, A. R. *Nat. Mater.* **2017**, *16*(6), 664–670.
25. Lu, H. H.; Thomopoulos, S. *Annu. Rev. Biomed. Eng.* **2013**, 15, 201–226.
26. Milz, S.; Tischer, T.; Buettner, a; Schieker, M.; Maier, M.; Redman, S.; Emery, P.; McGonagle, D.; Benjamin, M. *Ann. Rheum. Dis.* **2004**, *63*(9), 1015–1021.
27. Niyibizi, C.; Sagarrigo Visconti, C.; Gibson, G.; Kavalkovich, K. Biochem. *Biophys. Res. Commun.* **1996**, *222*(2), 584–589.
28. Fukuta, S.; Oyama, M.; Kavalkovich, K.; Fu, F. H.; Niyibizi, C. *Matrix Biol.* **1998**, *17*(1), 65–73.
29. Rufai, A.; Ralphs, J. R.; Benjamin, M. *J. Anat.* 1996, 189 (Pt 1), 185–191.
30. Oegema, T. R.; Carpenter, R. J.; Hofmeister, F.; Thompson, R. C. *Microsc. Res. Tech.* **1997**, *37*(4), 324–332.
31. Hu, Y.; Birman, V.; Demyier-Black, A.; Schwartz, A. G.; Thomopoulos, S.; Genin, G. M. *Biophys. J.* **2015**, *108*(2), 431–437.
32. Thomopoulos, S.; Birman, V.; Genin, G. M. *Structural Interfaces and Attachments in Biology*. (Springer Science+Business Media New York, **2013**).
33. Matyas, J. R. *The Structure and Function of the Insertions of the Rabbit Medial Collateral Ligament* [dissertation]. Medical Science: University of Calgary; **1990**.
34. Spalazzi, J. P.; Boskey, A. L.; Pleshko, N.; Lu, H. H. *PLoS One* **2013**, *8*(9), 1–16.
35. Biewener, A. A.; Fazzalari, N. L.; Konieczynski, D. D.; Baudinette, R. V. *Bone* **1996**, *19*(1), 1–8.
36. Zhao, L.; Thambyah, A.; Broom, N. D. *J. Anat.* **2014**, *224*(6), 624–633.
37. Clark, J.; Stechschulte, D. J. *J. Anat.* **1998**, *192*(Pt 4), 605–616.
38. Redler, I.; Mow, V. C.; Zimny, M. L.; Mansell, *J. Clin. Orthop. Relat. Res.* **1975**, *112*, 357–362.
39. Genin, G. M.; Kent, A.; Birman, V.; Wopenka, B.; Pasteris, J. D.; Marquez, P. J.; Thomopoulos, S. *Biophys. J.* **2009**, *97*(4), 976–985.

40. Wopenka, B.; Kent, A.; Pasteris, J. D.; Yoon, Y. J.; W, P. S. B.; Louis, S. *Appl. Spectrosc.* **2008**, *62*(12), 1285–1294.
41. Liu, Y.; Schwartz, A. G.; Birman, V.; Thomopoulos, S.; Genin, G. M. *Biomech. Model. Mechanobiol.* **2013**, *13*(5), 973–983.
42. Sevick, J. L.; Abusara, Z.; Andrews, S. H.; Xu, M.; Khurshid, S.; Chatha, J.; Hart, D. A.; Shrive, N. G. *J. Orthop. Res.* **2018**, *36*(9), 2506–2515.
43. Chen, M.-H.; Chen, W.-L.; Sun, Y.; Fwu, P. T.; Dong, C.-Y. *J. Biomed. Opt.* **2007**, *12*(6), 064018.
44. Mansfield, J. C.; Peter Winlove, C. *J. Anat.* **2012**, *220*(4), 405–416.
45. Green, E. M.; Mansfield, J. C.; Bell, J. S.; Winlove, C. P. *Interface Focus* **2014**, *4*(2), 20130058.
46. Henninger, H. B.; Valdez, W. R.; Scott, S. A.; Weiss, J. A. *Acta. Biomater.* **2015**, *25*, 304–312.
47. Chen, G.; Chen, J.; Zhuo, S.; Xiong, S.; Zeng, H.; Jiang, X.; Chen, R.; Xie, S. *Br. J. Dermatol.* **2009**, *161*(1), 48–55.
48. Zhuo, S.; Chen, J.; Luo, T.; Zou, D.; Zhao, *J. Opt. Exp.* **2006**, *14*(17), 7810–7820.
49. Wei, X.; Messner, K. *Anat. Embryol.* (*Berl*). **1996**, *193*(1), 53–59.
50. Gao, J.; Messner, K.; Ralphs, J. R.; Benjamin, M. *Anat. Embryol.* (*Berl*). **1996**, *194*, 399–406.
51. Nawata, K.; Minamizaki, T.; Yamashita, Y.; Teshima, R. *J. Orthop. Res.* 2002.
52. Galatz, L.; Rothermich, S.; VanderPloeg, K.; Petersen, B.; Sandell, L.; Thomopoulos, S. *J. Orthop. Res.* **2007**, 1621–1628.
53. Blitz, E.; Sharir, A.; Akiyama, H.; Zelzer, E. *Development* **2013**, *140*(13), 2680–2690.
54. Sugimoto, Y.; Takimoto, A.; Akiyama, H.; Kist, R.; Scherer, G.; Nakamura, T.; Hiraki, Y.; Shukunami, C. *Development* **2013**, *140*(11), 2280–2288.
55. Killian, M. L.; Thomopoulos, S. *FASEB J.* **2016**, *30*(1), 301–311.
56. Beredjiklian, P. K.; Favata, M.; Cartmell, J. S.; Flanagan, C. L.; Crombleholme, T. M.; Soslowsky, L. *J. Ann. Biomed. Eng.* **2003**.
57. Schwartz, A. G.; Long, F.; Thomopoulos, S. *Development* **2015**, *142*(1), 196–206.
58. Schwartz, A. G.; Galatz, L. M.; Thomopoulos, S. *Development* **2017**, *144*(7), 1159–1164.

59. Thomopoulos, S.; Kim, H. M.; Rothermich, S. Y.; Biederstadt, C.; Das, R.; Galatz, L. M. *J. Orthop. Res.* **2007**, *25*(9), 1154–1163.
60. Ploetz, E. *Zeitschrift für Orthop.* **1938**, *67*, 212–234.
61. Pauwels, F. Z. *Anat. Entwicklungsgesch.* **1960**, *121*, 478–515.
62. Matyas, J. R.; Anton, M. G.; Shrive, N. G.; Frank, C. B. *J. Biomech.* **1995**, *28*, 147–157.
63. Thomopoulos, S.; Marquez, J. P.; Weinberger, B.; Birman, V.; Genin, G. M. *J. Biomech.* **2006**, *39*(10), 1842–1851.
64. Sano, H.; Saijo, Y.; Kokubun, S. J. *Shoulder Elb. Surg.* **2006**, *15*(6), 743–749.
65. Spalazzi, J. P.; Gallina, J.; Fung-Kee-Fung, S. D.; Konofagou, E. E.; Lu, H. H. *J. Orthop. Res.* **2006**, *24*, 2001–2010.
66. Moffat, K. L.; Sun, W. H. S.; Chahine, N. O.; Pena, P. E.; Doty, S. B.; Hung, C. T.; Ateshian, G. A.; Lu, H. H. In *Annual International Conference of the IEEE Engineering in Medicine and Biology — Proceedings*, **2006**, pp. 2366–2369.
67. Liu, Y.; Thomopoulos, S.; Chen, C.; Birman, V.; Buehler, M. J.; Genin, G. M. J. *R. Soc. Interface* **2013**, *11*(92), 20130835.
68. Deymier, A. C.; An, Y.; Boyle, J. J.; Schwartz, A. G.; Birman, V.; Genin, G. M.; Thomopoulos, S.; Barber, A. H. *Acta Biomater.* **2017**.
69. Liu, Y. X.; Thomopoulos, S.; Birman, V.; Li, J.-S.; Genin, G. M. *Mech Mater.* **2012**, *44*, 130–134.
70. Greszczuk, L. B. *Interfaces Compos.* **1969**, *ASTM STP 4*, 42–58.
71. LeRoy, A. L.; Peter, G. *J. Proc.* **1967**, *64*(11), 711–721.
72. Paxton, J. Z.; Barr, K.; Grover, L. M. *Orthop. Muscular Syst.* **2012**, *S1*, 1–13.
73. Chen, C.-H. *Sports Med. Arthrosc. Rehabil. Ther. Technol.* **2009**, *1*(1), 21.
74. Rodeo, S. A.; Arnoczky, S. P.; Torzilli, P. A.; Hidaka, C.; Warren, R. F. *J. Bone Joint Surg. Am.* **1993**, *75*(12), 1795–1803.
75. Holmes, P. F.; James, S. L.; Larson, R. L.; Singer, K. M.; Jones, D. C. *Am. J. Sports Med.* **1991**, *19*(6), 596–599.
76. Aglietti, P.; Buzzi, R.; Zaccherotti, G.; De Biase, P. *Am. J. Sports Med.* **1994**, *22*(2), 211–217; discussion 217-218.
77. Corry, I. S.; Webb, J. M.; Clingeleffer, A. J.; Pinczewski, L. A. *Am. J. Sports Med.* **1999**, *27*(3), 444–454.

78. Keays, S. L.; Bullock-Saxton, J. E.; Keays, A. C.; Newcombe, P. A.; Bullock, M. I. A. *Am. J. Sports Med.* **2007**, *35*(5), 729–739.
79. Webster, K. E.; Feller, J. A.; Hameister, K. A. Knee Surgery, *Sport. Traumatol. Arthrosc.* **2001**, *9*(2), 86–91.
80. L'Insalata, J. C.; Klatt, B.; Fu, F. H.; Harner, C. D. *Knee Surg. Sports Traumatol. Arthrosc.* **1997**, *5*(4), 234–238.
81. Steiner, M. E.; Hecker, A. T.; Brown, C. H.; Hayes, W. C. *Am. J. Sports Med.* **1994**, *22*(2), 240–247.
82. Wang, J.; Xu, J.; Fu, W.; Cheng, W.; Chan, K.; Yung, P. S.; Qin, L. *Sci. Rep.* **2017**, *7*(January), 40369.
83. Sumner, D. R.; Galante, J. O. *Clin. Orthop. Relat. Res.* **1992**, *274*, 202–212.
84. Cutright, D. E.; Hunsuck, E. E. *Oral Surg., Oral Med. Oral Pathol.* **1971**, *31*(1), 134–139.
85. Weiler, A.; Peine, R.; Pashmineh-Azar, A.; Abel, C.; Südkamp, N. P.; Hoffmann, R. F. G. *Arthroscopy* **2002**, *18*(2), 113–123.
86. Weiler, A.; Hoffmann, R. F. G.; Bail, H. J.; Rehm, O.; Südkamp, N. P. *Arthroscopy* **2002**, *18*(2), 124–135.
87. Yamakado, K.; Kitaoka, K.; Yamada, H.; Hashiba, K.; Nakamura, R.; Tomita, K. *Arthroscopy* **2002**, *18*(1), 82–90.
88. Chen, C.-H. *Chang Gung Med. J.* **2009**, *32*(5), 483–493.
89. Rodeo, S. A.; Suzuki, K.; Deng, X. H.; Wozney, J.; Warren, R. F. *Am. J. Sports Med.* **1999**.
90. Zhang, W.; Pan, W.; Zhang, M.; Wei, Y. *Biotechnol. Lett.* **2011**, *33*(4), 837–844.
91. Lim, J.-K.; Hui, J.; Li, L.; Thambyah, A.; Goh, J.; Lee, E.-H. *Arthroscopy* **2004**, *20*(9), 899–910.
92. Hashimoto, Y.; Yoshida, G.; Toyoda, H.; Takaoka, K. *J. Orthop. Res.* **2007**, *25*(11), 1415–1424.
93. Hashimoto, Y.; Naka, Y.; Fukunaga, K.; Nakamura, H.; Takaoka, K. *J. Orthop. Res.* **2011**, *29*(12), 1923–1930.
94. Ma, J.; Goble, K.; Smietana, M.; Kostrominova, T.; Larkin, L.; Arruda, E. M. *J. Biomech. Eng.* **2009**, *131*(10), 101017.
95. Ma, J.; Smietana, M. J.; Kostrominova, T. Y.; Wojtys, E. M.; Larkin, L. M.; Arruda, E. M. *Tissue Eng. Part A* **2012**, *18*(1–2), 103–116.

96. Shahab-Osterloh, S.; Witte, F.; Hoffmann, A.; Winkel, A.; Laggies, S.; Neumann, B.; Seiffart, V.; Lindenmaier, W.; Gruber, A. D.; Ringe, J.; Häupl, T.; Thorey, F.; Willbold, E.; Corbeau, P.; Gross, G. *Stem Cells* **2010**, *28*(9), 1590–1601.
97. Wen, C. Y.; Qin, L.; Lee, K. M.; Chan, K. M. *J. Biomed. Mater. Res. — Part B Appl. Biomater.* **2009**, *89*(2), 466–474.
98. Kanazawa, T.; Soejima, T.; Noguchi, K.; Tabuchi, K.; Noyama, M.; Nakamura, K.-I.; Shiba, N. Muscles. *Ligaments Tendons J.* **2014**, *4*(2), 201–206.
99. Ahlfeld, S. K.; Larson, R. L.; Collins, H. R. *Am. J. Sports Med.* **1987**, *15*(4), 326–330.
100. Mascarenhas, R.; MacDonald, P. B. *McGill J. Med. MJM* **2008**, *11*(1), 29–37.
101. Smith, L.; Xia, Y.; Galatz, L. M.; Genin, G. M.; Thomopoulos, S. *Connect. Tissue Res.* **2012**, *53*(2), 95–105.
102. He, P.; Ng, K. S.; Toh, S. L.; Goh, J. C. H. *Biomacromolecules* **2012**, *13*(9), 2692–2703.
103. He, J.; Zhang, W.; Liu, Y.; Li, X.; Li, D.; Jin, Z. *Mater. Sci. Eng. C* **2015**, *50*, 12–18.
104. Spalazzi, J. P.; Doty, S. B.; Moffat, K. L.; Levine, W. N.; Lu, H. H. *Tissue Eng.* **2006**, *12*(12), 3497–3508.
105. Mosher, C. Z.; Spalazzi, J. P.; Lu, H. H. *Methods* **2015**, *84*, 99–102.
106. Spalazzi, J. P.; Dagher, E.; Doty, S. B.; Guo, X. E.; Rodeo, S. A.; Lu, H. H. *J. Biomed. Mater. Res. — Part A* **2008**, *86*(1), 1–12.
107. Li, X.; Xie, J.; Lipner, J.; Yuan, X.; Thomopoulos, S.; Xia, Y. *Nano Lett.* **2009**, *9*(7), 2763–2768.
108. Phillips, J.; Burns, K. L.; Le Doux, J. M.; Guldberg, R. E.; García, A. *J. PNAS* **2008**, *105*(34), 12170–12175.
109. Kim, B. S.; Kim, E. J.; Choi, J. S.; Jeong, J. H.; Jo, C. H.; Cho, Y. W. *J. Biomed. Mater. Res. — Part A* **2014**, *102*(11), 4044–4054.
110. Spalazzi, J. P.; Vyner, M. C.; Jacobs, M. T.; Moffat, K. L.; Lu, H. H. *Clin. Orthop. Relat. Res.* **2008**, *466*(8), 1938–1948.
111. Thomopoulos, S.; Das, R.; Birman, V.; Smith, L.; Ku, K.; Elson, E. L.; Pryse, K. M.; Marquez, J. P.; Genin, G. M. *Tissue Eng. Part A* **2011**, *17*, 1039–1053.

https://doi.org/10.1142/9789811204630_0006

Chapter 6

Italian Experience of the Use of *LARS* Synthetic Ligament for ACL Reconstruction: 15 Years Follow-Up

Giacomo Placella[*,¶], Gianpiero Cazzato[*], Salvatore Morello[†], Enrico Sebastiani[‡], Valerio Pace[§], Matteo Maria Tei[*], and Giuliano Cerulli[*]

[*]*Fondazione Policlinico Agostino Gemelli, Istituto di Clinica Ortopedica Traumatologica, Università Cattolica del Sacro Cuore di Roma, Largo Agostino Gemelli, 1 Policlinico Gemelli di Roma, 00135 Rome, Italy*
[†]*Policlinico P. Giaccone, Clinica Ortopedica e Traumatologica, Università degli Studi di Palermo, Palermo, Italy*
[‡]*Ospedale S. Maria della Misericordia, Clinica Ortopedica e Traumatologica, Università degli Studi di Perugia, Perugia, Italy*
[§]*Royal National Orthopedics Hospital, Stanmore, London, UK*
[¶]*giacomo.PLAcella@gmail.com*

Abbreviations

ACL	Anterior cruciate ligament
C.o.P.	Center of pressure
EBM	Evidence-based medicine
IKDC	International Knee Documentation Committee
PLA	Polylactic acid
PTFE	Polytetrafluoroethylene
R.O.M.	Range of motion

1. Introduction

Anterior cruciate ligament (ACL) lesions are very common, accounting for 80% of ligamentous injuries involving the knee.[1] Its surgical reconstruction aims to restore knee stability, preventing meniscal and chondral lesions by reducing the risk of osteoarthritis. It has been shown that the articular surface's wear can lead to degenerative arthritic manifestations, which in turn will require surgical intervention; within approximately 10 years.[2]

Three classes of graft are currently used for ACL reconstruction: autologous, allograft and synthetic ligaments.[3]

The autologous graft is considered the gold standard, with the option of using patellar tendon or hamstrings for reconstruction. These tissues have the advantage of being an effective scaffold for the collagen fibers ingrowth without the rejection risk. The disadvantages of this method are: complications at the explant site and prolonged rehabilitation time. The allograft, however, does not present the risk of problems related to the operation site, but they have the potential risk of developing a viral reaction.

The first attempt to reconstruct the ACL with synthetic material was in 1918 by Alwyn-Smith; the results were disappointing with a failure after 3 months. Since then, many things have changed, but many prejudices remain. At the beginning, the focus was the strength of the structure; prosthesis ensured stability for a limited time due to wear they were subjected to. An attempt was undertaken to build a structure that would guide and stimulate the growth of autologous tissue, which was not only sufficiently resistant to mechanical stress, but would also preserve its integrity.

It was seen that by protecting the tissue regeneration from tensile and compressive forces, the fibers grew in a disorganized manner, thus generating an unsuitable tissue with low resistance. Since the 1970s, synthetic devices have been available for use in the management of the cruciate-injured knee.[4]

These devices have the intended benefits of avoiding donor-site morbidity, providing a strong stabilizing construct. This would allow relatively rapid rehabilitation and a return to sport activity without the risks of disease transmission and rejection.[4]

The attempt at reconstruction with a prosthetic ligament made of polytetrafluoroethylene (PTFE) with embedded carbon or aluminum oxide fibers (Proplast) has been reported in 1973.[5] The results have shown prosthetic ligament lesion within just over 1 year.

In 1977, Jenkins *et al.* were the first to use a flexible carbon fiber implant, and suggested that the carbon fiber induced the formation of tendon in animals and humans.[6] However, subsequent studies reported the formation and migration of carbon fiber wear particles into the joint space and regional lymph nodes following implantation of the neoligament.[6] To solve this problem, the researchers tried to coat the carbon fiber with collagen and absorbable polymers. One of the most interesting attempts was a system with carbon fiber suggested by Alexander *et al.* coated with a co-polymer of polylactic acid (PLA) and polycaprolactone.[7] The carbon filaments would have to act as a scaffold for the tissue, distributing and reducing the interfacial stress between implant and soft tissues, while the PLA and polycaprolactone would help to protect the fiber during implantation. Despite the improving results, this technique was abandoned due to the high rate of complications such as re-lesion.

The Gore-Tex ligament prosthesis is composed of a long single fiber of expanded PTFE arranged into loops.[8]

Another device has been developed by Dacron, composed of four tightly woven polyester strips wrapped in a sheath of loosely woven velour, designed to minimize abrasion of the graft and act as a scaffold for fibrous tissue ingrowth.[8]

The Leeds-Keio artificial ligament was similar in composition: a polyester mesh like structure anchored to the femur and tibia with bone plugs.

Other devices were tried over the years, but the initial enthusiasm was tempered by the numerous complications related to use: failure, synovitis, non-infectious swelling, synthetic material accumulation into the knee, autoimmune reactions, osteolysis and premature development of osteoarthritis.

In the second half of the 1990s, technological growth in design of synthetic materials has led to a new series of devices that, although greeted with initial skepticism, were gradually adopted with great popularity from a broader community of orthopedics not only in Italy but also all over the world.[1]

The increasingly widespread use of these ligaments, the growth of clinical records of patients treated, the problems related to compliance with the instructions and a special surgery characterized, make it essential to analyze the results of these synthetic materials in view of modern evidence-based medicine (EBM).[1]

Therefore, the aim of this chapter is to present clinical and biomechanical results of ACL ligament reconstruction with a synthetic graft with a careful analysis of the most recent literature according to EBM criteria to evaluate critically and scientifically efficiency and safety.

2. Methods

After reviewing the archives, the researchers retrospectively contacted 50 patients (31 males and 19 females) who underwent ACL anatomic intra-articular arthroscopic reconstruction with LARS™ synthetic ligaments in the Santa Maria della Misericordia Hospital in Perugia between 2000 and 2001. All operations were performed by the same surgeon (G.C.), using the same fixation technique (femoral and tibial metal interference screws); no other graft was used during these operations. The post-operative protocol was the same in every case.

Mean age at surgery was 54.4 years (range: 41–66 years). Of the 50 patients contacted, 19 (38%: 12 males and 7 females), with a mean age of 54.1 years (range: 45–66 years) agreed to undergo clinical, biomechanical, and radiographic examination, with a mean follow-up of 10.4 years (range: 8.7–13 years). Informed consent was obtained from all individuals included in the study.

All patients were administered the International Knee Documentation Committee (*IKDC*) Scoring System, the Lysholm Knee Scoring Scale, and the Tegner Activity Scale. The level of satisfaction, sporting activity, and further complications eventually occurred after surgery were also evaluated.

The clinical assessment was performed through *IKDC* objective evaluation measured by the senior surgeon (G.C.). Two-projections radiographies of the knee under monopodalic load were also performed to evaluate articular deterioration (Figure 1); all patients underwent biomechanical tests at the "IRTAL-Nicola Cerulli-Let People Move" laboratory in Perugia, Italy.

Arthrometric evaluation was performed using KT-1000 arthrometer — MED metric, San Diego, CA, USA — at 15, 20, 30 pounds, and at manual maximum displacement, assessing side-to-side difference. In six cases, we could compare KT-1000 current absolute values with preoperative and postoperative ones, as recorded in our

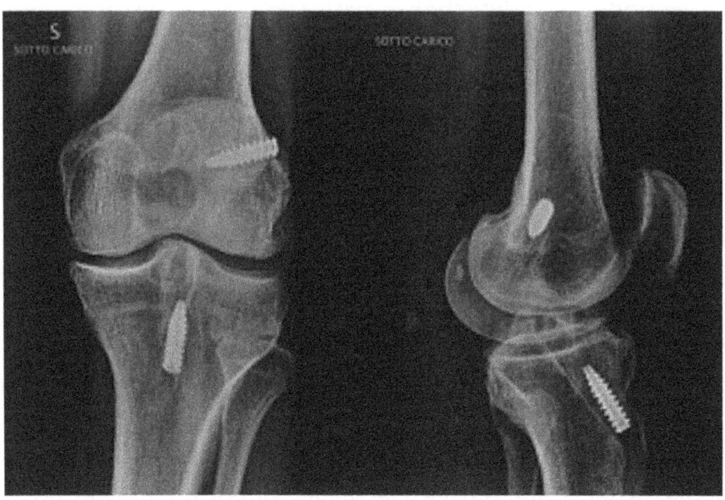

Figure 1. Two projections radiographies of the knee showing the evaluation of articular deterioration

database; the investigator was unaware of the results obtained by previous measuring.

Through an isokinetic evaluation performed with Kin-Com — Chattanooga Group, Hixson, Tennessee, USA — at 90°/s with an articular excursion between 10° and 90°, we assessed muscular strength of flexors and extensors compared to contralateral.

By using a 40 × 60 cm force plate — Bertec Corporation, Columbus, Ohio, USA — hidden in the floor, they performed a monopodalic stabilometric evaluation with the knee slightly flexed, keeping the position for 10 seconds' eyes wide open. The repositioning of the center of pressure (C.o.P.) was recorded and compared with the contralateral side. At a later stage, patients were subjected to Gait analysis.

3. Results

The IKDC Score showed a mean value of 87.78 (range: 57.5–100 points); the mean Lysholm Score was 94.47 (range: 85–100 points); the Tegner Score improved from 4.27 (range: 2–6 points) preoperatively to 6.00 (range: 4–9 points) postoperatively. No cases of synovitis or infections were detected in patients' clinical histories. None of the 19 patients underwent further surgery on the operated knee.

A high level of satisfaction was recorded, since only 3 patients (15.7%) were dissatisfied/very dissatisfied with their outcomes. Six patients out of 19 (31%) are currently practicing sport activities at the same level experienced before surgery; all remaining patients are doing sport at inferior levels, 3 of them because of their age, 2 because of work obligations. A second-look arthroscopy of the artificial ligament (Figure 2) was also performed for the only patient who sustained a meniscal tear.

Clinical assessment performed through the objective evaluation of the IKDC Score showed good outcomes in terms of stability and functionality (Table 1). Mild-moderate joint effusion was detected in 4 patients, while none showed articular range of motion (R.O.M.) deficit.

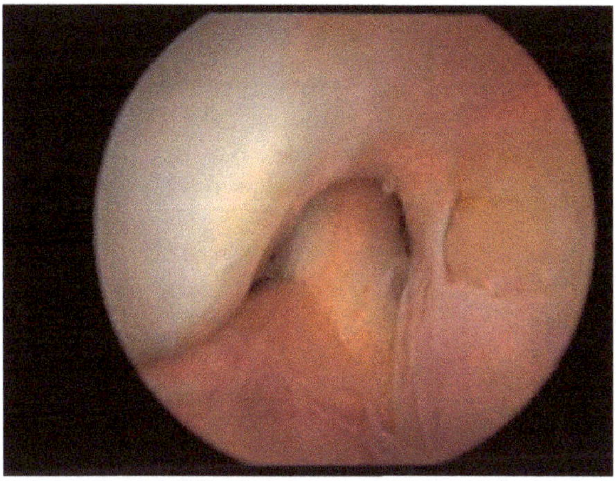

Figure 2. Arthroscopy of the artificial ligament

Anteroposterior translation of the tibia relative to the femur at 25° of flexion (Lachman test) was graded A in 10 patients, B in 5, C in 4, while no case of grade D was documented. Pivot-shift test showed a grade A in 10 patients (same as in the contralateral leg), a grade B (mild) in 5, a grade C in 3 patients and a grade D (severe) in 1 subject. Mild articular crepitus was detected in 9 patients. The One-leg Hop test of the affected leg was higher than 90% compared to the contralateral leg in 10 patients, between 76% and 89% in 7, between 75% and 50% in 3. Solely considering the patients with the lowest scoring grade at the endo of follow up, 4 (21%) reached group C, 10 (53%) group B, and 4 (21%) group A.

Results obtained from the KT-1000 test showed that side-to-side difference was less than 3 mm in 11 patients (58%), 3–5 mm in 5 (26%), and more than 5 mm in 3 (16%); mean side-to-side difference was 1.45 mm at 15 lbs, 1.87 mm at 20 lbs, 2.32 mm at 30 lbs, and 3.22 mm at manual maximum displacement. In six cases, data have been compared from the 10 years follow up with those measured 6–12 months after surgery (Table 2), thus recording the mean difference in absolute values at manual maximum displacement of 0.9 mm (–0.2 to +4; SD 2.3).

Table 1. IKDC knee examination form. The final evaluation is the worst group grade for each patient

	A Normal	B Nearly normal	C Abnormal	D Severely abnormal
1. Effusion	15	3	1	0
2. Passive motion deficit				
Lack of extension	19	0	0	0
Lack of flexion	19	0	0	0
3. Ligament examination				
Lachman 25° (134N)	13	3	3	0
Lachman 25° (manual max)	12	3	4	0
Anterior endpoint	13	4	2	0
Total AP translation (25°)	10	5	4	0
Total AP translation (70°)	11	5	3	0
Posterior drawer test (70°)	19	0	0	0
Med joint opening	16	3	0	0
Lat joint opening	15	4	0	0
External rotation test (30°)	18	1	0	0
External rotation test (90°)	18	1	0	0
Pivot shift	10	5	3	1
Reverse pivot shift	10	5	3	1
4. Compartment findings				
Crepitus ant.	10	9	0	0
Crepitus med.	18	1	0	0
Crepitus lat.	18	1	0	0
5. Harvest site pathology	19			
7. Functional test				
One leg hop	10	6	3	0
Final evaluation	4	10	4	1

The side-to-side difference changed over the time between the postoperative measurements and the most recent follow-up (Table 3), with a mean difference of 1.1 mm (–1.5 to +6; SD 2.1). Isokinetic

Table 2. Comparison of the side-to-side difference (mm) from six patients during post-op and the 10 years follow-up

Patient	Post-op (mm)	10-rs follow-up (mm)	Difference between post-op and 10-rs
1	16	20	+4
2	14	13.8	−0.2
3	13.5	15	+1.5
4	11.7	11.7	0
5	12.2	12.2	0
6	13.3	13.5	+0.2
Mean	13.4	14.3	0.9

Table 3. Comparison of the side-to-side difference (mm) over the time between the postoperative measurements and the most recent follow-up from 6 patients

Patient	Post-op (mm)	10-rs follow-up (mm)	Difference between post-op and 10-rs
1	4	10	+6
2	2	1.8	−0.2
3	1.7	4.7	+3
4	2.4	1	−1.4
5	1.7	0.2	−1.5
6	3.3	4.5	+1.2
Mean	2.5	3.7	1.1

evaluations highlight the mean strength reduction of 5.3% (−23 to +14; SD 11.1) of the extensors, and a mean strength reduction of 7.6% (−22 to +14; SD 11.9) of the flexors compared to the contralateral side. Stabilometry showed a slightly reduced proprioceptive control of the affected leg compared to the values of the contralateral leg; the ellipse area enclosing C.o.P. oscillations measured an average 584.1 mm^2 at the operated side, and an average 337.1 mm^2 at the contralateral side. Gait Analysis showed a mild reduction in the load acceptance of the injured side in 14 patients (73.6%). Following plain radiographs follow-up at 10 years show that all patients were graded stage I according to Ahlbäck classification.

4. Discussion

This current study is the only case of research on patients treated with LARS™ synthetic ligament for ACL reconstruction with such a long-term follow-up.

No major complications related to first-generation synthetic grafts — synovitis, infections, or traumatic ruptures of the graft — were recorded. Even though literature reports a unique documented example of foreign-body synovitis[3,7] following ACL reconstruction with synthetic ligaments (0.47% of total cases),[1] skepticism on the biocompatibility of the synthetic ligaments used for the reconstruction is widely recognized.

Ventura *et al.*[9] re-evaluated 51 patients treated with synthetic ligament with an even longer follow-up (18.75 years). However their group of patients was heterogeneous: three different types of synthetic ligament were used (all made of PET), and furthermore a bone–patellar–tendon–bone graft augmentation was used in 40 cases. Moreover, surgeries were performed with the "over-the-top" technique, and patients mean age at surgery was 24.85 years. The mean KOOS score was good (81.91), while the IKDC grades were not satisfactory, as 14 patients (27%) scored D, 25 (49%) C, 11 (22%) B, and 1 (2%) A. The grade of osteoarthritis increased if compared to pre-operative radiographs, and these findings were considered statistically significant; most of the patients (20) were considered grade III according to Ahlbäck classification. These results appear to be worse than those the researchers obtained, but the team mentioned that these patients' mean age at surgery was much higher, and that they used an anatomic ACL reconstruction technique.

Parchi *et al.*[10] recruited 26 patients treated with LARS™ synthetic ligament, 8 years after surgery. Mean age at surgery was 38.5 years. The level of satisfaction was substantial (8.1 on a range from 1 to 10), mean KOOS score was 84, mean Cincinnati Knee Rating Scale score was 89, with just 2 overall not satisfactory results. Articular stability was satisfactory in 24 patients out of 26, and only 1 case of mechanical graft failure after 58 months from the surgical procedure — occurred during high-level sporting activity — was recorded. No cases of synovitis or infections were detected.

Liu *et al.*[11] compared the results after ACL reconstruction using a four-strand hamstring ligament (32 patients) vs LARS™ artificial ligament (28 patients) with a mean follow-up of 4.08 years (range: 48–52 months). Patients treated with LARS™ ligaments obtained excellent results, with a mean Lysholm score of 92.1, and a mean Tegner score of 6.2. KT-1000 arthrometer showed a side-to-side difference less than 3 mm in 26 patients (92.8%), and 3–5 mm in 2 patients (7.2%). Mean age at surgery was 36 years (range: 18–54 years).

In a multicenter study, Gao *et al.*[12] evaluated 156 patients with a mean follow-up of 4.16 years (range: 36–62 months), obtaining further encouraging results. The mean Lysholm score was 94.5 (range: 65–100 points), and the Tegner score was 6.1 (range: 1–9 points). According to the IKDC scale, 81 patients (52%) were graded A, 65 (41.4%) were graded B, 9 (6%) were graded C, and 1 patient (0.6%) was graded D. KT-1000 arthrometer showed a side-to-side difference less than 3 mm in 121 patients (78%), 3–5 mm in 31 (20%), more than 5 mm in 4 (2%). 93% of patients were satisfied/very satisfied with their outcomes, resulting in a high overall level of satisfaction. The authors recorded 3 graft ruptures (2%), 1 case of infection, and 1 synovitis (the only case currently documented in literature).

Ye *et al.*[13] enrolled in a retrospective study with 53 patients with a mean age of 31.2 years (range: 22–51 years), and follow-up of 3.75 years (range: 36–52 months). The mean Lysholm score was 93.1 (range: 89.8–96.6 points). *IKDC* grades showed 0 patients in group D, 2 (3.8%) in group C, 23 (43.4%) in group B, and 28 (52.8%) in group A.

Huang *et al.*[14] reviewed 43 ACL reconstructions with LARS™ synthetic ligament performed on patients with a mean age of 27.5 years (range: 17–48 years), with a mean follow-up of 2.45 years (range: 10–49 months). The mean Lysholm score was 82.8 (range: 80–85 points); IKDC grades showed 27 patients (63%) in group A, 14 (32%) in group B, 2 (5%) in group C, none in group D. No graft rupture or infection was reported. KT-1000 arthrometer also showed good results, with a side-to-side difference of less than 2 mm in 40 patients (75.5%), 3–5 mm in 11 (18.9%), more than 6 mm in 2 (5.7%). No complications, such as infections, synovitis, or further ruptures, were recorded during the follow-up.

Two studies evaluated knee stability by performing TELOS stress radiographs: Nau *et al.*[15] and Lavoie *et al.*[16] The first research group recorded a mean difference at KT-1000 of 4.86 mm (SD 3.8), while the second one recorded a difference of 7.3 mm (0–17; SD 4.22).

Five studies evaluated knee stability using KT-1000 arthrometer (Table 4). The study conducted by Derricks *et al.*[17] documented, in wider terms, that with a mean follow-up of 2.5 years (range: 4.5 years to 4 months), 90% of treated patients show a tibial translation equal to the contralateral. Four additional studies,[8,11,13,18] with similar follow-up periods, report more thoroughly that the side-to-side difference was less than 3 mm in 75–92% of the patients, 3–5 mm in 7–20%, 5–10 mm in 0–10%. By adding up all the data the researchers obtained, they can assert that the side-to-side difference of patients treated with LARS™ synthetic ligament, recorded through KT-1000 arthrometer, is less than 3 mm in 77% of the cases, 3–5 mm in 18.8%, 5–10 mm in 4.2%.[19]

Table 4. Knee stability using KT-1000 arthrometer

Kt-1000	Gao K. 2010	Liu ZL. 2010	Ye JX. 2013	Pan X. 2013	Derricks G. 1995	Team's study	Total
< 3 mm	121 (77.6%)	26 (92.8%)	40 (75.5%)	24 (75%)	90% of patients	11 (58%)	222 (77%)
3–5 mm	31 (19.9%)	2 (7.2%)	11 (20.7%)	5 (15%)		5 (26%)	54 (18.8%)
5–10 mm	4 (2.5%)	0	2 (3.8%)	3 (10%)		3 (16%)	12 (4.2%)
> 10 mm	0	0	0	0		0	0
Mean (mm)	1.5 ± 1.6	1.2 ± 0.3	2.35 ± 2.28	2.29 ± 2.03		3.22	

Comparing out results to those obtained in the above-mentioned works, they noticed a higher percentage of patients with a side-to-side difference greater than 5 mm and lesser percentage of patients with a side-to-side difference less than 3 mm. The researchers hypothesized that this discrepancy was caused by the extent of their follow-up period, which is definitely longer (10 years vs 4) compared to the rest of the studies.

It is important to highlight that, even though in only 6 patients, the results in absolute values and the side-to-side difference recorded by the KT-1000 at manual maximum displacement are similar to the data obtained through the postoperative evaluation, since they respectively increase by a mean of 0.9 mm and 1.1 mm. If the patient 1 was not included in Tables 2 and 3 (clearly an unstable knee), the researchers would state that the synthetic ligaments appropriately hold the initial tension, even after 10 years. Therefore, the researchers would conclude that the 6 patients with a side-to-side difference greater than 4 mm already presented with ligamentous laxity prior to the study, and the recorded instability is not linked to the duration of the follow-up.

The researchers are convinced that strict compliance to the correct recommendations is of paramount importance in order to obtain good results using synthetic ligaments. According to some authors, it is essential that enough ACL stump is left, so that the new-ACL can pass through it and be sutured.[8,12] Parchi *et al.*[10] recommend this graft in patients with symptomatic ALRI, older than 30 years, strongly motivated and needing a fast recovery. Regarding the opinion of the researchers, the age limit should be raised at least up to 40 years, restricting the use on younger patients just for exceptional cases, when in the presence of relevant work or sport requirements. Analyzing the data of the long-term follow-up period, they noted that even if a tibial translation greater than 3 mm was recorded in 42% of the patients, the researchers think that they had a very high level of satisfaction (84.3%) among the patients. This is due to the inevitable fact that patients lowered their functional request over the years, even if carrying on with sporting activities.

5. Conclusion

Using synthetic ligaments for ACL reconstructions can be considered a suitable surgical option if used with due precautions. Promising results were obtained in the short, medium, and long term, but further studies (to be conducted with an even more accurate methodology) are necessary in order to provide additional and definitive evidence. Extreme caution is needed when using synthetic ligaments to perform ACL reconstruction. Furthermore, the surgical procedure should be preceded by extensive discussion with patients in order to distinctly clarify pros and cons of this choice and his appropriateness.

References

1. Cerulli, G.; Antinolfi, P.; Bruè, S.; Placella, G.; Sebastiani, E.; Potalivo, G.; Zamarra, G. *GIOT* **2011**, *37-S1*(4), 159–166.
2. Giannotti, S. M.; Marshall, S. W.; Hume, P. A.; Bunt, L. *J. Sci. Med. Sport.* **2009**, *12*, 622–627.
3. Machotka, Z.; Scarborough, I.; Duncan, W.; Kumar, S.; Erraton, L. *SMART* **2010**, *2*, 29.
4. Batty, L. M.; Norsworthy, C. J.; Lash, N. J.; Wasiak, J.; Richmond, A. K.; Feller, J. A. *Arthroscopy* **2015**, *31*(5), 957–968.
5. Ahlfeld, S. K.; Larson, R. L.; Collins, H. R.; *Am. J. Sports Med.* **1987**, *15*(4), 326–330.
6. Jenkins, D. H. R. *J. Bone Joint Surg. Br.* **1978**, *60-B*(4), 520–522.
7. Alexander, H.; Weiss, A. B.; Parsons, J. R. *Aktuelle Probl. Chir. Orthop.* **1983**, *26*, 78–91.
8. Mascarenhas, R.; MacDonald, P. B. *McGill J Med* **2008**, *11*, 29–37.
9. Ventura, A.; Terzaghi, C.; Legnani, C.; Borgo, E.; Albisetti, W. *The Knee* **2010**, *17*, 108–113.
10. Parchi, P. D.; Ciapini, G.; Dolfi, L.; Baluganti, A.; Nicola, P.; Chiellini, F.; Lisanti, M. *SICOT* **2013**, *37*, 1567–1574.
11. Liu, Z. L.; Zhang, X.; Jiang, Y.; Zeng, B. F. *SICOT* **2010**, *34*, 45–49.
12. Gao, K.; Chen, S.; Wang, L.; Zhang, W.; Kang, Y.; Dong, Q.; Zhou, H.; Li, L. *Arthroscopy* **2010**, *26*(4), 515–523.
13. Ye, J. X.; Shen, G. S.; Zhou, H. B.; Xu, W.; Xie, Z. G.; Dong, Q. R.; Xu, Y. J. *Eur. Rev. Med. Pharmacol. Sci.* **2013**, *17*, 1438–1446.

14. Huang, J. M.; Wang, Q.; Shen, F.; Wang, Z.; Kang, Y. *Chin. Med. J.* **2010,** *123*(2), 160–164.
15. Nau, T.; Lavoie, P.; Duval, N. *J. Bone Joint Surg.* (*Br*) **2002**, *84-B*, 356–360.
16. Lavoie, P.; Fletcher, J.; Duval, N. *The Knee* **2000**, *7*, 157–163.
17. Dericks, G. Jr. *Op. Tech. Sport Med.* **1995**, *3*(3), 187–205.
18. Pan, X.; Wen, H.; Wang, L.; Ge, T. *Eur. J. Orthop. Surg. Traumatol.* **2013**, *23*, 819–823.
19. Newman, S. D. S.; Atkinson, H. D. E.; Wills-Owen, C. A. *SICOT* **2013**, *37*, 321–326.

https://doi.org/10.1142/9789811204630_0007

Chapter 7

LARS Ligament: 10 Years' Chinese Experience

Shiyi Chen

Department of Orthopaedic Sports Medicine, Huashan Hospital, Fudan University Sports Medicine Centre, Shanghai 200040, China
cshiyi@163.com

Abbreviations

ACL	Anterior cruciate ligament
CALSG	Artificial Ligament Study Group
LARS	Ligament augmentation reinforcement system
PET	Polyethylene terephthalate
SFDA	State Food and Drug Administration

1. Introduction

The clinical application of artificial ligaments in the anterior cruciate ligament (ACL) reconstruction is controversial because of early backfire. In literature, there were two waves regarding artificial ligament related papers published over the past 40 years. The first came into being in the early 1990s. Then, after muffling of nearly 20 years, the papers focusing on the artificial ligaments in the ACL reconstruction raised again. Between 2011 and 2015, the resurgence developed into the second wave. Then why two waves of published papers happen in this area of time? To answer this question, a brief retrospect of the artificial ligaments applied in the ACL reconstruction will be helpful.

In dialectics, each coin has two sides. Over the past 5 years, studies on artificial ligaments applied in the ACL reconstruction were widely reported.[1–17]

In the ACL reconstruction using certain artificial ligament, satisfactory outcomes were seen in the short and mid-term follow-ups.[2,4,14,18] Furthermore, confident of the practical experience from over 10 years' clinical application in China, the researchers hold the viewpoint that current efficacy of artificial ligaments is satisfactory. Outcomes of the ACL reconstruction with new generation artificial ligament was different from those with early products, which were substantial fiascos as literature recorded.

In this chapter, the researchers reviewed the application of artificial ligaments in the ACL reconstruction in China. Then, new generation artificial ligaments as well as their current application in the ACL reconstruction are introduced, in which the issue of surgical failure and post-operative complications are of high concern. In addition, the author also introduce a Chinese organization associated with the application of artificial ligaments, especially in the ACL reconstruction. Particularly, they shared here their rethinking of the artificial ligaments applied in the ACL reconstruction, which involves three aspects:

(1) the reason of early failure,
(2) the rate of surgical failure and complication,
(3) the meaning of artificial ligaments in the ACL reconstruction.

Given the tight connection between the prognosis and the surgical techniques, surgical essentials of the ACL reconstruction with artificial ligaments is stressed in the following content. A technique essential, "isometric like reconstruction", is illustrated. In the end, the development of new kind artificial ligaments and relevant fundamental studies are briefly introduced.

2. Current Application of Artificial Ligament: New Generation

The artificial ligaments currently adopted in the ACL reconstruction includes the ligament augmentation reinforcement system (LARS Surgical Implants and Devices, Arc-sur-Tille, France) and Neoligaments (Neoligaments, Leeds, England).

The LARS is consisted of a series of new generation artificial ligaments made of polyethylene terephthalate (PET). The LARS used for the ACL reconstruction was called "LARS-ACL". With cleaning process to remove potential residues and oils during manufacturing, it was supposed that the LARS was able to encourage tissue in-growth and lower the potential risk of severe complications like synovitis, especially for the ACL reconstruction.[19] Compared with other types of artificial ligaments, the intra-articular portion of the LARS was unique. It abandoned the cross-linked structure and was woven in parallel PET fibers that were pre-twisted at 90°. The twist orientation was dependent on the side of joint. Why such design? Derick *et al.* explained that "knitted (cross-linked) fibers tend to chew on themselves with rotational torsional motions, much the way tennis racket strings wear out by rubbing against each other when hitting the ball". It is likely that by adopting the parallel fibers woven fashion, wearing particles and debris of materials could be prevented. Besides the cruciate ligaments' reconstruction, the coverage of LARS includes the rotator cuff repair, acromioclavicular joint dislocation, patellar tendon rupture and lateral ligament reconstruction of ankle and etc. In fixation, titanium cannulated interference screws were used for press fixation. Edges of the screws were blunt, which can share the ligament from damage during screwing.

3. Chinese Experience

3.1. *The Status of the ACL Reconstruction with Artificial Ligaments in China*

The miserable failure from the large-scale application of artificial ligaments in the ACL reconstruction in the US during the 1980s and 1990s was not experienced by surgeons in China. In the ACL reconstruction, the using of artificial ligaments was initiated from the LARS in 2004. At 2005, Ao *et al.* reported the ACL reconstruction increased with the Leeds-Keio artificial ligament and obtained satisfactory outcomes.[20] However, no related reports were published ever after. Since approved by the State Food and Drug Administration

(SFDA) in 2004, the LARS artificial ligament has been applied for almost 12 years in the mainland of China and its distribution has covered all the provinces throughout the country. So far, an estimated of over 10,000 cases were performed. Until December 2015, surgeons all over the country published over 100 related papers in Chinese, and some studies also have been published on international journals.[2–4,8,10,11,14,17,18,21–23]

3.1.1. *Middle-term follow-ups*

From the reports of different centers, the short- and middle-term clinical outcomes of the ACL reconstruction with the LARS were satisfactory and the incidence of complication and surgical failure all remained at low levels. In 2010, Gao *et al.* firstly reported a multi-center follow-up study, in which a total of 159 cases receiving the ACL reconstruction with the LARS between August 2004 and July 2006 were included, and the mean follow-up period was 50 months.[4] In overall results, rupture of grafts was only seen in three cases, and one of them developed synovitis. The cause of rupture was re-injury in all three cases. Laxity was demonstrated in another four cases (side-to-side difference > 5 mm), with the failure rate being 4.4%. In three cases, the loosening screws were found by protruding out of tibial or femoral tunnels, with rate of 1.9%. In remaining cases, joints stability was maintained. Satisfaction was obtained in 93% patients. Notably, most of the surgical failure occurred in one center, and this might be relevant to the technique manipulation and patient's selection. In another middle-term retrospective follow-up study by Liu *et al.*, the outcomes demonstrated that in the ACL reconstruction, the joint stability in the LARS group was higher than the 4-strand hamstring autograft group.[18] In addition, there was no significant difference in general outcomes evaluation between the two groups. In another middle-term follow-up study, Pan *et al.* compared the clinical efficacy of the LARS to the BPTB autograft in the ACL reconstruction, both showed "similarly good clinical results".[14] In a prospective randomized study, Chen *et al.* investigated the ACL reconstruction using the LARS in young active adults of either acute or chronic condition.

The final outcome of the 5 years follow-up study demonstrated that "performing ACL reconstruction soon after injury using a LARS graft could provide an advantage for treating and rehabilitating".[3]

3.1.2. *Long-Term Follow-Up*

There was only one study of long-term follow-up period; Wang *et al.* from Taiwan reported a long-term (8–15 years) follow-up study of the ACL reconstruction with the LARS. [21] Among a total of 28 patients included, graft rupture was seen in two cases. In remaining cases, one case was confirmed as laxity (side-to-side difference > 5 mm), and synovitis was occurred in two. For the two cases of synovitis, one developed the condition 2 months post-operative and symptoms released after conservative method; in the other case, severe condition developed 2 years post-operative and had to accept arthrocentesis and other conservative method. The investigator maintained that the ACL reconstruction with LARS demonstrated good results in improving life function and activity at a mean of 11.4 years.

3.1.3. *Complications*

In a follow-up study by Li *et al.*, 58 patients receiving the ACL reconstruction with the LARS were included and divided into acute and chronic groups.[21] Follow-up period ranged from 3–7 years. Biopsy was made in four cases needing the second arthroscopy. In result, according the IKDC standard, only four patients were graded as C and D, with the failure rate of 6.9%. For the complications, infection and synovitis was no seen in any patients, but the screw raising symptoms cannot be ignored. Bursitis caused by protruding screws in the tibial side was seen in 11 cases with one of them needing surgical intervention. On the femoral side, protruding screws were seen in two cases, and both accepted related surgical treatment because of symptoms. Those symptoms caused by loosening screws were termed as "screw protruding syndrome" by the investigators. In addition, bone tunnel enlargement was also obvious in the research. Among 41 cases fulfilled final radiographic exam, tunnel enlargement was observed in 25, with an average enlargement rate of 30% (2.7 mm). The researcher concluded that bone tunnel enlargement did exist to some extent in the ACL reconstruction with the LARS artificial ligaments, but it did not affect the knee joint stability. Data evaluation in acute and chronic groups was similar and normal fibrous tissues ingrowth was found in the LARS artificial ligaments. For the issue of bone tunnel enlargement in the LARS-ACL reconstruction, Huang *et al.* investigated 43 cases receiving surgery between 2004 and 2007 because of isolated ACL injury.[7] The follow-up period was 40 months and radiographic evaluation methods included X-ray and tomography (CT). The assessment was made in six sequential time points respectively at 1, 3, 6, 12, 24, and 36 months post-operative. The condition of bone tunnel enlargement was classified into four degrees according to the Peyrache standard. The final outcome demonstrated that three cases were finally ranked as level one (≥ 2 mm and < 4 mm), all appearing at the femoral tunnels near articular surface with an average width of 2.5 ± 0.3 mm; in 40 cases of level zero, the average width of enlargement was 0.8 ± 0.3 mm in the tibial tunnels and 1.1 ± 0.3 mm in the femoral tunnels. No patients revealed level two (≥ 4 mm and < 6 mm) or level three (≥ 6 mm) tunnel enlargement. In this study, laxity was not observed, and subjective evaluation was satisfactory. Just from the two reports, perhaps it could be maintained that in the LARS-ACL reconstruction, bone tunnel enlargement did exist to some extent, but the joint stability was not therefore influenced.

Li *et al.* reported a case of synovitis.[11] A young male patients received the LARS-ACL reconstruction at another hospital, obtaining good joint function after rehabilitation program. Twenty-eight months post-operative, he suddenly suffered a twisting injury of the operated joint during sports. By conservative treatment, the recurrent symptoms like swollen and pain were not relieved. Then he came to the author's hospital where physical exam demonstrated recurrent laxity. Taking his injury history and symptoms into consideration, the author suggested the rupture of the graft. Following the second opinion, he received the revision surgery, during which the synovitis was severe and the intra articular segment of the LARS artificial ligament was ruptured near the tibial tunnel orifice. Notably, in this case, the position of femoral tunnel was too anteriorly located. Considering reported causes of failure from other reports and the explicit injury history in this case, the author held the viewpoint the malposition of the femoral tunnel was the root cause leading to the surgical failure.

3.1.4. *Specialists' consensus from China artificial ligament study group (CALSG)*

With the clinical application of artificial ligaments, the subject is taken more into consideration. As a matter of fact, the cases of the ACL reconstruction with such devices grows each year on the mainland. To evaluate effectively the artificial ligaments as well as the communication and experience exchange among specialists from different districts, an organization focusing on the clinical application of artificial ligaments in China was founded at 2014 that is named CALSG. After fully exchanging views of the characteristics of artificial ligaments and related surgical indications, sports medicine specialists reached this following consensus.

On the characteristics of artificial ligaments:

- No harvest side morbidity;
- Operation convenience, short time of operation, relatively minor operation wound;
- Good mechanical properties, and immediate tensile strength after surgery;
- Early function recovery was the highlight compared with traditional methods;
- Surgical essential in successful ACL reconstruction with artificial ligaments was the isometric reconstruction principle. (Surgical failure was largely due to the incorrect indication and the violation of isometric principle).

On the surgical indications:

- Acute ACL injury (optimal indication: ideal remnant preservation);
- Multiple ligament injuries of knee;
- Athlete, requiring early return to the fields and to sports activity;
- Middle- or old-aged patients, requiring fast return to sports or daily activity;
- Special patients asking fast recovery of sports activity;
- Patients rejecting autografts or of allergic constitution;
- Patients rejecting allografts because of religion, economy, disease, legitimacy and so on;
- Cases of bone neoplasms needing limb salvage as well as repair or reconstruction surgery.

3.2. *Multi-center Follow-up Program: Study Focusing on Failure Cases and Causes*

From the outcomes in related reports at home and abroad, the long-term outcome of the LARS-ACL reconstruction was still controversial. Focusing points mainly fall on the long-term failure rate and post-operative complications. In response, the CALSG held two meetings respectively in Shenzhen and Chongqing in 2015, launching a mass trans-regional research program, namely, "Long-term failure rate investigation in the ACL reconstruction with the LARS artificial ligaments: a multi-center follow-up study". The purposes of this research were to clarify three questions in the ACL reconstruction with the LARS artificial ligaments: (1) How much failure actually happened in long-term after surgery in China? (2) What was the reason of failure and which factor played a major role? (3) What was the complications rate and how to deal with that in different conditions? A total of 19 orthopedics sports medicine centers from both the mainland and Taiwan have been included to participate in this program, and the follow-up investigation is currently carrying out according to a unified registry approach in China.

4. Rethinking: Value of Artificial Ligaments in the ACL Reconstruction

The outcome of the ACL reconstruction with artificial ligaments was decided by both external forces and internal reasons. There are many influential factors and any one of them could be powerful enough to break the balance of success and failure. The factors the team highly valued were the patient selection and indication, grasping of technique essential, mechanical and biological properties of grafts, compliance of rehabilitation and patients' overall condition, regained activity intensity and accident. After that, what they realized is that no graft was perfect with each kind of both advantages and disadvantages, therefore the researchers think that they should not attribute the cause of a surgical failure all to the graft *per se*. For those reporting high surgical failure and post-operative complications, they should look for reasons elsewhere, such as in methods and techniques. To rethink on why studies from other investigators demonstrated high success rates, while other cases failed. To rethink on if there is any experience leading to success. To rethink on this issue and in each step of the whole surgical process.

4.1. *Analysis of Early Failure in ACL Reconstruction with Artificial Ligaments*

In the ACL reconstruction, the early application of artificial ligaments was largely proved a failure. There are several reasons the researchers think that lead to failure.

4.1.1. *Defects of graft structure and design*

Function was born in structure. Therefore, the design of artificial ligament should mimic the native ACL as much as possible, to realize the so-called bionics design. Taking the Gore-Tex artificial ligament for example, the researchers found that it looked like a girl's twisted braid, which was far away from the native not only in contour but also in structure. While the Kennedy and the Leeds-Keio artificial ligament didn't specialize their intra-articular portion and still adopted crossing woven pattern, in which the crossing fibers would chew on each other and therefore the forming of wearing particles were inevitable. Derick *et al.* figuratively expounded this mechanism by using the analogy between the crossing fibers and the strings of a racket.[19]

4.1.2. *Defects of graft materials*

To choose an ideal material for artificial ligaments, two elements must be taken into consideration: (1) meeting the mechanical requirement for the ACL reconstruction; (2) being non-toxic or adverse effect on human body.

The artificial ligament using carbon fiber demonstrated high tensile strength, but it was breaking slowly in animal model according to Jenkins' research.[24] In addition, the carbon particles also could be found in regional lymph nodes. And clinical practice also demonstrated that it could break in human body. Finally, people realized that even though the carbon fibers had a dense structure and a high tensile strength, the capacity to resist torsion was the weakness so that it cannot meet the requirement of the ACL reconstruction despite some advocating reports.[25] Gore-Tex artificial ligament was fabricated by the PTFE fibers, which also demonstrated high tensile strength.[26] However, severe synovitis was reported in following studies and the free PTFE particles were regarded as the direct cause. [27] The Travira, the Leeds-Keio, and the Dacron artificial ligaments all made of the PET fibers; they were proved with high rupture rates long-term after surgery and therefore should not be applied in the ACL reconstruction according to some investigators.

The LARS was also made of the PET fibers. Although related clinical studies largely revealed satisfactory outcomes and the intra articular free fibers theoretically could avoid abrasion and forming of debris, considering the material aging process, which is the natural character of macromolecule, it still need long-term follow-ups to collect more evidence in the future.

4.1.3. *Key problems: Indication and surgical technique*

Correct structural design and appropriate materials were essential conditions for the success of one kind artificial ligament. The two factors were similar to the double wheels of one chariot, which means that they are equally important, and none is dispensable. While for a hurtling Roman chariot, a well-trained driver also plays a crucial role. In other words, the ACL reconstruction with artificial ligament in most cases cannot be successful without seasoned surgeons. From the aspect of the surgeon, correct indication and "isometric" principle were key points for the surgical success.

In terms of indication, beside several aforementioned points, for the patients of chronic ACL condition and poor remnant quality, the research team do not recommend the application of LARS artificial ligament. At this point, the author agrees with Prof. Cerulli's opinion, which suggests that the LARS artificial ligament was only an intra-articular brace having mechanical transmission property, and it need the wrapping of remnant and ingrowth from self-tissue to reach the so-called "biological reconstruction".

In terms of surgical technique, the isometric point is pivotal. Over the past 30 years, surgical technique progressed rapidly and became more and more elaborate. The position of bone tunnels, especially the femoral tunnel, was consistently evolving. The prefixes used before the "ACL reconstruction" was various and consisted of "over the top", "anatomical", "double bundle", "single bundle", "ribbon", "isometric" and "Isometric-like". When discussing failure reasons, the inaccurate location of bone tunnels was sometimes ignored; however, the main cause of a failed surgery was always due to the intra articular malposition of the artificial ligament. For the LARS, because the artificial ligament lacks viscoelasticity, the isometric principle is indispensable. Mr. Laboureau, the inventor of LARS artificial ligament, and Derick *et al.* all clearly pointed out that the application of LARS in the ACL reconstruction must abide the isometric principle, and the accurate tunnel position was utterly important. However, through various follow-up studies, the research team found that the incorrect tunnel position was not a rare phenomenon. According to the two case reports in which synovitis developed due to ruptured grafts, femoral tunnels were both to some extent anteriorly positioned, and it was worthy of high attention.

Notably, the researchers began to hold the viewpoint that the theoretical isometric point might not really exist in clinical practice, and what the surgeons could do was to find a point, by which the relative movement between the graft and the bone tunnel was as little as possible. And the so-called isometric reconstruction was also based on this idea. In their practice, the researchers have already found a point, by which the bone tunnels and the graft can remain relatively static during knee flexion of 90 degrees to full extension. It was termed as "isometric-like" point and more details are introduced in following text.

4.2. *Rate of Surgical Failure and Complications*

Regarding the LARS-ACL reconstruction, the research team was not pessimistic about the current rate of surgical failure and post-operative complications.

On one hand, it was based on the outcomes of most clinical reports as well as the successful experiences in China over the last 10 years, which also included the outcomes from long-term follow-up study focusing on the cases of our own department. On the other hand, it was based on the comparison between the outcome of the LARS and that of traditional grafts regarding the long-term surgical failure rate of the ACL reconstruction. In 2015, Bottoni *et al.* reported a prospective randomized trial.[28] The result revealed that the long-term (≥ 10 years) failure rate in the ACL reconstruction was 8.3% for hamstring autografts and it was up to 26.5% for the posterior tibialis allograft. In 2013, Crawford reviewed the long-term failure rate of the ACL reconstruction.[29] The outcome revealed that "At least 1 in 9 patients undergoing the ACL reconstruction will have re-rupture or clinical failure at long-term follow-up". Currently, it seems that the surgical failure rate of the LARS was lower than traditional grafts in the ACL reconstruction. In the ACL reconstruction using the LARS artificial ligaments, there were two major problems: (1) the difficulty in flexing knee joints ranging from 90° to 120° in early rehabilitation; (2) the recurrent laxity and loosening screws. The main cause of these two problems was the trouble of isometric point.

4.3. *The Significance of the Artificial Ligament Applied in the ACL Reconstruction*

"Function supreme" was the final objective in sports medicine. Early recovery of knee function, early return to the field, and no harvest side morbidity were the pearls of the application of artificial ligaments in the ACL reconstruction. The serving objects of sports medicine were mass sports enthusiasts and professional athletes; therefore, the functional return at the maximum level was the ultimate goal between doctors and patients to satisfy the demands for sports activities. In other words, the work of sports medicine doctors would be a little bit different from that of the general orthopedists, whose patient population was largely consisted of ordinary people without specific demand for athletic, and the function or capacity of daily life was the therapeutic goal in most cases. Furthermore, in terms of graft used in the ACL reconstruction, the team thinks they should take the requirement of patients into full consideration. In this way, the researchers can realize the goal of precise treatment.

In comparing different grafts in the ACL reconstruction, the team cannot just focus on the long-term surgical failure rate, joints stability, and various evaluation questionnaires. In contrast, the team thinks they should pay more attention to whether the patients can return to sports or not, when and at which level. For the patients receiving the ACL reconstruction with the LARS artificial ligaments, early return to sports was the biggest highlight. Averagely, patients can return to light physical activity and jogging 4–5 weeks post-operative, heaven physical activity allowed in 6–8 weeks post-operative and contact athletic exercise or competition in 8–10 weeks post-operative. Whilst the return to athletic sports and exercise would take at least 24–36 weeks or even longer in the ACL reconstruction using autografts.

The actual situation might be even worse. Ardern *et al.* investigated the situation of return to sports in patients receiving the ACL reconstruction with autografts.[30] Among 5770 included athletes, only 63% of them could return to the pre-injury sport events, no more than 30% athletes could return to the athletic games in 37 months post-operative. Moreover, in Ardern *et al.*'s other report, in the Australian rules football players who received the ACL reconstruction with the autografts, only 42% of them could return to the full competition sports, and nearly 21% of them could not even make attempts on training or modified competition.[31] This situation was even worse in the patients participating in other sports events like soccer, basketball, and netball. Although the autografts in the cases looked intact, these athletes were not able to return to these activities at pre-injury level or other related sports. Did the surgery succeed on this case? European sports medicine specialists encountered the same problem.[32] The athletes receiving the ACL reconstruction using autografts could not return to sports activity at pre-injury level. Even though the muscle function fully recovered, most athletes reported that it was the poor outcomes of knee function and knee related quality of life that mainly block their homeward journey to sports instead of the fear of re-injury.

5. Research of a New Kind of Artificial Ligament: Current Progress and Future Orientation

5.1. *Backgrounds of Research*

Many orthopaedic departments and sports medicine centers around the world have applied artificial ligaments, especially the LARS. Though the long-term efficiency was still in dispute, many renowned experts in their clinical researches favored the application of artificial ligaments.[11] Of course, as synthetic implants, the artificial ligament holds a much shorter research history than the joint prosthesis. Even up until now, the research team thinks that the scientific community still fail to manufacture a joint prosthesis that can be equally compared with the native one. Therefore, the intrinsic defects of artificial ligaments including the LARS, the Neoligaments *et al.* are to some extent reasonable and relatively acceptable, and it is the defects that still need further improvement. To solve this problem, sports medicine physicians and related enterprises around the world, especially in China, devoted their efforts and funds to ameliorate current artificial ligament products in different aspects, expecting to bring about new kind artificial ligaments, which can meet clinical requirement.

5.2. *Purpose and Meaning of Research and Development*

Artificial ligaments were used to permanently replace ruptured ligaments in joint. An ideal product should have the following properties:

(1) Artificial ligament is supposed to show great mechanical property, including high intensity, proper viscosity, and visco-elasticity to some extent, of which the prosthesis can bear high tension. In addition, great anti-fatigue property is also indispensable.
(2) Material used to fabricate the ligament should be hydrophilic, ensuring excellent biocompatibility. The biocompatibility may be illustrated as good cellular compatibility *in vitro* and autologous tissue in-growth naturally *in vivo*, the latter phenomenon is obvious to observe in intra-articular part. Tissue in growth leads to thorough synovium coverage around the intra-articular artificial ligament, promoting autologous changing process in artificial ligaments.
(3) In addition to biocompatibility, artificial ligament material calls for good osteoconduction and osteoinduction to achieve better graft-bone healing within bone tunnel.
(4) As a well-developed implant, the structure and fixation methods should not block self-tissue ingrowth. In a word, the ideal artificial ligament is the ligament that resembles natural ligament anatomically and physically, which is now named as new kind biological artificial ligament.

5.3. *Current Progress in Research and Development*

Various researches focusing on the improvement of current artificial ligaments were conducted regarding the requirements of new kind artificial ligaments. Relevant programs consisted of material science research, products design and manufacture, and other studies involving advanced techniques such as tissue engineering, biological drug delivery technique to ameliorate the artificial ligament in use.

5.3.1. *Surface coating and modification of polyethylene terephthalate material*

The PET was widely applied in artificial ligaments manufacturing and demonstrated hydrophobicity as a polyester. In addition, it does not have the capacity of osteoinduction and osteoconduction property. Therefore, they came up with an idea that the intra-articular part of artificial ligament was coated with hydrophilic components leading to fiber tissue ingrowth, and the extra-articular part was coated with components leading to osteogenesis. Based on that, a segmental multi-functional coating biological artificial ligament is obtained. Results show that surface coating in intra-articular part with bioactive protein like fibroin and some growth factors, may induce autogenous synovial tissues covering.[33] Outcomes of researches proved that it was an effective method to improve material cellular compatibility *in vitro* and promote ligaments incorporation into auto-tissue *in vivo*. As for extra-articular part, numerous researches have proven that coating PET surface with hydroxyapatite, bioglass and silicon dioxide results in mineralized coating forming with osteoinduction and osteoconduction ability.[33,34] The mineralized coatings not only improve cellular compatibility and osteogenesis ability *in vitro*, but also promote tendon–bone healing and new bone growth into tendon–bone interface *in vivo*. Based on the tentative results, attention is paid to the stability and adhesion enhancement of the coating surface. Biomimetic mineralized coating or plasma spraying techniques are put into use to improve coating results. The author's research team has tried several functional coatings in the surface modification research and published about 30 articles in domestic and foreign journals up to now.

5.3.2. *Modification on artificial ligament material*

Currently, artificial ligaments were mainly made of polyester with some limitation of knowledge. One kind of artificial ligament manufactured in Israel called Tavor even use nitinol as primary material, though its viscosity is in doubt. The research team is focusing on applying latest material such as carbon nanotube and ultrahigh molecular weight polyethylene into artificial ligament material innovation process. Another research hotspot was the tissue engineering artificial ligament, which consisted of a supporting scaffold made of biodegradable materials like natural silk fibers, and relevant effective growth factors for cellular introducing. The growth factors included polylactic acid, polyglycolic acid, *et al.*[35,36] Among those materials, degradation product of polylactic acid and polyglycolic acid are acidic, which may have irritation effect on human body. Unlike the former two kinds of acid, natural silk does not degrade into acidic products. Artificial ligaments made from silk have been used in animal ACL reconstruction experiments like rabbits, beagle dogs, and pigs. The results were satisfactory.[36] Silk artificial ligaments were applied in clinical trials abroad, but the experimental results were still not clear.

5.3.3. *Improvements on artificial ligament structure and fixation*

The LARS ligament adopted a fixation method named press fit, which fixes the ligament prosthesis with two interference screws.[12] The defects of this method are listed as following:

(1) The screws press the part of ligament in bone tunnel mechanically or even flatten the ligament due to press fit method, thus destroying the porous structure designed to promote autologous tissue ingrowth, eventually impeding autologous bone growth normally, which may lead to post-operative prosthesis loosening. (2) Press fit method relies heavily on strength of the fixation screw to form screw-implant-bone tunnel stability system in the early to middle post-implantation period. In long term or even life-span implanted prosthesis system like artificial ligaments, due to drawbacks of internal fixation method screws tend to loosen or even retreat from tunnel especially in the case that graft–bone healing is not firm enough, weakening operation results greatly and making the surgery in vain. Given the defects discussed above, finding a better biological fixation method instead of press fit method is an inevitable trend.

The research team led by Professor Chen Shiyi introduced endobutton® suspensory fixation method which has been in use successfully for nearly 20 years around the world into artificial ligament reconstruction. Besides, the appearance of press-fit type artificial ligament has been changed as well and ultimately designed several types of artificial ligament granted with patents in China in the light of suspensory fixation method.[12] The new type artificial ligaments avoid defects of press fit fixation as mentioned in the previous discussion. Meanwhile, Neoligament Company and Corin Group, which supplies LARS ligament, are engaged in suspensory ligament research and manufacture as well.

5.3.4. *Other related research*

The hotspots of artificial ligament research shift quickly. Some scientists are doing "hybrid" research. They take artificial ligament as augmentation and make a combination of artificial ligament and autograft as a union. Based on this concept, products like Neoligament are designed and produced. Besides, biological proteins and various growth factors proven to be beneficial for artificial ligament autologous changes and osteogenesis are introduced in local treatment via drug carriers like virus vehicle, nanoparticle vehicle and hydrogel vehicles, which is a hot issue in recent years.

5.4. *Future Research Orientation*

Having summarized the current artificial ligament research hotspots as shown above, the team think that the future research orientation includes the following aspects:

(a) Improvements of materials:
Both in material innovation and in surface modification, the hybrid application of autograft and artificial ligament; it is promising for researchers spending their effort in searching for biomimetic material with viscoelasticity based on the mechanical properties of native anterior cruciate ligament.

(b) Optimizing of fixation method:
A new fixation method with proximal suspensory fixation and distal press/suspensory fixation in order to maintain cushion to a certain extent will be the new trend in products update.

(c) Optimizing of surgical techniques:
The precise controlled repeatable location method, especially isometric reconstruction, will ensure the success of surgery.

(d) Application of biomimetic design:
Researchers try to mimic natural ligament anatomy and physical characteristics by different ways, including regional biological therapy to introduce bioactive particles into surgical sites and improvements in manufacturing procedures so as to make ligament accord with natural biological and biomechanical features.

Acknowledgment

The National 863 Hi-tech Project (2015AA033703), National Natural Science Foundation of China (NO.81271958, NO. 81572108 and NO.81370052), supported this work.

References

1. Batty, L. M.; Norsworthy, C. J.; Lash, N. J. *et al. Arthroscopy* **2015**, *31*(5), 957–968.
2. Chen, C. P.; Lin, Y. M.; Chiu, Y. C. *et al. Orthopedics* **2012**, *35*(6), e800–806.
3. Chen, J.; Gu, A.; Jiang, H. *et al. Arch. Orthop. Trauma Surg.* **2015**, *135*(1), 95–102.
4. Gao, K.; Chen, S.; Wang, L. *et al. Arthroscopy* **2010**, *26*(4), 515–523.
5. Giannotti, S.; Dell'osso, G.; Bugelli, G. *et al. Eur. J. Orthop. Surg. Traumatol.: Orthopedie Traumatologie* **2013**, *23*(8), 873–876.
6. Hamido, F.; Misfer, A. K.; Al Harran, H. *et al. The Knee* **2011**, *18*(6), 373–378.

7. Huang, J. M.; Liu, H. Y.; Chen, F. R. *et al. Chin. Med. J.* **2012**, *125*(22), 3961–3965.
8. Huang, J. M.; Wang, Q.; Shen, F. *et al. Chin. Med. J.* **2010**, *123*(2), 160–164.
9. Ibrahim, S. A.; Ghafar, S.; Salah, M. *et al. Arthroscopy* **2013**, *29*(4), 733–741.
10. Ji, T.; Tang, X.; Guo, W. *The J. Arthrop.* **2013**, *28*(6), 892–894.
11. Li, H.; Yao, Z.; Jiang, J. *et al. Arthroscopy* **2012**, *28*(4), 583–586.
12. Machotka, Z.; Scarborough, I.; Duncan, W. *et al. Sports Med. Arthro. Rehabil. Therapy Technol.: SMARTT,* **2010**, *2*(29).
13. Mulford, J. S.; Chen, D. *ANZ J. Surg.* **2011**, *81*(11), 785–789.
14. Pan, X.; Wen, H.; Wang, L. *et al. Eur. J. Ortho. Surg. Traumatol.: Orthopedie Traumatologie* **2013**, *23*(7), 819–823.
15. Parchi, P. D.; Gianluca, C.; Dolfi, L. *et al. Int. Orthop.* **2013**, *37*(8), 1567–1574.
16. Smith, C.; Ajuied, A.; Wong, F. *et al. Arthroscopy* **2014**, *30*(1), 111–120.
17. Ye, J. X.; Shen, G. S.; Zhou, H. B. *et al. Eur. Rev. Med. Pharmacol. Sci.* **2013**, *17*(11), 1438–1446.
18. Liu, Z. T.; Zhang, X. L.; Jiang, Y. *et al. Int. Orthop.* **2010**, *34*(1), 45–49.
19. Dericks, G. Jr. *Op Tech Sports Med.* **1995**, *3*, 187–205. doi: 10.1016/S1060-1872(95)80009-3.
20. Ao, Y.; Wang, Y.; Qu, M. *et al. Chin. J. Sports Med.* **2005**, *6*, 42–45.
21. Wang, C.-L.; Hsiao, C.-K.; Ku, M.-C. *et* al. *J. Mech. Med. Biol.* **2013**, *13*(02), 1350046.
22. Shen, G.; Xu, Y.; Dong, Q.; *et al. The J. Surg. Res.* **2012**, *173*(1), 75–82.
23. Lu, N.; Zhu, L.; Ye, T. *et al. Knee Surg Sports Traumatol Arthrosc.* **2014**, *22*(9), 2223–2227.
24. Jenkins, D. H. *The J. Bone Joint Surg. Brit. Vol.* **1978**, *60-b*(4), 520–522.
25. Claes, L.; Neugebauer, R. *Clin. Orthop. Relat. Res.* **1985**, *196*, 99–111.
26. Bolton, C. W.; Bruchman, W. C. *Clin. Orthop. Relat. Res.* **1985**, *196*, 202–213.
27. Paulos, L. E.; Rosenberg, T. D.; Grewe, S. R. *et al. Am. J. Sports Med.* **1992**, *20*(3), 246–252.

28. Bottoni, C. R.; Smith, E. L.; Shaha, J. *et al. Am. J. Sports Med.* **2015**, *43*(10), 2501–2509.
29. Crawford, S. N.; Waterman, B. R.; Lubowitz, J. H. *Arthroscopy* **2013**, *29*(9), 1566–1571.
30. Ardern, C. L.; Webster, K. E.; Taylor, N. F. *et al. Brit. J. Sports Med.* **2011**, *45*(7), 596–606.
31. Ardern, C. L.; Webster, K. E.; Taylor, N. F. *et al. Am. J. Sports Med.* **2011**, *39*(3), 538–543.
32. Thomee, R.; Kaplan, Y.; Kvist, J. *et al. Knee Surg. Sports Traumatol Arthrosc.* **2011**, *19*(11), 1798–1805.
33. Jiang, J.; Hao, W.; Li, Y. *et al. Biotechnol. Lett.* **2013**, *35*(4), 657–661.
34. Li, H.; Wu.; Y, Ge, Y. *et al. Appl. Surf. Sci.* **2011**, *257*(22), 9371–9376.
35. Cho, S.; Li, H.; Chen, C. *et al. Int. Orthop.* **2013**, *37*(3), 507–513.
36. Jiang, J.; Ai, C.; Zhan, Z. *et al. Artif. Org.* **2016**, *40*(4), 385–393.

https://doi.org/10.1142/9789811204630_0008

Chapter 8

Achilles Tendon Injuries Reconstruction with LARS

Luigi Corso*, Giovanni Frezza†, and Frederico Mela‡

Orthopedics and Traumatology Pordenone, Santa Mara degli Angeli Hospital, via Montereale 24 Pordenone, PN, Italy

**Luigi.corso@aas5.sanita.fvg.it*
†Giovanni.frezza@aas5.sanita.fvg.it
‡Federico.mela@aas5.sanita.fvg.it

Abbreviations

ACL	Anterior cruciate ligament
AOFAS	American Orthopaedic Foot Ankle Society
LARS	Ligament advanced reinforcement system
MRI	Magnetic resonance imaging

1. Introduction

Achilles tendon partial or complete rupture may be caused by a traumatic event — direct or indirect — or may occur with no trauma, whereas the patient feels severe pain and an immediate functional impotence while walking without effort or without functional overload.

Clinical framing of tendon injuries, with the distinction between chronic and acute, is of utmost importance. Different genesis of tendon injuries of this type necessarily involves patients with different age and different functional request.[1] Nevertheless, clinically and in everyday surgical practice, in the discussion of the reconstruction technique, a common factor emerges: Achilles tendon is subjected to degenerative phenomena and its rupture, as well as its repair, must be studied and carried out taking into account the rupture tissue quality.

Tendon tissue quality must be tested at the beginning of the surgical operation. A good quality tissue will be utilized in the reconstruction. Moreover, it will have to be performing during physiotherapy and when returning to sports activities or simply to everyday life.

2. Choice of Surgical Technique

Different techniques to repair Achilles tendon are still being discussed and even the simple conservative method is considered and is used when examining patients.

Find Table 1, hereafter, summarizing the approach to the problem scheme. The two authors have classified the lesions of Achilles tendon and showed how the severity is essentially linked to the size of the loss of tissue. They show how at any increasing gap, created by

Table 1. Classification of Achilles tendon lesions with preferred treatment per authors in Refs. 2 and 3

		MYERSON
I:	**gap 1-2 cm**	→ end-to-end tenorrhaphy
II:	**gap 2-5 cm**	→ V-Y plasty
III:	**gap > 5 cm**	→ tendon transfer + V-Y plasty
		KUWADA
I:	**partial rupture**	→ non operative treatment
II:	**complete rupture**	→ end-to-end tenorrhaphy gap < 3 cm
III:	**3–6 cm**	→ biological graft +/– augmentation with artificial graft
IV:	**> 6 cm**	→ gastrocnemius recession, biological/artificial graft

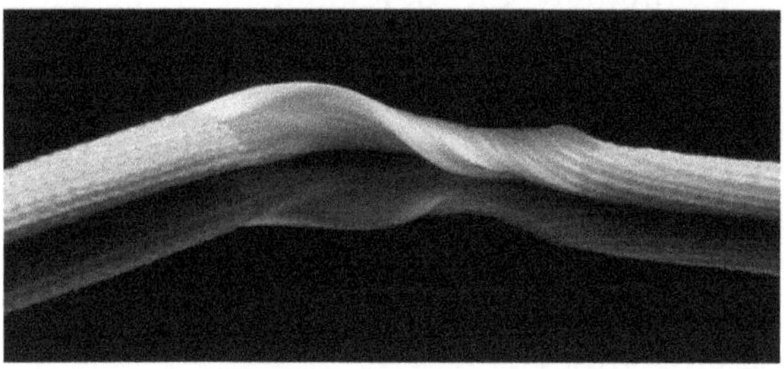

Figure 1. The ligament advanced reinforcement system (LARS ligament)[5]

the injury, corresponds to an increasing complexity of surgical treatment necessary for tendon repair.

Prior to performing this type of surgery, medical history, clinic and diagnostic imaging of the patient are to be analyzed.

As mentioned above, determining the type of injury — acute or chronic — has to be the first step. As a matter of fact, in the past, chronic injuries of Achilles tendon were treated with the ligament advanced reinforcement system (LARS) as illustrated below in Figure 1.

Undoubtedly, LARS reconstructions have proved to be of fundamental importance in repairing inveterate injuries re-ruptures or in revising previously operated tendons.[4]

Although LARS technique used in chronic injuries is the most widely documented in literature, some types of acute injuries may need LARS treatment as well. Such injuries may include degenerated injuries or injuries presenting such tendon material loss as to cause important tendon shortening if termino-terminal sutures are used. Both lesions it is difficult to obtain a valid tenorraphy, if we mean a surgical suture of a divided tendon.

Achilles tendon degeneration symptoms are not uncommon since ruptures that occur without trauma are a sign of degeneration; they often manifest themselves earlier than observed under surgery. Therefore, it is not surprising that, in the history of orthopaedic surgery, the following main problems had to be dealt with:

- Analysis of remaining tendon tissue and analysis of present peritenon and accordingly the development of percutaneous techniques and the use of Tenolig or Achillon devices.[6]
- Pursuit of better methods to perform reinforced plastics, among which V–Y skin incision, Bosworth techniques, hallux long flexor tendon reinforcement, with short peroneal tendon, with fingers long flexor, have to be mentioned (Table 2).
- Search for materials and technologies to be exploited in this field and clinical outcomes evaluation

In the most recent years, Achilles tendon reconstruction has given solutions to the problems that have been discussed so far.[8] Artificial

Table 2. Achilles tendon salvage procedures (Ref. 7)

Autograft
Flaps reversed/advancement
• V–Y advancement flap (Abraham, Pankovich)
• Proximal reversed flap (Bosworth)
Tendon transfer
• Peroneus brevis tendon (Teuffer, Turco, Spinella)
• Flexor longus hallucis tendon (Wapner)
Free tissue transfer
• Fascia lata (Bugg, Boyd)
• Gracilis tendon (Maffulli)
• Semitendinousus tendon (Sarzaeem)

Table 3. Implantable ligament in allograft augmentation technique

Allograft
Artificial tissues • Carbon fibers • Dacron • Marlex mesh • *LARS*
Allograft tendon (tissues bank)

ligaments, as reported in Table 3, seem to represent, more and more frequently, the suitable option to reinforce injured tendon as well as to obtain fast functional recovery. Moreover, they represent a less invasive surgical treatment in that technique and materials improvement involve final follow-up, showing, through magnetic resonance imaging (MRI) cells and vital tissue restoration in artificial fiber skeleton.[9]

3. Ligament Advanced Reinforcement System LARS

LARS ligament (Figure 1) is a well-known artificial ligament among knee surgery specialists owing to its consolidated use in anterior cruciate ligament reconstruction. It is made of terephthalic polyethylene polyester fibers, built using a technology meant to prevent or to reduce reactive phlogosis and keeping a high resistance capacity under traction.[10]

As far as Achilles tendon repair is concerned, LARS has historically been the leading strategy in chronic injuries. Nevertheless, in examining acute injury, it is common to observe in degenerated tissue — that is the real cause of the rupture — difficulty in performing a termino-terminal suture or a poor strength of suture itself, or a tendon tissue deficit higher than 3 cm. This is the gap size commonly used to consider a termino-terminal suture at risk of re-ruptures according to the classification of Kuwada [as reported in Table 1].

Table 4. Indication to implanted LARS

LARS in acute rupture	LARS in chronic lesion
• Tendon degeneration	• Re-ruptures
• Not possible end-to-end suture	• Inveterate lesions
• Reinforcing plasty	
• Bilateral rupture	

A third case has to be mentioned which, though less frequent, is reported in literature. The acute bilateral ruptures that are treated with LARS, benefits of shorter recovery time in patients whose rehabilitation, if treated with traditional surgery, would be longer and psychologically more traumatic.[11]

In any case, as it is indicated in Table 4, LARS is still recommended in such chronic injuries as re-ruptures, treatment of previously operated Achilles tendon, and inveterate injuries with stumps diastasis.

Since this surgical technique involves an anchorage of the artificial ligament at the level of myotendon junction; if this area appears to be injured and compromised, LARS is absolutely contraindicated.

4. Surgical Technique

Prior to LARS implant and tendon repair, Achilles tendon has to be examined through usual access technique for injury assessment (Figure 2). Although experienced orthopaedic surgeons can easily learn LARS technique, it is recommended to initially perform some implants with open technique and later, to use LARS with minimally invasive techniques. After medial peritendinous access to tendon and injury evaluation, the myotendinous junction has to be located and afterwards, the two ends of the artificial ligament have to be passed inside the two stumps.

If minimally invasive technique is being used, three incisions will definitely be done. Ligament insertion must maintain its central portion where free fibers are present at the injury level. The flat proximal portion is located through his dedicated pipe (Figure 3) and is

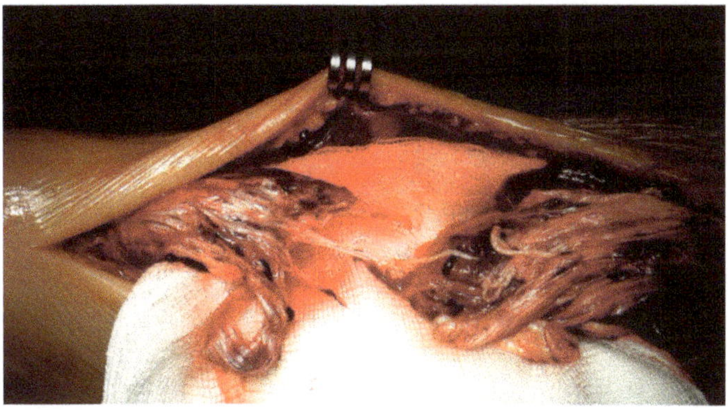

Figure 2. The surgical open-approach shows the whole tendon loss of tissue

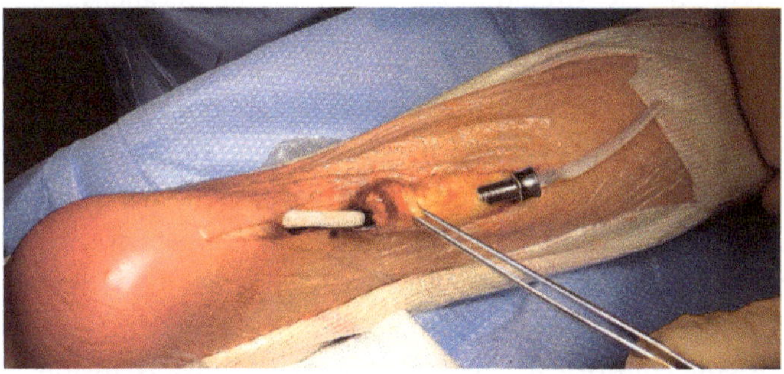

Figure 3. LARS proximal portion insertion

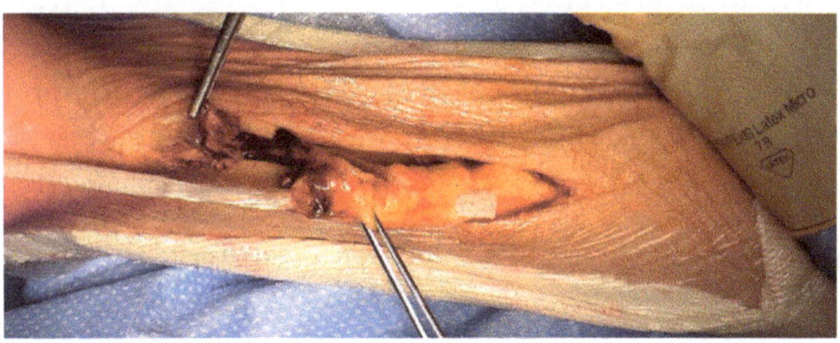

Figure 4. Myotendinous junction

anchored at the myotendinous level and care is taken so that its end does not go out of tissue plane also avoiding micro-traumatisms or friction with above planes (Figure 4).

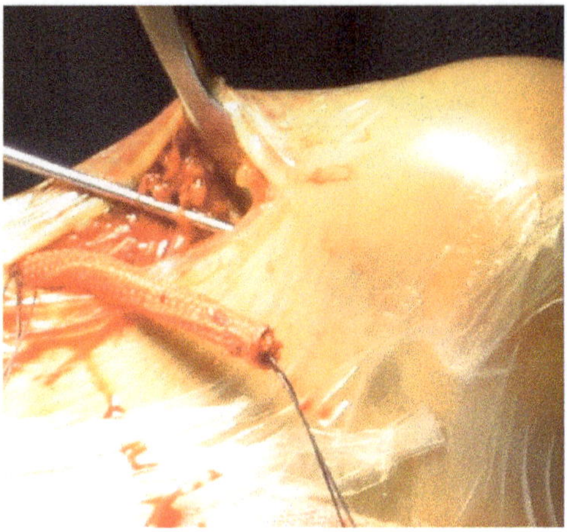

Figure 5. K-wire positioning through the calcaneus bone

The next step is operating distally from the injury (Figure 5). The direction and the insertion site of new tendon are prepared with the aid of a metal holed guide-wire. The wire is positioned proximo-distally at about 50° (Figure 6) in the posterior tuberosity of the calcaneus. Through this wire, the preparation of half-tunnel is performed with appropriate reamer (Figure 7)

The distal cylindrical portion has to be passed inside the half-tunnel and first tests showing the neo-tendon tension rate are carried out. Finally, an interference screw distally blocks the LARS implant (Figure 8).

After usual fluoroscopic control (Figure 9), peritenonium and surgical access are carefully sutured (Figure 10).

5. Imaging

Clinical elements in Achilles tendon complete injuries are mostly important and they are generally considered as sufficient information to make a diagnosis.

The most significant signs appear to be immediate functional impotence associated with a clear depression in tendon palpation. Nevertheless, it is good practice to document through imaging techniques the lesion, even for legal purposes.

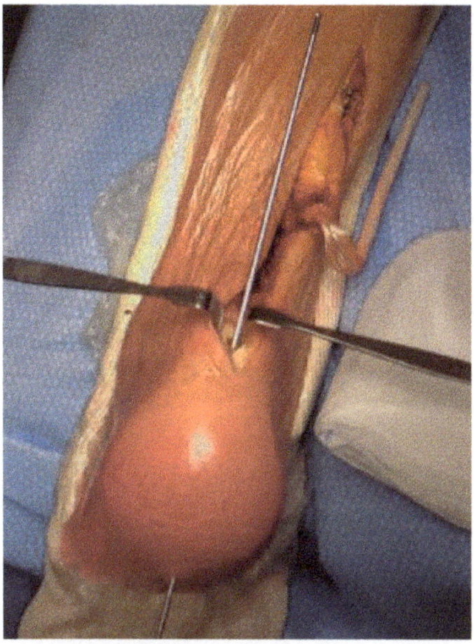

Figure 6. K-wire 50° direction in posterior calcaneus apophasis

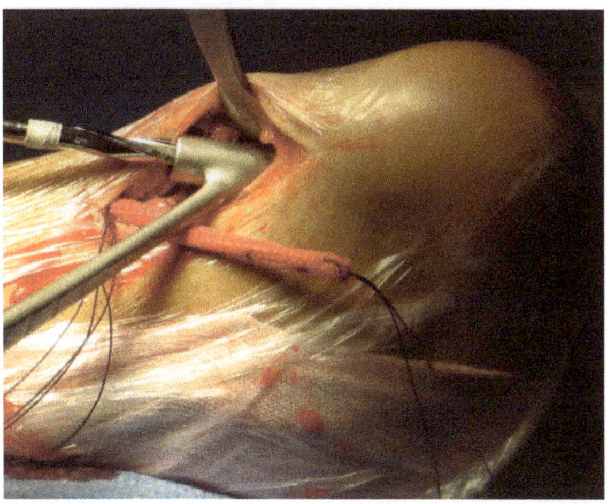

Figure 7. Reaming the tunnel for dedicated screw

The first exam to be performed is myotendinous echography to evaluate lesion severity (complete or partial) and the exact lesion level.

Ultrasound elastography and ultrasound tissue characterization can be used to evaluate tendinous tissue quality.[8]

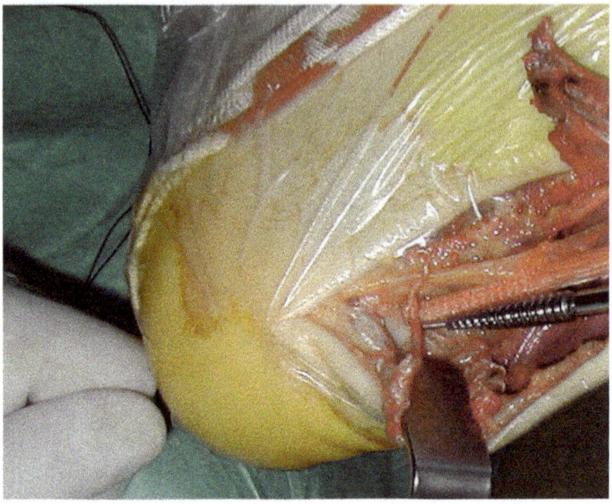

Figure 8. Screw dedicated positioning

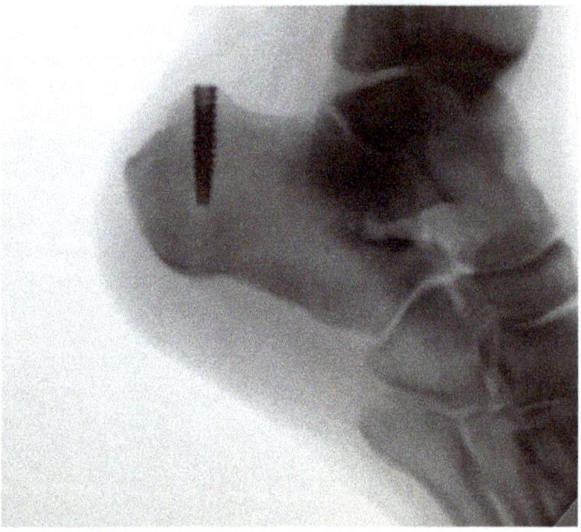

Figures 9. Screw correct position

MRI is hardly ever indicated. In the case of complete lesions, Echography represents the gold standard for diagnosis. MRI would be useful while evaluating degenerative lesions[9,10] which tend to lead to complete rupture. Since in this stage of the injury the patient is asymptomatic, *MRI* cannot have a clear role for tendon disease.

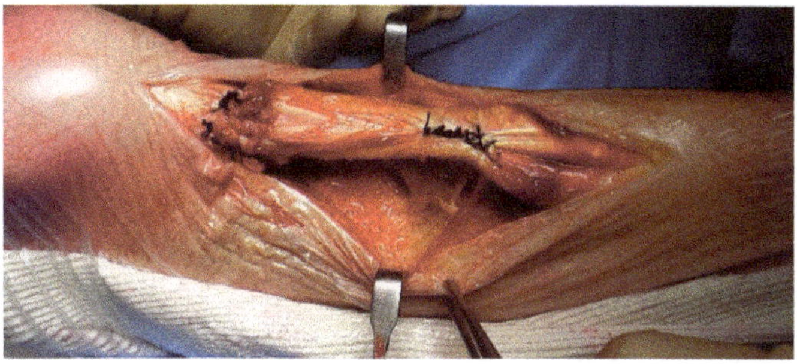

Figure 10. Peritenonium suture

6. Aftercare

Post-operative treatment requires the following indications:

- Ankle Walker Boot at 90° for 2 weeks;
- At the third and fourth week, removal of the Ankle Walker Boot for 20 minutes, 4 times per day and active mobilization (with only dorsal extension);
- Fifth week, free load (depending on pain);
- Sixth week, gradual restart of sports activity.

7. Complications

Complications associated with Achilles tendon reconstruction with LARS include foreign body rejection[11] and low tolerance of the calcaneal screw. Wound recovery delay is a common complication in all reconstruction techniques.

In the authors' study, they report two wounds recovery delay and two calcaneal screw removals due to intolerance.

8. Discussion

The authors' group treated 131 patients in 10 years (from 01/01/2008 to 01/03/2018). The age of patients who present this kind of lesion is increasing[12] and in their study, the average age is 56 years. This study shows that the treatment of Achilles tendon with LARS delivers good clinical results combined with very low re-rupture and surgical complication rates in chronic and acute injuries, at every age. Other studies have reported that reconstruction with LARS decreases post-operative complications, but most importantly, patients have improved functional outcomes.[3]

All the outcomes were significantly correlated with patient satisfaction. The American Orthopaedic Foot Ankle Society (AOFAS) scores were satisfactory in those patients with an average score of 93, but Achilles-tendon-specific problems, such as decreased jumping ability and muscle atrophy have not been taken into consideration in the AOFAS score and seem to be not so reliable in athletes.

Acute Achilles tendon ruptures mainly occur in sports like soccer and basketball, which are popular sports in Italy, and for young patients. The goal of treatment is a return to play at the pre-injury level.[13,14]

The authors interviewed the group of patients they treated with LARS reconstruction who play sport at an agonistic level and most of them affirmed they returned to play at the same level as before the operation. Rehabilitation has a key role in this kind of patients.[14] The authors' main concern is a quick return to competitive play and to recreational activities. Reconstruction with LARS technique seems to have better results compared to most of the other techniques for this specific kind of patients. Although good clinical results have been reported also for the other techniques and for non-operative treatments,[15–18] long-lasting functional deficits may occur, such as reduction in plantar flexion strength, a reduced range of motion, or a limited plantar flexion moment due to increased tendon stiffness,[19–23] which do not appear in the authors' study.

Low re-rupture rates and surgical complication rates are prerequisites for any reliable surgical technique. Re-rupture rate of the Achilles tendon in the authors' study was less than 2%, while no Sural nerve lesions nor infections were observed. These data are comparable to the complication rate of most reviews about minimally invasive and percutaneous reconstruction techniques.[24]

Wound irritation is a common complication after tendon reconstruction if LARS is anchored too superficially in the proximal part.

Based on the authors' experience, they did not find any differences in distinct timing of surgery: patients who were operated on later than 2 days had the same outcomes than those who underwent immediate surgery within the first 48 h after trauma.

References

1. Atkinson, T. S.; Easley, M. *Medscape Orthopaed.* **2001**, *5*(3).
2. Kuwada, G. *The J. Foot Ankle Surg.* **1993**, *32*(6), 611–616.
3. Myerson, M. *Instr. Course Lect.* **1999**, *48*, 219–230.
4. Ibrahim, S. *The J. Foot Ankle Surg.* **2009**, *48*(3), 340–346. doi:10.1053/j.jfas.2009.02.007.
5. https://www.coringroup.com/legacy/medical_professionals/products/lars_ligaments/overview/index.html.
6. Carmont, M.; Rossi, R.; Scheffler, S.; Mei-Dan, O.; Beaufils, P. *Sports Med. Arthrosc. Rehabil. Ther. Technol.* **2011**, *3*, 28. doi:10.1186/1758-2555-3-28.
7. Feibel, J.; Bernacki, B. *Foot Ankle Clin.* **2003**, *8*(1), 105–114.
8. Fernández-Fairén, M.; Gimeno, C. *Am. J. Sports Med.* **1997**, *25*(2), 177–181. doi:10.1177/036354659702500206.
9. Soo, C.; Mungovan, S.; Kwa, A. *Ortho. Proc.* **2018**.
10. Viateau, V.; Manassero, M.; Anagnostou, F.; Guérard, S.; Mitton, D.; Migonney, V. *Arthroscopy.* **2013**, *29*(6), 1079–1088. doi:10.1016/j.arthro.2013.02.025.
11. Dimitrios, P.; Dimitrios, N.; Dimitrios, S.; Efstathios, C.; George, C. *Orthop. J. Sports Med.* **2016**, *4*(6), 2325967116653359. doi:10.1177/2325967116653359.
12. Dhillon, M.; Chauhan, D.; Kumar, V.; Saini, U. *Foot (Edinb).* **2010**, *20*(4), 154–157. doi:10.1016/j.foot.2010.09.008.
13. Washburn, N.; Onishi, K.; Wang, J. *J. Ortho. Trans.* **2018**, *15*, 9–20. doi:10.1016/j.jot.2018.06.003.
14. Zeiss, J.; Saddemi, S.; Ebraheim, N. *AJR Am. J. Roentgenol.* **1992**, *159*(5), 1031–1034. doi:10.2214/ajr.159.5.1414770.
15. Kannus, P.; Józsa, L. *J. Bone Joint Surg. Am.* **1991**, *73*(10), 1507–1525.

16. Henry, J.; Konarski, A.; Joseph, L.; Pillai, A. *J. Surg. Case Reports* **2018**, *2018*(1). doi:10.1093/jscr/rjx258.
17. Lantto, I.; Heikkinen, J.; Flinkkilä, T.; Ohtonen, P.; Leppilahti, J. *Scand. J. Med. Sci. Sports.* **2015**, *25*(1), E133–138. doi:10.1111/sms.12253.
18. Józsa, L.; Kvist, M.; Bálint, B.; Reffy, A.; Järvinen, M.; Lehto, M.; Barzo, M. *Am. J. Sports Med.* **1989**, *17*(3), 338–343. doi:10.1177/036354658901700305.
19. Parekh, S.; Wray, W.; Brimmo, O.; Sennett, B.; Wapner, K. *Foot Ankle Spec.* **2009**, *2*(6), 283–286. doi:10.1177/1938640009351138.
20. Khan, R.; Carey Smith, R. *Cochrane Database Syst. Rev.* **2010**, *9*, CD003674. doi:10.1002/14651858.CD003674.pub4.
21. Willits, K.; Amendola, A.; Bryant, D.; Mohtadi, N.; Giffin, J.; Fowler, P.; Kirkley, A. *J. Bone Joint Surg. Am.* **2010**, *92*(17), 2767–2775. doi:10.2106/JBJS.I.01401.
22. Del Buono, A.; Volpin, A.; Maffulli, N. *Br Med Bull.* **2014**, *109*, 45–54. doi:10.1093/bmb/ldt029.
23. Khan, R.; Fick, D.; Keogh, A.; Crawford, J.; Brammar, T.; Parker, M. *J. Bone Joint Surg. Am.* **2005**, *87*(10), 2202–2210. doi:10.2106/JBJS.D.03049.
24. Ebinesan, A.; Sarai, B.; Walley, G.; Maffulli, N. *Disabil. Rehabil.* **2008**, *30*(20–22), 1721–1725. doi:10.1080/09638280701786815.

https://doi.org/10.1142/9789811204630_0009

Chapter 9

Reconstruction of Anterior Cruciate Ligament and Anterolateral Ligament with Looped Hamstrings

Márcio de Castro Ferreira

Knee Surgeon at the Knee Institute, Hospital do Coração, Hcor, São Paulo, Brazil
marciojoelho@gmail.com

Abbreviations

ACL	Anterior cruciate ligament
ALL	Anterolateral ligament
GR	Gracilis tendon
IKDC	International Knee Documentation Committee
MRI	Magnetic resonance imaging
PCL	Posterior cruciate ligament
ST	Semitendinosus tendon

1. Introduction

The treatment of anterior knee instability through reconstruction of the anterior cruciate ligament (ACL) presents good clinical results. However, the failure rate for this operation is estimated to range from 1.8% to 14%.[1,2] The persistence of anterolateral instability assessed by the pivot-shift test post-operatively is described as one of those factors.[2,3]

After the anatomical "re-discovery" and biomechanical studies of the anterolateral ligament (ALL) demonstrated that this structure is important in anterolateral knee stability, it was observed that insufficiency of this ligament may contribute to the functional failure of isolated ACL reconstructions.[4] This study aimed to present a reproducible technique of anatomical ACL and ALL reconstruction with the hamstring tendons, using three interference screws

The following description is based on a technique developed by the author at the Center for Orthopedics and Rehabilitation in Sport at the Hospital do Coração using hamstring grafts and three interference screws for ACL and ALL fixation.

2. Indication

The reconstruction of the anterior cruciate ligament associated with the anterolateral ligament has not fully established criteria. It is important to repeat the knee examination with the patient under anesthesia to assess the degree of instability, preferably before inflating the pneumatic tourniquet.

After spinal anesthesia, a clinical examination must be performed to estimate ALL sufficiency. The anterior asymmetry of the lateral plateau with internal rotation of the tibia in 30–60° (see Ref. [5]) of flexion relative to the contralateral knee and increased positivity of the pivot-shift maneuver may be a clinical sign of failure of the ALL.[4]

We used the classification for the pivot-shift maneuver determined by the International Knee Documentation Committee (IKDC) 2000,[6] which describes four grades: 0 — normal, 1 — glide, 2 — clunk, 3 — gross shift.

The criteria used for ALL reconstruction associated with ACL injuries were:

1. Injury in the ALL substance identified at a magnetic resonance imaging (MRI), termed second-like injury;
2. Second fracture[7];
3. Pivot-shift classified as grade II/III;
4. ACL reconstruction review in which patients had residual pivot-shift during the post-operative period and evolved with graft injury;
5. Asymmetrical anterior lateral plateau visible with knee internal rotation in flexion between 30° and 60°;
6. Lateral femoral notch sign[8];
7. Isolated Anterolateral complex lesion.

3. Surgical Setup

The patient is operated in the same position as routinely the reconstruction of the ACL is performed.

The patient is positioned in supine dorsal decubitus under spinal anesthesia. A support is placed on the side of the surgical table, lateral to the pneumatic tourniquet placed in the thigh of the patient (Figure 2(a)), to facilitate the application of valgus stress in the knee and allow the opening of the medial femorotibial compartment to observe the posterior horn of the medial meniscus.

After applying antiseptic methods, the pneumatic tourniquet is inflated. The arthroscopy is performed with the knee positioned in 90° flexion and hanging on the side of the table as shown in Figure 2(a).

The anatomical points that serve as a reference for tunnel positioning (fibular head, Gerdy tubercle, articular line, anterior tibial tuberosity and lateral epicondyle) can be marked with a skin marking pen to facilitate surgery.

4. Graft Harvesting and Preparation

The excision of the semitendinosus tendon (ST) and gracilis tendon (GR) is made through a 4-cm anteromedial oblique incision in the tibia over the pes anserinus.

The GR used to rebuild the ALL is prepared to form a double graft. Each end is sutured with Krackow stitches. One end of the G*R* is passed as a "handle" during the preparation of the triple or quadruple ST graft, which will be used for ACL reconstruction, so that the double GR graft has the same size in its two parts and the triple or quadruple ST graft has a Krackow suture in one end and the other end is anchored in the GR (Figures 1(a)–1(c)).

After preparation and measurement of graft diameters (usually 8mm for the triple *ST* graft and 5mm for the double *GR*), the femoral and tibial tunnels are prepared.

5. Artroscopic ACL Reconstruction

ALL tunnels are performed by the outside-in technique and the author uses the conventional guide routinely used for the tibial tunnel.

It is important to observe the positioning of the lower limb during the choice the locations of the femoral and tibial tunnels.

The lower limb should be at 90° of flexion to determine the femoral tunnel site. If the position of the femoral tunnel is determined with the knee "extended" (less than 90° of flexion) the graft will be anterior to the anatomical center of the ACL, as well as the graft can

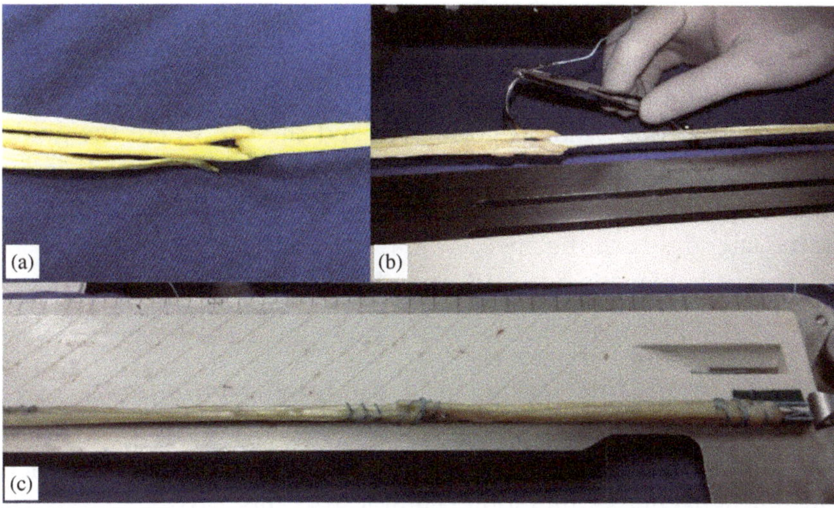

Figure 1. (a) Tensioned triple semitendinosus graft and double gracilis graft; intertwined, ready for suturing. (b) Triple semitendinosus graft (LCA) and double gracilis graft (LAL), started suturing. (c) Finished grafts

be positioned posteriorly to the anatomic center of the ACL if the the femoral tunnel is determined with the knee flexed more than 90°. The arthroscopic visualization is performed through the anteromedial portal to allow introduction of the guide through the anterolateral portal.

The correct anatomical site of the tibial tunnel is less influenced by knee positioning and its preparation is performed anterior to the PCL medially the insertion of the anterior horn of the lateral meniscus with the arthroscopic visualization through the anterolateral portal and the guide positioned through the anteromedial portal.

The author avoids major debridement of the injured ACL by removing only the amount of tissue that makes it difficult to see the references for the choice of femoral and tibial tunnels site.

5.1. *Preparation of the Femoral Tunnel*

The femoral tunnel, common to the ACL and ALL, is made using the outside-in technique. A tibial ACL guide is placed so that its joint position overlaps the footprint of the anatomical insertion of the ACL in the intercondylar wall. A 65° opening is applied to minimize the "killer turn" of the graft.

After the ACL guide is positioned and the site where the guide wire will be introduced is assessed, the guidewire is removed, and a 4-cm longitudinal incision in the skin and iliotibial tract is performed on the lateral side of the knee.

The lateral epicondyle is identified by palpation; the guidewire is introduced 8mm (about one digital tip) posterosuperiorly in the lateral femoral cortex to mark the entry site.[9,10]

The ACL guide is then reattached and coupled to the guidewire, followed by the drilling of the path for the ACL footprint. Sequentially, one drill of the same diameter as the graft is used to make the tunnel, which is generally 35-mm long (Figures 2(a) and 2(b)).

5.2. *Preparation of the Tibial Tunnels*

The tibial tunnel is prepared with the same guide and similarly, but with an angle of 55° on the tibial ACL footprint.

After creating the tunnels for the ACL, the ST graft (ACL) is passed outside-in from the femur to the tibia, remaining in its final position (Figures 2(a) and 2(b)). An interference screw of the same diameter as the drilled tunnel, with 30–35mm length, is used for femoral fixation.

For the reconstruction and attachment of the ALL in the tibia, the ACL guide is positioned at 65°, so that the guidewire can be inserted 2 cm distal to the ACL tibial tunnel through the same incision made for graft removal. It exits halfway between Gerdy's tubercle and the head of the fibula, 9–13 mm distal to the surface of the lateral tibial plateau, the anatomical ALL tibial point.[9]

A 3-cm anterolateral skin and iliotibial tract incision is made (Figure 2(c)) and the tunnel is drilled with a 6-mm bit. A long Kelly forceps is introduced through the ALL tibial incision deep into the iliotibial tract until its output in the femoral ACL tunnel incision, where the *GR* graft is pulled and passed through the tibial ALL tunnel (Figures 2(d)–2(f)).

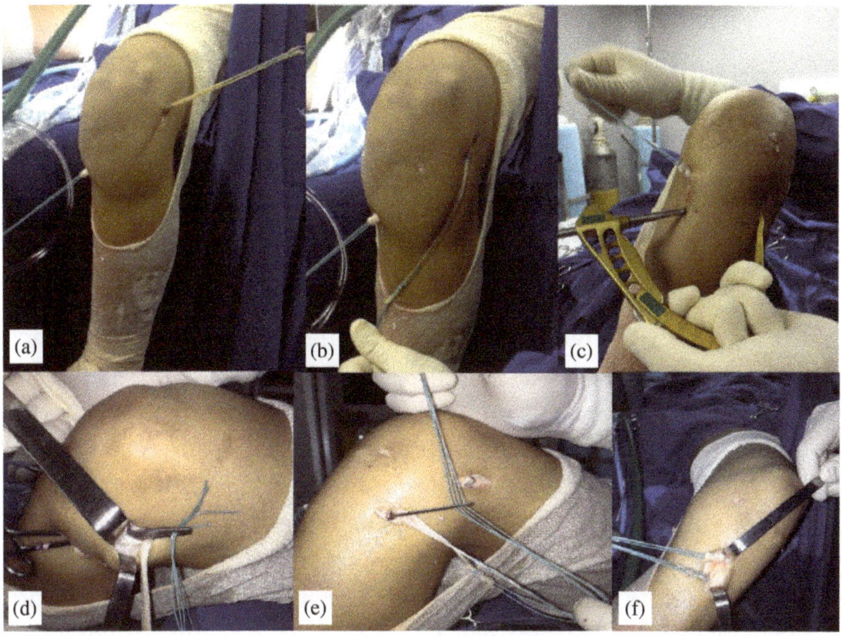

Figure 2. (a) ACL graft positioned in the femoral and tibial tunnels and ALL graft fixed in the femoral point; (b) double *GR* graft length to rebuild the ALL on the path it must follow; (c) positioning of the ACL guide at 65° and exit point halfway between Gerdy's tubercle and the fibular head, 13 mm from the surface of the lateral tibial plateau; (d) clamp passed deep into the iliotibial tract to drive the ALL graft into the tibial tunnel; (e) passage of the ALL graft through the tibial tunnel; (f) ACL and ALL grafts ready to be fixed with interference screw through the same incision

5.3. *Graft Positioning and Fixation*

The knee is then placed at 30° flexion for ACL fixation and ALL fixation with interference screws that are 2 mm larger than the drilled tunnels, both through the same anteromedial incision. If the ALL graft does not fill the entire tibial tunnel, the screw fixation is performed by the anterolateral entrance of the ALL tunnel. The suture grafts (ACL and ALL) can be tied to reinforce the fixation "post-like" (Figure 2(f)).

5.4. *Post-operative Care*

Post-operative rehabilitation follows the protocol for ACL reconstruction with hamstrings.

The author usually divides rehabilitation into three phases based on the main objectives.

- **First stage:** Complete restoration of normal limb function. The goal at this stage is to allow full range of motion and normal gait within 8 post-operative weeks, respecting the individuality of each patient.
- **Second stage:** Graft maturation. At this stage, it is necessary to maintain the rehabilitation with evolution for proprioception and muscular strengthening of the limb, however respecting the graft's fragility in this period. This phase corresponds to the period from the 8th to the 16th post-operative week.
- **Third stage:** Preparing for sports. This phase begins at the 16th post-operative week and will be extended until the patient has a maximum asymmetry of 15% in the isokinetic dynamometer test and presents without complaints to the plyometric activities compatible with the sport practiced.

During the first and second phases of the post-surgical recovery program, all patients are instructed to undergo rehabilitation activities assisted by a physiotherapist at least three times a week. The third phase is practiced mostly in the gym and the patient is accompanied by personal trainer and physiotherapists.

6. Discussion

The "rediscovery" of the ALL and its role in anterolateral knee stability is currently presented as one of the trends in knee ligament reconstructions.[11]

The facts that the ALL is not a structure routinely described in *MRI* reports and that the reconstruction criteria are not fully established contribute to the misdiagnosis and undertreatment of this injury.

Helito *et al.* showed that the ALL is fully visualized in 71.7% of the MRIs.[12] In turn, Taneja *et al.* have identified the full ALL view in 11%.[13] Spencer *et al.* showed that the anterolateral knee instability is accentuated when the ACL and the ALL are torn, emphasizing the pivot-shift maneuver.[14]

Sonnery-Cottet *et al.* recommend ALL reconstruction in Segond fractures, chronic ACL injuries, grade III pivot-shift, high-level athletes or those who practice sports that require rotation of the knee, and in the presence of lateral femoral notch sign.[11] However, the present authors do not consider chronicity and the patient's activities as criteria for empirical ALL reconstruction if the physical examination shows no evidence of its failure.

Regarding the described techniques for ACL and ALL reconstruction, Helito *et al.* used a quadruple graft (triple ST and one GR) for ACL and one GR for ALL[14]; tibial fixation was conducted with anchors. Sonnery-Cottet *et al.* used triple ST graft for ACL and double GR graft for ALL, with two tibial holes to rebuild the ALL.[11]

In the present technique, the method used for graft preparation creates a suspension effect similar to the Endobutton, added to the suture to reinforce this union, which also includes an interference screw. This allows the end of the ST graft to remain close to the articular femoral point, and there is no need to occupy the entire tunnel, which will be completed by the GR graft, thus facilitating the procedure in case of short grafts.

Studies have shown differences in the ALL femoral anatomical point. Caterine *et al.* and Kennedy *et al.* demonstrated that its origin is on average 3 mm posterior and proximal to the lateral epicondyle[9,10]; this point was used in the present technique. In turn, Helito *et al.* and Claes *et al.* demonstrated that the origin of the ALL is anterior to the lateral epicondyle.[15,16]

The option adopted in the present technique was to make the tunnel posterosuperior to the lateral epicondyle, in order to reduce the intraarticular "killer turn" of the graft; this point approaches the isometrics described by Kurosawa *et al.* for lateral tenodesis of the iliotibial tract.[17]

For the tibial point, Sonnery-Cottet *et al.* used two tunnels,[11] which does not appear necessary, since the ALL anatomical insertion has about 9 mm in the tibia.[9]

Although extra-articular reconstruction has been performed in association with the ACL for a long time, the importance of this structure for rotational joint stability is still questioned.

Most anatomical and biomechanical studies of the anterolateral knee complex are performed in cadavers, and unfortunately, they fail to reproduce the complex biomechanical motion of the knee as well as determine the role of ALL for joint rotational stability.

It is important to note that the reconstruction of ALL is not yet consensual, however, the importance of this structure for rotational instability of the knee can be demonstrated with this case report treated by the author.

A 24-year-old female suffered a knee sprain after being hit by a motorcycle at low speed. She complained of lateral proximal pain in her right leg at her first medical visit. After performing X-rays, the informed diagnosis at her first evaluation at other service was contusion of the proximal leg. The leg was immobilized for two weeks followed by rehabilitation.

Three months after the accident, she came to our outpatient clinic complaining of pain and instability of the right knee presenting frequent giving away episodes. During the clinical examination, she presented normal gait and normal range of motion. The Lachman test showed slight anterior translation with a firm endpoint as well as the anterior drawer test when compared to the normal side, being both classified as grade B (nearly normal). The pivot-shift test was positive and classified as grade C (abnormal).

An important finding was the positive ACL tests in the presence of an intact ACL when compared to the normal side. Although the drawer test and Lachman test were interpreted as nearly normal presenting a firm end point, the pivot-shift was rated abnormal. The anterior drawer and Lachman tests findings probably correspond just to an anterolateral knee instability and not a true anterior translation.

Knee radiographs revealed the Second fracture. The patient underwent an MRI and a computed tomography. Both exams showed the Second fracture. The MRI showed integrity of the ACL, PCL, medial collateral ligament, posterolateral corner structures and menisci.

Joint instability was eradicated with the isolated reconstruction of ALL with hamstring.[18]

References

1. Mariscalco, M. W.; Flanigan, D. C.; Mitchell, J. *et al. Arthroscopy* **2013**, *29*(12), 1948–1953.
2. Prodromos, C. C.; Joyce, B. T.; Shi, K.; Keller, B. L. *Arthroscopy* **2005**, *21*(10), 1202.el–1202.e9.
3. Mohtadi, N. G.; Chan, D. S.; Dainty, K. N.; Whelan, D. B. *Cochrane Database Syst. Rev.* **2011**, *9*, CD005960.
4. Spencer, L.; Burkhart, T. A.; Tran, M. N.; Rezansoff, A. J.; Deo, S.; Caterine, S.; Getgood, A. M. *Am. J. Sports Med.* **2015**, *43*(9), 2189–2197. doi: 10.1177/0363546515589166. Epub 2015 Jun 19. PMID: 26093007.
5. Parsons, E. M.; Gee, A. O.; Spiekerman, C.; Cavanagh, P. R. *Am. J. Sports Med.* **2015**, *43*(3), 669–674.
6. Irrgang, J. J.; Ho, H.; Harner, C. D.; Fu, F. H. *Knee Surg. Sports Traumatol. Arthrosc.* **1998**, *6*, 107–114.
7. Claes, S.; Luyckx, T.; Vereecke, E.; Bellemans, J. *Arthroscopy* **2014**, *30*(11). 1475–1482.
8. Herbst, E.; Hoser, C.; Tecklenburg, K.; Filipovic, M.; Dallapozza, C.; Herbort, M.; Fink, C. *Knee Surg. Sports Traumatol. Arthrosc.* **2015**, *23*(8), 2250–2258.
9. Kennedy, M. I.; Claes, S.; Fuso, F. A.; Williams, B. T.; Goldsmith, M. T.; Turnbull, T. L. *et al. Am. J. Sports Med.* **2015**, *43*(7), 1606–1615.
10. Caterine, S.; Litchfield, R.; Johnson, M.; Chronik, B.; Getgood, A. *Knee Surg. Sports Traumatol. Arthrosc.* **2015**, *23*(11), 3186–3195.
11. Sonnery-Cottet, B.; Thaunat, M.; Freychet, B.; Pupim, B. H.; Murphy, C. G.; Claes, S. *Am. J. Sports Med.* **2015**, *43*(7), 1598–1605.

12. Helito, C. P.; Helito, P. V.; Costa, H. P.; Bordalo-Rodrigues, M,; Pecora, J. R.; Camanho, G. L.; Demange, M. K. *Skeletal Radiol.* **2014**, *43*(10), 1421–1427.
13. Taneja, A. K.; Miranda, F. C.; Braga, C. A.; Gill, C. M.; Hartmann, L. G.; Santos, D. C.; Rosemberg, L. A. *Skeletal Radiol.* **2015**, *44*(3), 411.
14. Helito, C. P.; Bonadio, M. B.; Gobbi, R. G.; Albuquerque, R. F. M.; Pécora, J. R.; Camanho, G. L.; Demange, M. K. *Arthro. Tech.* **2015**, *4*(3), e239–e244. https://doi.org/10.1016/j.eats.2015.02.006.
15. Helito, C. P.; Demange, M. K.; Bonadio, M. B.; Tirico, L. E.; Gobbi, R. G.; Pecora, J. R; *et al. Am. J. Sports Med.* **2014**, *42*(10), 2356–2362.
16. Claes, S.; Vereecke, E.; Maes, M.; Victor, J.; Verdonk, P.; Bellemans, J. *J. Anat.* **2013**, *223*(4), 321–328.
17. Kurosawa, H.; Yasuda, K.; Yamakoshi, K.; Kamiya, A.; Kaneda, K. *Am. J. Sports Med.* **1991**, *19*(4), 384–388.
18. Ferreira, M. C.; Zidan, F. F.; Miduati, F. B.; Fortuna, C. C.; Franciozi, C. E. D. S. *et al. MOJ Sports Med.* **2017**, *1*(6): 0031. doi: 10.15406/mojsm2017.01.00031.

https://doi.org/10.1142/9789811204630_0010

Chapter 10

Anterior Cruciate Ligament Repair with LARS Artificial Ligament Augmentation

Nicolas Duval

Duval Orthopaedic Clinic, 1487 Boulevard des Laurentides,
Laval (Québec), Canada H7M 2Y3
nicolasduval@duvalclinic.com

Abbreviations

ACL	Anterior cruciate ligament
LARS	Ligament advanced reinforcement system

PCL	Posterior cruciate ligament
PET	Polyethylene terephthalate

1. Introduction

Once a sub-acute rupture of the anterior cruciate ligament (ACL) is diagnosed in an active person, the orthopaedic surgeon must decide which option is in the patient's best interest. However voluminous the literature concerning ruptures of the ACL, data remain scarce on their long-term outcome so that even today, deciding remains problematic. Because of the biomechanical importance of the ACL, the surgeon is often inclined to favor surgery as the best option. It has been shown that the ACL contains mechanoreceptors near the surface of the ligament which provide information concerning joint position and interaction between the joint and the muscles.[1,2] Their presence which contribute to the dynamic stability of the knee, combined with the mechanical stability provided by the menisci and collateral ligaments support the idea that the knee can function well following successful ACL repair. It has been shown that morphologically normal mechanoreceptors remain in the ACL stump for 3 months after a complete tear.[3] Therefore, a repair could possibly restore the mechanical and proprioceptive function of the knee by acting on the neuromuscular system.

Most orthopedic surgeons believe a torn ACL cannot heal if repaired because the intra-articular location is associated with poor blood supply and hostile biological synovial reaction. Animal models[4,5,6] have documented the healing potential of the repaired ACL augmented by an artificial ligament. The artificial scaffold helps protect the repair and support fibrous growth between the torn end of the ligament and the femoral bone. When supported, the ACL does not undergo the processes of necrosis and ligamentization.

The Ligament Advanced Reinforcement System (LARS™, Arc-sur-Tille, France) Terresuisse — polyethylene terephtalate (PET) ligament can support the biological healing of the newly ruptured ACL (Figure 1).[7,8] The LARS™ intra-osseous segment is composed

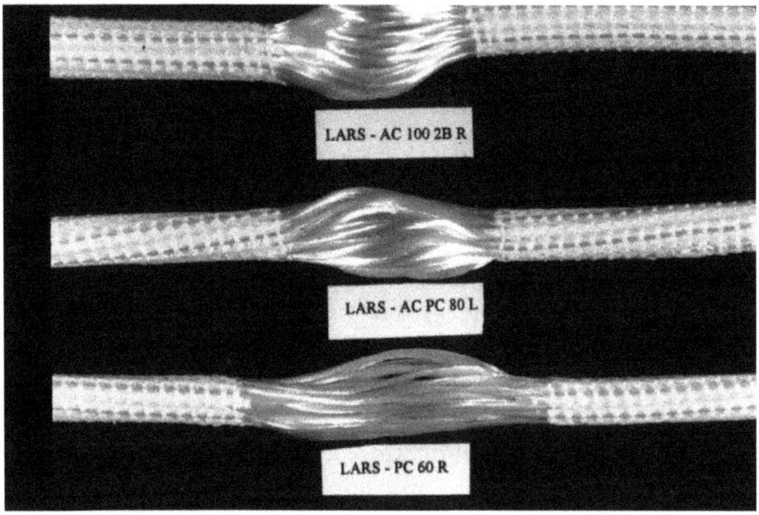

Figure 1. LARS artificial ligaments

of longitudinal fibers bound together by a transverse knitted structure while an intra-articular segment is composed of parallel longitudinal fibers twisted at 90° clockwise or counter-clockwise for use in right and left knees, respectively. The main innovation of this artificial ligament lies in its ability to mimic the natural ligamentous structure and reduce shearing forces by orientating the free fibers of the intra-articular portion of the graft.[9,10] Therefore, every time a knee flexion occur, the LARS™ ligament unwinds instead of twisting, reducing considerably the combined loading of traction, flexion and torsion, while reducing abrasion.[11] Furthermore, the PET fibers of the intra-articular segment are designed to encourage tissue formation due to the porosity of the material, helping the healing process and creating a stronger and more reliable synthetic graft.[12] Growing tissue around the ligament fibers may contribute to the viscoelasticity of the graft and protect against friction at the opening of the bony canal.

Therefore, this chapter aims to present the author current technique of ACL repair augmented by a LARS™ artificial ligament. Dr. Nicolas Duval started to use LARS™ in 1993 and this technique, presented below, was performed from 2004 on every knee when decision was made to perform ACL surgery and a good quality remnant could be stitched to the femur. It was found that most ACL remnants could be repaired within 3 months following rupture or later when healing has taken place between the ACL and the posterior cruciate ligament (PCL).

2. Surgical Technique

2.1. *Placement of the Guide Pin*

After arthroscopic evaluation of the knee joint and assessment of the ACL tear, the technique described by Laboureau[13] is used. With the knee in flexion, as shown in Figure 2, a double-pointed K-wire is inserted via an antero-medial portal, aiming at 10 o'clock for the right knee or at 2 o'clock for the left knee and driven just anterior to the over-the-top position in front of the femoral posterior cortical bone. Fluoroscopy is used to check its location. It then goes through the femur and exits the anterolateral skin. The motor is switched to the proximal part to move it further proximal until the distal end of the pin is intra-articular. The knee is brought back to 45° and the pin is driven distally through the posterior tibial insertion of the ACL,

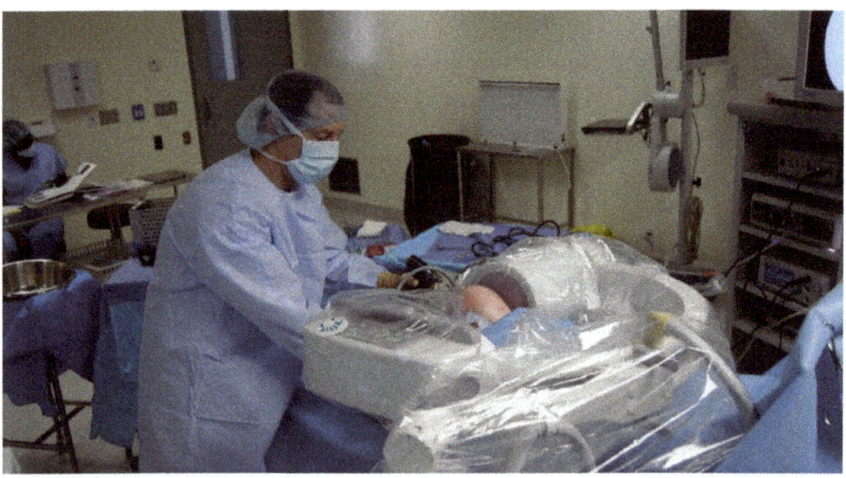

Figure 2. Mini C-arm is used to check location of the K-wire

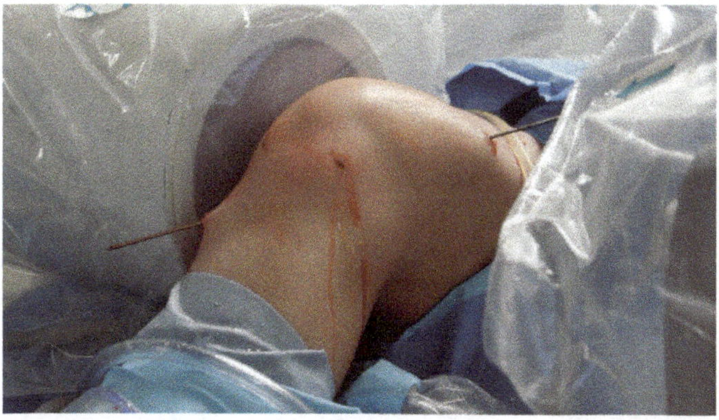

(a)

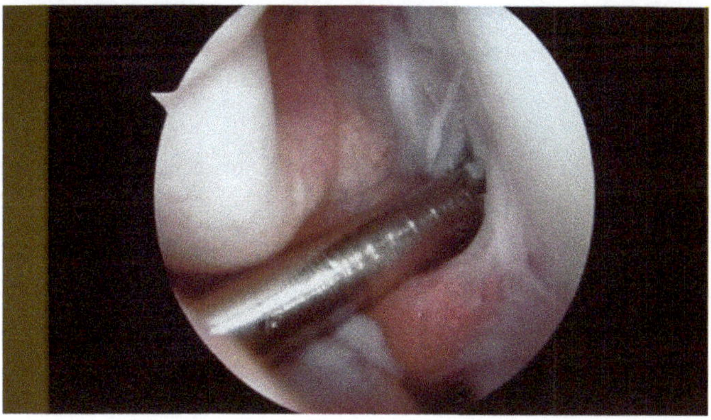

(b)

Figure 3. (a) Knee is brought back to 45° and the pin is driven distally through the posterior tibial insertion of the ACL. (b) Final position of the guide pin

just behind the middle of the tibial plateau on a fluoroscopic lateral view (Figure 3(a)). It then goes through the tibia and exits the antero-medial skin. The cannulated drill is passed over the guide pin in the tibia and the femur (Figure 3(b)).

2.2. *ACL Repair*

The ACL remnant is stitched to the femur with three or four 2-0 non-resorbable sutures with the Arthrex® Meniscal Viper (Figures 4 and 5).

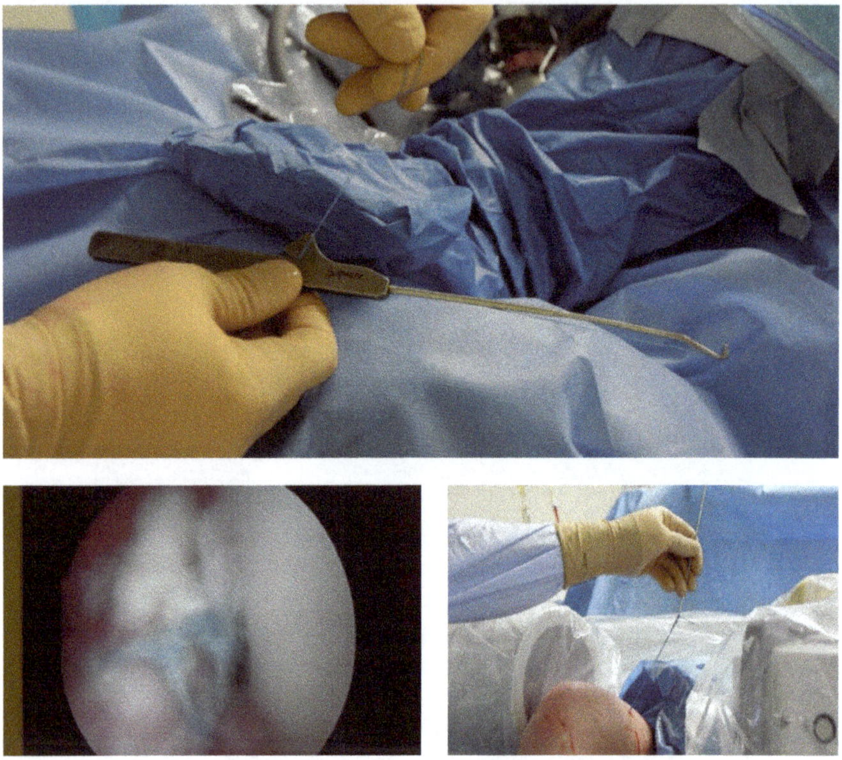

Figure 4. ACL repair Arthrex® Meniscal Viper

Then the LARS™ ligament is passed through the tibial and femoral tunnel posterior to the ACL remnant. The LARS™ and the sutures are fixed with outside-in metal screws.

2.3. *Postoperative Protocol*

Postoperatively, all patients used crutches weight bearing as tolerated. They are allowed immediate motion without a brace. They are starting physiotherapy at 2 weeks focusing on closed kinetic chain exercises. They are allowed running in straight line at 2 months, figure of 8 at 3 months and hard pivot at 4 months. Return to specific training is started at 4 months and competing is allowed at 6 months.

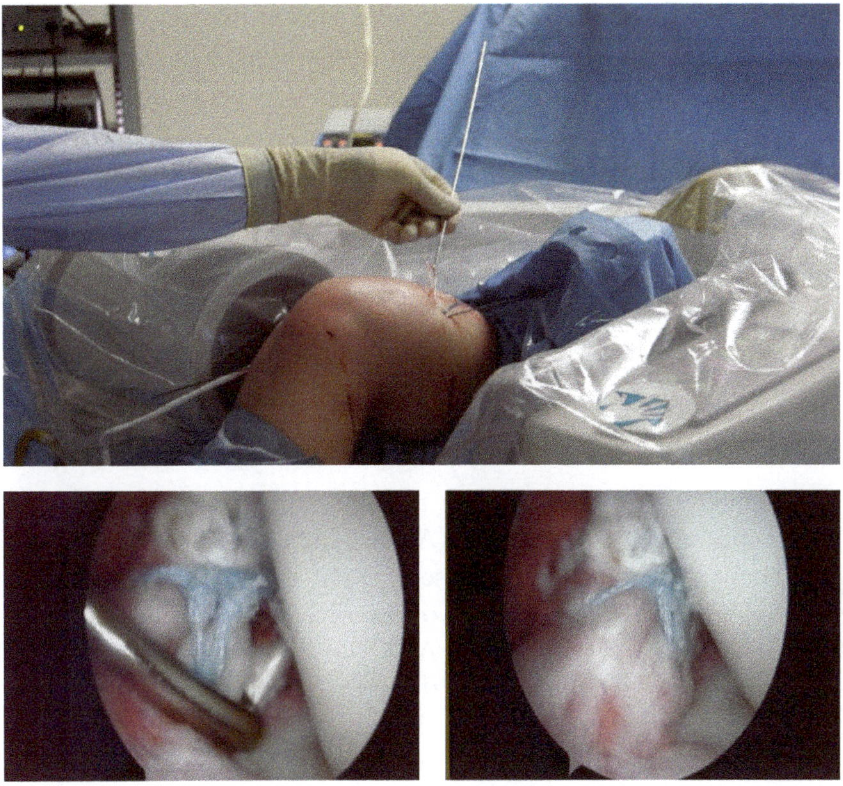

Figure 5. LARS™ augmentation through tibial and femoral tunnel

3. Results

Patient satisfaction was high and most patients demonstrated a significant improvement of their knee after surgery.[7,8] The results compared with ACL reconstruction using a standard autograft or allograft technique. Dr Duval's technique obviously avoids potential graft harvesting complications such as patellar fracture, anterior knee pain, hamstring weakness or rupture of the remaining tendon(s), and potential allograft reduced healing, rejection, and disease transmission.[14–19] Full range of motion was the norm, the most common complaint being occasional residual pain around the tibial screw. No patient experienced knee synovitis.

Failure rate was a little less than 10%. Half of the failures were not related to a new injury and all occurred within 2 or 3 years after repair. Not one knee failed beyond 4 years. In all cases, the rupture was between the ACL-LARS™ structure and the femoral tunnel. Revision surgery using fluoroscopic guidance was usually easy as bone grows on the outer surface but never inside the LARS™. It was easy to pull it out when the screws were removed. The tibial and femoral tunnels, usually 6 or 7 mm wide, were intact and easily enlarged to adapt the new reconstruction graft. Finally, all usual autograft tendons were available for the revision procedure.

4. Discussion

The analysis of the outcomes in patients afflicted by an ACL sub-acute rupture proved fascinating. A constellation of elements concurs in certain patients treated conservatively to produce satisfactory results whereas in others, the evolution leads to chronic instability and thence to surgery. Once an ACL has ruptured, the purpose of surgery in the sub-acute stage is the stabilization of a not yet unstable knee, to prevent instability, should the conservative treatment fail. Yet, however abundant the published material devoted to the ACL, the lack of knowledge concerning the proprioceptive factors conducing to a functional stability in spite of a ruptured ACL, it is impossible to conceive a selective, objective prevention of instability. The orthopaedic surgeon is limited to a subjective experience-based prevention.

As Dye proposed,[20] the goal of treatment is to maximize a knee's envelope of function as safely and predictably as possible and encourage patient to stay within the range of loading the knee can accept. The natural history of a ruptured ACL is still not clear. Surgical stabilization of a knee, which would remain stable after a conservative treatment, represents an unnecessary surgery that submits the patient to the complications that may ensue.

A meta-analysis of the literature demonstrates the extent to which the emphasis is directed towards technical surgical details as well as to short-term outcomes.[21] Few prospective randomized studies have looked at the long-term functional impact. Moreover, data analysis is complicated by a lack of uniformity in reporting of the results, by a large number of patients being lost to follow-up and by the fact that treatment success or failure — as assessed by the surgeon — does not necessarily match that of the patients.[7,22]

Long-term ACL reconstruction revision rates have ranged from 5% to 15%/[23] An Australian prospective study documented autograft rupture rate of 17% for hamstring tendon and 8% for patellar tendon at 15 years.[24] Young cadets at the United States Military Academy (USMA) who undergone ACL reconstruction before entrance to service experienced a failure rate of 12% following autograft reconstruction and 44% following allograft less than 2 years on average from matriculation.[25]

A large number of past reports disapproved of the utilization of artificial ligaments.[26–28] Dr. Duval's experience support the view that an appropriate implant, like the LARS™, supporting ACL healing can provide good results while ACL prosthetic replacement, the presumed role granted artificial ligaments in the past, is unable to offer adequate biofunctionality and biodurability.[29,30] LARS™ ligaments, made of "de-enzymized" polyester, set in multiple intra-articular fibers may be better tolerated than other materials such as carbon fibers and other textile structures like braids. Clinical synovitis, occasionally reported by other surgeons,[31] was not observed in Dr. Duval's practice, although one cannot exclude microscopic alterations of the synovial membrane. Early stabilization of the knee may favor protection from the mechanoreceptors and the secondary stabilizers of the knee, during the critical period identified as the first 2 years, when most of the failures take place.

Based on Dr. Duval's results, the future lie in helping the repair and healing of the ACL. The development of bioactive ligaments[32] to enhance cell growth, where nanofibers of PET and bioactive groups attached on the synthetic ligament can link the growth factors, the adhesive proteins, the type I collagen and the fibroblasts is in progress. Other ACL repair techniques were recently developed adding local factors enhancing the biological repair process[33,34,35,36] or using a synovial graft wrap around the repair.[37] The traditional ACL surgery is still an autograft reconstruction but that may change in a near future.

5. Conflict of Interest Statement

Dr Duval LARS® work was supported by a grant from LARS, 5 rue de la Fontaine 21560 Arc sur Tille, France. LARS was not involved in the study design, in the collection, analysis and interpretation of data, in the writing of the chapter and in the decision to submit this chapter for publication.

Acknowledgments

Dr. Duval thanks Dr. Pauline Lavoie, MD, LMCC, MSc (Epidemiology and Biostatistics) for her help in following patients, Professor L'Hocine Yahia and student Michèle Voyer for help with preparing this chapter.

References

1. Yahia, L.; Newman, N. *Anat. Anz. Bd.* **1991**, *173*(4), 233–238.
2. Yahia, L.; Newman, N.; St-Georges, M. *Anatomia, Histologia, Embryologia* **1992**, 21(1), 1–8.
3. Denti, M.; Monteleone, M.; Berardi, A.; Schiavone Panni, A. *Clin Orthop.* **1994**, *308*, 29–32.
4. Ng, G. Y.; Oakes, B. W.; McLean, I. D.; Deacon, O. W.; Lampard, D. *Am. J. Sports Med.* **1996**, *24*, 109–117.
5. Richter, M.; Duerselen, L.; Ignatius, A.; Missler, F.; Claes, L. *J. Mat. Sci.* **1997**, *8*, 855–859.
6. Seitz, H.; Menth-Chiari, W. A.; Lang, S.; Nau, T. *Knee Surg. Sports Traumatol. Arthrosc.* **2008**, *16*, 1087–1093.
7. Lavoie, P; Fletcher, J.; Duval, N. *Knee* **2000**, *7*, 157–163.
8. Nau, T.; Lavoie, P.; Duval, N. *J. Bone Joint Surg. [Br].* **2002**, *84-B*, 356–360.
9. Yahia, L'H.; Hagemeister, N.; Drouin, G. *et al. Biomimetics* **1994**, *2*, 309–330.

10. Sati, M.; de Guise, J. A.; Larouche, S.; Drouin, G. *The Knee* **1996**, *3*(4), 179–190.
11. Gely, P.; Drouin, G.; Thiry, G. P.; Tremblay, G. R. *J. Biomech. Eng.* **1984**, *106*(4), 285–294.
12. Trieb, K.; Blahovec, H.; Brand, G.; Sabeti, M.; Dominkus, M.; Kotz, R. *Eur. Surg. Res.* **2004**, *36*(3), 148–151.
13. Laboureau, J. P.; Marnat-Perrichet, F. Isometric reconstruction of the anterior cruciate ligament: femoral and tibial placement. In: Yahia, H. (ed.), *Ligaments and Ligamentoplasties.* (Berlin: Springer-Verlag, **1997**), pp. 209–225.
14. Hughston, J. C. *Orthop Clin North Am.* **1985**, *16*, 237–240.
15. Clancy, W. J. *Tech. Orthop.* **1988**, *2*, 13–23.
16. Anderson, C.; Odensten, M.; Good, L.; Gillquist, J. *J. Bone Joint Surg.* [*Am*]. **1989**, *71-A*, 965–974.
17. Daniel, D. M.; Stone, M. L.; Dobson, B. E.; Fithian, D. C.; Rossman, D. J.; Kaufman, K. R. *Am. J. Sports Med.* **1994**, *22*, 632–644.
18. Fox, J. A.; Nedeff, D. D.; Bach, B. R. Jr.; Spindler, K. P. *Clin. Orthop.* **2002**, *402*, 53–63.
19. Fithian, D. C.; Paxton, E. W.; Stone, M. L.; Luetzow, W. F.; Csintalan, R. P.; Phelan, D.; Daniel, D. M. *Am. J. Sports Med.* **2005**, *33*, 335–346.
20. Dye, S. *Clin Orthop.* **1996**, *323*, 10–186.
21. Casteleyn, P. P.; Handelberg, F. *J. Bone Joint Surg. [Br].* **1996**, *78-B*, 446–451.
22. Lavoie, P.; Fletcher, J.; Duval, N. *Knee* **2001**, *8*, 19–24.
23. Yabroudi, M. A.; Björnsson, H.; Lynch, A. D.; Muller, B.; Samuelsson, K.; Tarabichi, M.; Karlsson, J.; Fu, F. H.; Harner, C. D.; Irrgang, J. J. *Orthop. J. Sports Med.* **2016**, *4*(9)
24. Leys, T.; Salmon, L.; Waller, A.; Linklater, J.; Pinczewski, L. *Am. J. Sports Med.* **2012**, *40*(3), 595–605.
25. Pallis, M.; Svoboda, S. J.; Cameron, K. L.; Owens, B. D. *Am. J. Sports Med.* 2012, *40*(6), 1242–1246.
26. De Smedt, M. *Acta. Orthopaedica Belgica.* 1998, *64*(4), 422–433.
27. Mascarenhas, R.; MacDonald, P. B. *McGill J. Med.* **2008**, *11*, 29–37.
28. Legnani, C.; Ventura, A.; Terzaghi, C.; Borgo, E.; Albisetti, W. *Int. Ortho. (SICOT)* **2010**, *34*, 465–471.

29. Lukianov, A. V.; Richmond, J. C.; Barrett, G. R.; Guillquist, J. *Am. J. Sports Med.* **1989**, *17*, 380–386.
30. Sledge, S. L.; Steadman, J. R.; Silliman, J. F. *et al. Am. J. Sports Med.* **1992**, *5*, 65–70.
31. Glezos, C. M.; Waller, A,; Bourke, H. E.; Salmon, L. J.; Pinczewski, L. A. *Am. J. Sports Med.* **2012**, *40*(5), 1167–1171.
32. Chen, C.-S.; Shao, H.-J.; Lin, W.-C.; Chang, C.-H.; Wang, J.-H.; Young, T.-H. *J. Orthop. Surg. Taiwan* **2007**, *24*, 107–110.
33. MacKay, G.; Anthony, I. C.; Jenkins, P. J.; Blyth, M. *Orthop. Muscul. Syst.* **2105**, *4*, 2
34. DiFelice, G. S.; Van der List, J., P. *Arthrosc. Tech.* **2016**, *5*(5), e1057–e1061.
35. Vavken, P.; Fleming, B. C.; Mastrangelo, A. N.; Machan, J. T.; Murray, M. M. *Arthroscopy* **2012**, *28*(5), 672–680.
36. Eggli, S.; Hohlhof, H.; Zumstein, M.; Henle, H.; Hartel, M.; Evangelopoulos, D. S.; Bonel, H.; Kohl, S. *Knee Surg. Sports Traumatol. Arthrosc.* **2015**, *23*(4), 1215–1221.
37. Pritchett, J. W. *J. Knee Surg.* **2009**, *22*(4), 325–330.

https://doi.org/10.1142/9789811204630_0011

Chapter 11

Biomimetic Challenge of Anterior Cruciate Ligament Design

L'Hocine Yahia[*,†,‡], Ghislaine Bayade[*], and Jacques-Philippe Laboureau[†]

[*]*Laboratoire d'Innovation et d'Analyse de Bioperformance, Polytechnique Montréal, C.P. 6079, Succursale Centre-ville, Montréal, Québec, Canada H3C 3A7*

[†]*651-C Chemin de la Martourette, 06530 Le Tignet, France*

[‡]*lhocine.yahia@polymtl.ca*

Abbreviations

AAOS	American Academy of Orthopaedic Surgeons
ACL	Anterior cruciate ligament
ACP	Amorphous calcium phosphate
ACLR	ACL reconstruction
ALL	Anterolateral ligament
ALR	Anterolateral reconstruction
AM	Anteromedial
BLAs	Biologics license applications
CNTs	Carbon nanotubes
ECM	Extracellular matrix
F	Femoral isometric zone
FDA	Food and Drug Administration
FE	Flexion extension
HMWPE	High molecular weight polyethylene
LARS	Ligament advanced reinforcement
LR	Longitudinal rotation
MDR	Medical device reporting
MWNTs	Multi-walled CNTs
OA	Osteoarthritis
OI	Outside-in
510(k)	Premarket notification
PCL	Posterior cruciate ligament
PEI	Polyethyleneimine
PET	Polyethylene terephthalate

PL	Posterolateral
PN	Peripheral nerve
PolyNASS	Polystyrene sodium sulfonate
PRP	Platelet-rich plasma
PTFE	Polytetrafluoroethylene
RCT	Randomized clinical trial
RTS	Return to sport
SBF	Simulated body fluid
TLF	Thoracolumbar fascia
TP	Transportal
TT	Transtibial technique

1. Introduction

There was a time when clinicians published more successes than failures. Now things have changed. However, instead of learning from their failures, some clinicians quickly attribute these failures to a design flaw, i.e. to bioengineers.

The scientific community has a disappointing track record for dissemination of clinical trial results. Numerous factors may contribute to these poor publication rates, including some that are beyond the control of researchers.[1] Despite the best efforts of investigators, the results of some trials may never reach the threshold deemed necessary to merit the attention of journal editors and of readers. Even published results may focus only on the findings of most interest to the investigators. Other means to share such data are necessary because both real and potential harm can result from failure to fully disclose the results of clinical trials. Nonetheless, difficulty with achieving publication in scientific journals for negative results cannot be blamed entirely.

First, companies tend not to publish negative or inconclusive studies or secondary analyses for a number of reasons: such findings can be exploited by competing medical device companies; they can complicate a clean narrative for investors; and they can diminish off-label use of a licensed device. Similar pressures may deter academics from pursuing publication as well. Policymakers and funding bodies should pursue measures that promote unbiased and prompt publication for unsuccessful translation trajectories. Public funding agencies might also consider withholding the last installments of grants until all the relevant data have been made public, or they might offer small grants for publishing negative results. When hosting privately funded trials, academic medical centers could insist on using contracts that commit sponsors to sharing full datasets with local investigators, and that allow researchers to publish complete datasets when private sponsors do not.

Second, researchers and healthcare professionals should better exploit the information generated by unsuccessful translation trajectories. Researchers should pay more attention to negative and to inconclusive findings when they are published as researchers tend to cite positive findings more frequently than negative findings, even when there are no obvious differences in the quality of the studies,[2] and many clinical investigators perceive negative studies as uninformative.[3]

The Medical Device Reporting (MDR) regulation (21 CFR 803) contains mandatory requirements for manufacturers, importers, and device user facilities to report certain device-related adverse events and product problems to the US Food and Drug Administration (FDA). Patients, healthcare professionals and consumers who find a problem related to a medical device are encouraged to report medical device adverse events or product problems to the FDA through MedWatch, the FDA Safety Information and Adverse Event Reporting Program.

1.1. *Learning from Failures*

Artificial ligaments have been used for knee ligament reconstruction as far back as the 1970s[4] although most of the research has focused on anterior cruciate ligament (ACL) reconstruction. The first generation involved Teflon, carbon fiber, and polypropylene ligaments, but they were withdrawn because of high failure rates[5]. In the 1980s expanded polytetrafluoroethylene (PTEE) was used. It was thought to have a good biomechanical profile, but complication rates of up to 76%[6] have been reported. The complications include PTEE deposits in the distant lymph nodes.[7] PTEE soon fell into disuse thereafter. Woven Dacron ligaments were used in the 1990s. Although complication rates with Dacron were lower than those with previous synthetic ligaments, they were still high, and this product was withdrawn in 1994.[5]

This early enthusiasm was abruptly stopped by the poor long-term stability which often result in catastrophic failures of these structures. Indeed, several short to mid-term clinical retrospective studies revealed that despite appropriate initial behavior and rapid patient recovery, the vast majority of implanted ligaments were breaking down and had to be explanted. This ligamentous catastrophe is similar to that reported later for cardiovascular implants.[8] Most of these newly developed artificial ligaments were rated as inappropriate for clinical utilization. The reasons for this immense failure are multiple and are related to the biomaterials used in the process of fabrication of the ligament, which were not necessarily adequate for repetitive loading.

1.2. *Forensic Engineering*

Knowing the causes of these failures and conditions, they can all be prevented. Forensic engineering helped reveal how the design and use of the medical instruments could cause such failures. As a result, changes were made to the instrument design and the procedural protocols in ACL reconstruction.

Forensic engineering is the investigation of materials, products, structures or components that fail or do not operate or function as intended, causing personal injury or damage to property. The law of product liability deals with the consequences of failure. The field also takes part with retracing processes and procedures leading to accidents in operation of vehicles or machinery. The subject is applied most commonly in civil law cases, although it may be of use in criminal law cases. Generally, the purpose of a forensic engineering investigation is to locate the cause or causes of failure with a view to improve performance or life of a component, or to assist a court in determining the facts of an accident. It can also involve investigation of intellectual property claims, especially patents.

Most manufacturing models will have a forensic component that monitors early failures to improve quality or efficiencies. Insurance companies use forensic engineers to prove liability or nonliability. Most engineering disasters (structural failures such as bridge and building collapses) are subject to forensic investigation by engineers experienced in forensic methods of investigation.

The failure of medical devices is often safety-critical to the user, so reporting failures and analyzing them is particularly important. The environment of the body is complex, and implants must both survive this environment, and not leach potentially toxic impurities. Problems have been reported with breast implants, heart valves, and catheters, for example.

There are many examples of forensic methods used to investigate accidents and disasters. For artificial ligaments, Guidoin *et al.*[9] investigated the explanted failed ligaments and concluded that most of the ligaments failed at the bony interface, which engendered an acute inflammatory response. Guidoin *et al.*[9] analyzed polymer fiber-based replacements for the ACL;[9] they suggested that three elements played key roles in the artificial ligament failure: (1) inadequate fiber abrasion resistance against osseous surfaces; (2) flexural and rotational fatigue of the fibers; and (3) loss of integrity of the textile structure due to unpredictable tissue infiltration during healing.

This failure of synthetic ligament replacement will discredit ligament prostheses for more than two decades and push the American Academy of Orthopedic Surgeons (AAOS) to recommend only transplants or autografts as an alternative. Thus, the FDA guidelines for ligament prostheses have not been updated for more than 20 years.

In recent years, two new paradigms have emerged for ACL repair: improvement healing with platelet-rich plasma (PRP) and ligament regeneration. However, because of the biological complexity, these two new approaches require a lot of research in order to transfer them to the clinic.

1.3. *Platelet-Rich Plasma* (*PRP*)

PRP is the blood plasma loaded with platelets. It has been quite some time since PRP has been in use as a treatment option for musculoskeletal disorders, for chronic conditions, and for sports injuries including acute ligamentous injuries.[10] In general, the FDA approves a new drug, a biologic or a device, for its safety and for its efficacy before they are introduced into the market. PRP is a biologic substance.

Clinical PRP, used by the health care providers, also needs an FDA approval. The biologics may be approved by the Biologics License Applications (BLAs), or by the Premarket Notification (510(k)). For BLAs approval, a clinical review needs to be done; making it a time-consuming and a costly procedure. The FDA has not given an approval of using PRP in sports injury. Regardless of this disapproval, PRP is being used in the management of sports injuries as it leads to an early healing. As discussed, PRP is not an artificial treatment; it is produced in fact naturally. Many studies have been conducted which show the efficiency of PRP injections in tendonitis. Currently, the FDA approval is awaiting, however, such injections are considered exception in use, as they are prepared from the patient's own blood. FDA has also approved the use of PRP as allograft or as autograft in orthopedic surgery and in non-healing diabetic ulcers. Therefore, it seems that the FDA has no objection in the application of PRP in both medical and surgical management. However, health care providers need to stay updated with the recent changes in PRP approval by the FDA.

Animal studies, case reports, case series and a single-blinded randomized controlled trial have suggested a beneficial effect of PRP injections on both healing and return to play duration following muscle injury.[11–13] However, a double-blind randomized controlled trial in amateur athletes conducted by Reurink *et al.* in 2014 failed to reproduce this finding, and high-quality studies in professional athletes are lacking.[14]

In a randomized controlled trial involving predominantly professional football athletes suffering an acute hamstring injury, Hamilton *et al.*[15] found that a single PRP injection in combination with an intensive rehabilitation program did not reduce the return to sport (RTS) duration when compared with rehabilitation only. In contrast, a single PRP injection in combination with intensive rehabilitation reduced the RTS duration when compared with a single PRP injection and rehabilitation.

There remain many unanswered questions when considering the use of PRP for muscle injuries in athletes. While this study fails to show any benefit of a single injection of PRP, it remains a possibility that further injections, or injections delivered at a different time period or location, may have had some impact. Furthermore, there is a known variation in the white cell and red cell concentrations in different PRP formulations, which could potentially affect the outcome. All these elements require further evaluation before PRP can be routinely recommended for use in acute muscle strain injuries. Moreover, the development of a qualified tissue-engineered ligament is still full of challenges.

1.4. *Tissue Engineering*

Tissue-engineered ligaments are promising devices in future clinical work. However, limited by the current knowledge in such fields, there is still plenty of work to do to transfer a qualified product from the laboratory to the operation theatre.

It is undeniable that tissue-engineered ligament researches have progressed in the past decades.[16] In some respects, the increasing understanding can be literally claimed as breakthroughs. However, the difficulties to conceive an ideal product are still challenging owing to the insufficient understanding of natural ligament healing process and its *in vivo* development, specifically for the ACL — the most focused tissue-engineered ligament research area.

Hence, in contrast to the huge amount of preclinical reports dealing with cellular therapeutic or tissue engineering approaches in ligament repair, clinical trials are still rare up to date. There is a need to generate high-quality evidences before recommending and applying cellular therapy or tissue engineering to patients. Very often, standard protocols and reliable data are still missing, which makes clinical decisions difficult. Nevertheless, a continuing progress in the research of tissue-engineered ligaments will lead to a viable product in the future especially if, studying the properties of nature, a systematic scientific approach is used to better reproduce them by imitating nature.

In the meantime, artificial ligaments (ligament advanced reinforcement system (LARS), Leeds-Keio) and grafts remain the only available options for ACL reconstruction.

1.5. *Biomimetic Approach*

The innovative concept of "biomimetic prosthetics" envisages that, once implanted in the patient's body in place of the damaged tendon or ligament, this represents the structural support on which new ligament tissue is formed. Therefore, a biomimetic prosthesis should be manufactured from a material capable of promoting cell adhesion and proliferation, without its subsequent degradation compromising cell metabolism and eliciting an abnormal inflammatory response from the host.

The mechanical characteristics of the biomimetic prosthesis must guarantee functional continuity between the implant and the surrounding tissues *in vivo*. Furthermore, the porosity and geometry of the pores must be such as to also allow cellular migration within the structure and promote the passage of oxygen, metabolites and growth factors.

Particularly, a biomimetic prosthesis for the regeneration of the ACL must satisfy the following characteristics:

- Mechanical properties comparable to those of the human ACL, which possesses a mean rupture load value of approximately 2000 N;
- The ability to allow cell colonization and the formation of new tissue in all its parts (fibroblasts and tenocytes);
- Such a rate of degradation as to guarantee the gradual transfer of load onto the new ligament and ensure the mechanical stability of the joint until tissue regeneration is complete.

Yahia *et al.* have been among the first to suggest a biomimetics approach to improve the design of the artificial ligaments.[17]

Engineers who emphasized the Nature design developed the first generation of artificial ligaments. Indeed, at that time the knowledge of the ligaments was incomplete. For example, in nature, it is known that most tissues or organs have not only one function; but also, more than one.

Thus, this updating chapter on the ACL has the aim of addressing some of the most interesting current topics in this field.

1.5.1. *Can the Natural Ligament be Successfully Copied?*

Morphology is basically the science of reverse engineering; it looks at how a body is assembled and tries to figure out how it's supposed to function. The bioengineer is faced with a similar reverse engineering problem. He/she is given a solution and tries to find the parameters that were contained in the problem definition. By looking at natural ligaments, it is distinctly possible to derive an optimal design for the prosthesis. However, in the past, prosthetic ligaments have been simple cylindrical elements. Replacing a very complex structure that sustains extreme loading, such as the ACL, by a simple element, is bound to failure. A prosthetic ligament design should take into consideration the normal structural hierarchy of the natural ligament, since the biomechanical performance of this tissue is related to its architecture. For example, crimping of tendons and ligaments is an essential feature for auxeticity. On one side, this chapter will present the biomechanical and the functional results of the current replacement procedures and, on the other side, the demands of the biomechanics of the knee. This will bring the possibility to display the most important mechanical properties, the prosthesis should have to respond to the requirements of the biomechanics of the knee. The challenge will be to achieve a design that makes the best use of synthetic materials in order to reproduce the function of the natural ligament.

1.5.2. *Trying to Copy Nature with Synthetic Fibers*

LARSLARS was developed by Laboureau in 1992 and was originally designed for posterior cruciate ligament (PCL) reconstruction.[18]

LARS ligaments are made from polyethylene terephthalate with a varying intra- and extra-articular structure. It appeared from trials of different ligaments structures on knee simulator, reproducing the *in vivo* stresses by combining tension, flexion, and torsion, that the fibers, which were crossing each other, were cutting each other, particularly during torsion. This torsion is what happens at the femoral insertion during flexion, clockwise for the right knee, counter-clockwise for the left knee. These shearing forces between crossing fibers were leading to abrasion, to production of micro particles and finally to rupture. The obvious conclusion was that any intra-articular synthetic ligament must avoid structures like knitting, braiding, weaving which all have crossing fibers. The "free fibers" of the LARS ligament were patented by Laboureau in 1992. Intraosseous section of LARS ligament is formed from longitudinal fibers bound together by a knitted structure, and the intra-articular portion is made of purely unlinked longitudinal fibers. In order to mimic anatomy and biomechanics of the natural ligament, the fibers are orientated in a 90° spiral clockwise for the right knee and counter-clockwise for the left knee.[19,20] The intra-articular structure resembles the normal anatomy of the ACL compared with earlier attempts, helping to avoid shearing forces. The porosity of this structure and the special chemical treatment of the polyethylene terephthalate fibers allow tissue ingrowth, reducing friction and theoretically avoiding tunnel enlargement. Although tunnel enlargement seems to be due to several factors, one of them being the mobility of the synthetic material inside the tunnel, depending on the type of fixation. This suggests that when using synthetic material, the ligament must be absolutely blocked into the tunnels. One of the common solutions today is to use of a non-resorbable interference screw.

Brulez and Laboureau *et al.* patented a new biomimetic prosthetic ligament in 2004.[21] The first pre-clinical results show a better adhesion of the fibroblasts on the synthetic fibers and a better collagenic tissue ingrowth.

There is still a long way to improve design and development of anisotropic bioengineered systems with potential to review the hierarchical architecture and organization of tendons and ligaments from nano to macro scale.

2. Natural Design of ACL

2.1. *Hierarchical Organization of ACL*

Ligaments and tendons are composed primarily of water and fibrillary type I collagen, which is hierarchically organized into complex structures that span multiple physical scales. Forces at the macroscopic joint level are transmitted via interactions at the mesoscale, the microscale and the nanoscale. Tissue repair and growth is mediated by fibroblasts and tenocytes, which are subjected to a unique microscale mechanical environment.

2.1.1. *Ligament Level*

A ligament consists of collagen fibrils of 0.4–1.4 μm in diameter, which are responsible for the ligaments' resistance to elongation.[22] Therefore, arrangement and ultimate elongation of the collagen fibrils result in 8–9% ultimate elongation of the ligament (see Figure 1(a)).[23,24] Several fibrils form a fiber. Fibers are organized into fascicles, which are surrounded by a thin sheath, which allows slipping between adjacent fascicles (see Figures 1(b) and 1(c)).[24,25] Another useful observation of the natural ligament is that the ligament fans out near its ends and forms a "foot" region. This is believed to give the ligament a wide basis for torsional resistance. Furthermore, the merging of fascicles toward the middle of the natural ligament provides cross-linking.

2.1.2. *Fascicle Level*

It is well known that the ACL comprises two main fiber bundles, one anteromedial (AM bundle) and one posterolateral named PL bundle (see Figure 2),[26,27] which behave differently throughout the flexion-extension range.[28] *In vitro* studies have found that the PL bundle is taut in full extension, while the AM bundle is taut across the flexion–extension range.[29–31] The PL bundle relaxes during knee flexion, allowing the tibia to rotate internally during quadriceps muscle contraction. This pattern supports the knee weight bearing in extension and allows movement during knee flexion.[32]

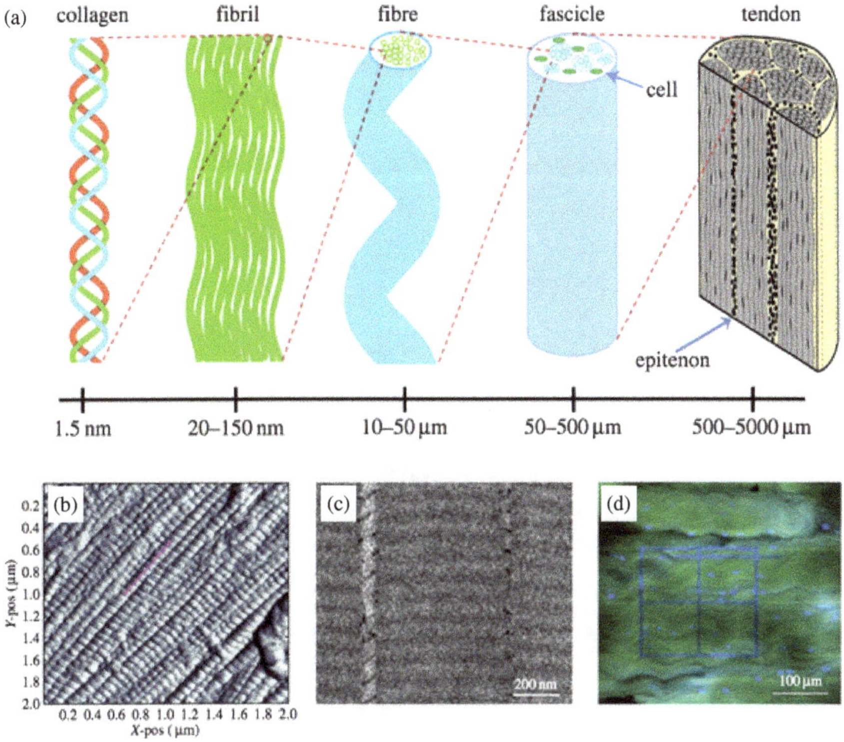

Figure 1. (a) Schematic of the multiscale tendon hierarchical structure; (b) Atomic force microscopy showing D-period (red line) in collagen fibrils from mouse supraspinatus tendon; (c) Micrograph from transmission electron microscopy showing stained collagen fibrils and GAGs in native tendon[25]

The AM and PL bundles control the anterior translation of the tibia at any degree of knee flexion. At high degrees of knee flexion, the AM bundle is more effective in controlling the anterior translation compared to the PL bundle. On the other hand, the PL bundle is more efficient from 0° to 20° of knee flexion.[33]

The ACL bundles also play different roles in controlling rotational motion and stability of the knee joint due to the differences in their attachment areas and orientation.[34] The AM bundle is almost vertically oriented in the intercondylar notch in the coronal plane, thus having little ability to restrain axial tibia rotation. On the other hand, the PL bundle slants across the intercondylar notch to a more

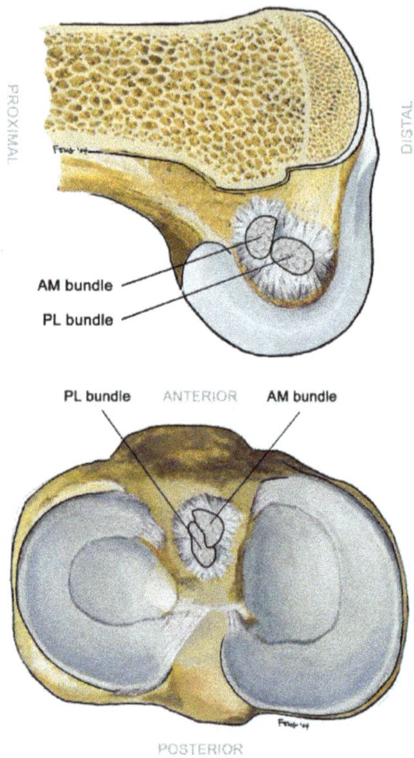

Figure 2. Attachment areas of the ACL[27]

distal–lateral femoral attachment (see Figure 3). It has a more horizontal orientation, which suggests a further position from the axis of axial tibia rotation, implying by this a higher ability to control rotations of the tibia compared to the AM bundle.[35,36]

In the past, attempts have been made to decompose the ligament into its basic structural elements. A study from Clark *et al.* proposes a new approach, which does not attempt to break the ACL into such divisions.[37] Clark *et al.* observed that the interrelationship of the collagen fiber bundles changed as the ligament approached to the bone.[37] At the ligament–bone interface (or fibrocartilage region), the grouping into fascicles became more apparent because spaces between fascicles became wider and the sheaths became thicker. Toward the middle of the ligament, this distinction was no longer present.

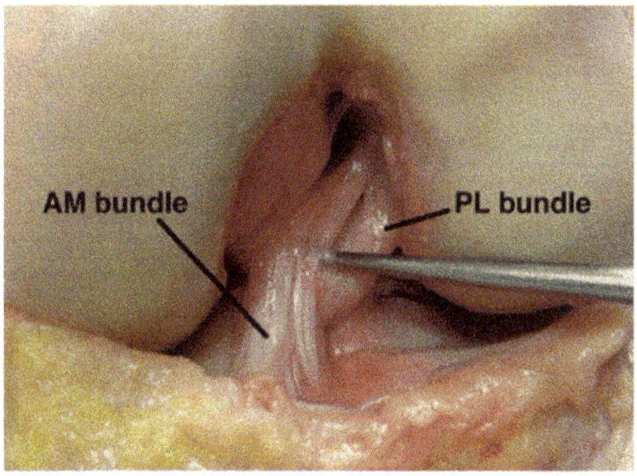

Figure 3. Bundles of the ACL[36]

This might explain the difficulty researchers have had in distinguishing the basic structural strands of the ACL. It was also well known that the stiffness of the natural ligament increases when it approaches the bone insertion.[38] This gradual change in cross-sectional area reduces the stress concentration at bone insertion.

In the natural ligament, deformations are shared between many individual elements, each of which undergoes minimal deformation. Since the single element prosthetic ligament must tolerate enormous load in elongation, bending, and torsion, it will often fail prematurely, because it is not a proper design to sustain the loading conditions.

Current reconstructive procedures usually reduce the distributed attachment to a single site. When augmentation is used with one more biological segment, the bands are usually not positioned in a way to simulate the original ACL insertion and may create a high stress concentration at the fixation sites.

The use of a single bundle leads to disappointing results even in the isometric tracking: A considerable loosening of all remaining structures was observed.[39] Better results were achieved mimicking the natural situation by using a "two-bundle prosthesis" resulting in negligible changes of the length pattern of the remaining ligaments.[39] The different mechanical properties of the two ACL bundles suggest further investigation into their different functions to establish if there is a need for a double bundle implant.[40]

Radford *et al.*[41] compared the biomechanical properties of a "double bundle" prosthetic ligament replacing the ACL in cadaver knees, with those of "single bundle," "over the top," and "through the condyle" techniques. The implant used in all types of repair was a multifilament polyester (Terylene) prosthetic ligament, consisting of 40,000 fibers, each of 15 μm in diameter (compared to 1–20 μm in diameter for the natural ACL) and secured by stainless steel cortical screws through loops at each end of the implant. They performed two clinical tests to measure anteroposterior movement: the Lachman test for ACL laxity at 20° of knee flexion and the anterior drawer test for ACL laxity at 90° of knee flexion. They found out that the "double bundle" repair approximates in function to the intact ACL at both 20° and 90° knee flexion angles; meanwhile, the other repairs only function like an intact ACL at either 20°or 90°. These results indicate that further investigation should be performed to replace the ligament by a prosthesis, reproducing at least two of the basic structural elements of the natural ligament. From a biomechanical point of view, this type of design seems to be interesting since the biomechanics of the knee is nearly respected, in comparison to braided or to wove single-element prosthetic ligaments. However, this study does not give any indication on the fatigue life of the "double bundle" prosthetic ligament. It appears that this type of replacement does not consider the stress concentration, which appears in the region of the insertion. This could lead to early failure. It seems to be important to develop a design reducing the stress concentration or shearing at the bone-prosthesis interface.[42]

A 2016 work of Moewis[43] focused exclusively on the rotational laxity of the knee joint in the axial plane during passive conditions. The fundament in this investigation is the now clear role played by the ACL in the rotational stabilization of the knee joint in the axial plane, a role that — despite being considered secondary in the literature — seems crucial for the proper function of the knee joint. Evidence for this statement are the founded significant differences in axial rotational laxity between the ACL-injured and the contralateral healthy knees observed preoperatively, differences that surprisingly remained significant at higher flexion angles suggesting that the contribution in rotational stabilization by the ACL is not only limited between extension and low flexion as previously assumed. Moreover, even if the affected subject could theoretically be able to compensate and to stabilize the knee joint through muscular contraction, the continuous post-operative recovery observed in the reduction of rotational laxity and energy dissipation as well as the increase in internal rotational stiffness strengthen the need of ligament reconstruction as the only way to achieve a proper recovery of function in the short term.[43] As the flexion angle increases, the axial rotation ("twisting") of the ACL bundles increases as well. At full extension, the ACL is internally twisted by approximately 10°. This internal twist increases to approximately 40° with the knee at 90°of flexion.[44]

2.1.3. *Kinematics of the Human Knee*

The kinematics of the human knee joint matches the elephant knee.[45–48] Any deviation of the helical axis from the horizontal flexion–extension axis indicates a compulsory rotation. This is true for the helical axis in extension, which runs from proximal–medial to distal–lateral and represents the screw-home motion. The only difference between the elephant and the human knee is that the human screw-home motion is smaller, i.e. 10° instead of 16° during flexion from 60° until maximal extension.[46,47] The cause of the screw-home motion is the oblique path of the PCL isometric bundle, which is attached to the inner side of the medial femoral condyle.[49] In higher mammals, the most anterior (cranial) PCL fibers usually originate from the roof of the inter-condylar fossa, and hence they are purely aligned in the sagittal plane. These fibers, however, are missing in the elephant knee. Thus, all PCL fibers are oblique, which explains the greater extent of screw-home rotation.

2.1.4. *Spiraling of Fascicles*

In collagen type I, repeating sequences of amino acids spontaneously form a left-handed helix of procollagen, with three of these helixes combining to form a right-handed helix of tropocollagen. Five tropocollagen molecules then coil in a staggered helical array, which lengthens longitudinally by the addition of more tropocollagen to form a microfibril, with higher arrangements forming fibrils, fibers and fascicles. Collagen appears at several different hierarchical levels within bones, tendons, ligaments and fascia.

Logarithmic spirals such as golden spirals (with a growth factor of $\varphi = 1.6180339887$, the golden ratio) are ubiquitous in Nature and are seen in arrangements of leaves, seeds, pinecones and many different arrangements in Nature. Such spiral patterns are frequently observed and utilized in a variety of phenomena including galaxies, biological organisms, as well as turbulent flows.

While Fibonacci spirals are everywhere in Nature, and indeed common in art and in architecture; in a laboratory setting, spontaneous assembly of such patterns has rarely been realized in mechanical tests, and never before on skin.

The helical architecture of collagen fascicles may be related to the alternative rotation of the pelvis during locomotion. As a matter of fact, two schools of thought have emerged over the years regarding locomotion. The first and oldest idea was that the legs played a primary role in human gait. Walking was simply a motion of the legs carrying its passive passenger, the trunk. In contrast, the theory of the spinal-engine held that the spine was the predominant machinery involved with gait as inherited from our ancestor, the fish. Since both legs and spine are involved in locomotion, the problem is to elucidate their respective roles.

Most studies of the knee ligaments were done using the pedestrian theory of human locomotion, which prioritizes the observation, and analysis of leg movement; this theory holds that the lower extremities are the primary tools by which humans ambulate; the trunk, head and upper extremities are considered "passengers".

Although the legs are obviously important factors in efficient locomotive activities, are they really the primary driving force behind body movement?

In the early 1900's, Robert Lovett, developed theories based on the assumption that a rotational component was essential to human movement. His research concluded that in the presence of normal lumbar lordosis, side bending produced an axial torque (side bending to one side and rotation to the other) which he labeled "coupled motion".

In 1988, Serge Gracovetsky, expounded on this idea in his book titled "Spinal Engine" by declaring that the legs were not responsible for gait but merely "instruments of expression." He theorized that during heel strike, kinetic energy was not displaced into the earth as in the pedestrian model, but efficiently transmitted up through the myofascial system causing the spine to resonate in the gravitational field.

Therefore, during right-legged weight bearing, the lumbar spine is pulled into right side bending (left rotation) by the multifidus, the longissimus, the iliocostalis and the thoracolumbar fascia (TLF). This action counter-rotates the pelvis as the sacrum is forced into left side bending and right rotation.

During the stance phase of walking, rotary motion is translated through the core causing storage of potential energy in deep collagen structures such as the annular disc fibers and the TLF. As the spine unwinds, a pulse of kinetic (movement) energy counter-rotates the torso and pelvis and with help from four major myofascial spring systems, propels the body forward in space.

Based on the conservation of angular momentum during the motion of the pelvis during gait, Gracovetsky[50] showed that the pelvis cannot be driven from below and must be driven from above. Somehow, the spine generates the necessary forces to drive the pelvis. He introduced the Spinal Engine Theory where he hypothesized that the motion of the spine first achieved locomotion and that legs came after as an improvement not as a substitute. Spirals are shown both in the shapes of the leg and the arm bones and in the interaction between them at the joints.

2.1.5. *Chinese Handcuffs as a Spring-Like Resilience Model*

These were tubes of woven straw, which expand when compressed and contract when elongated, allowing one's fingers to enter the tube from both ends but preventing the withdrawal of the fingers when they were pulled away. After either compression or elongation or twisting, the spiral double helix weave pattern will always return to its original shape by its own momentum. This model is closer to a spring than a lever/pull model and reflects the knee spring-like resilience.

A helix has the most efficient kinetic storage potential. It can integrate both angular and linear momentum separately or simultaneously. A coil spring is the most obvious example of this property. When returning to the physical design of the body, many things make much more sense. It becomes easier to picture walking as a spiraling action of the whole body rather than seeing it as powered by a sequential series of lever/pull actions.

Running, throwing, kicking, swinging objects such as baseball bats, golf clubs, skiing; all are exaggerations of the overall coiling, spiraling, and uncoiling, counter spiraling action of walking. In other words, walking is the warmup practice and the mild maintenance of the body's capacity for these larger actions. Let's look at what happens with the initiation of a step.[50] At the knee, the close-packed position of the support leg allows the tibia to counter the medial rotation of the femur with a lateral rotation or, more precisely, a torque. Therefore, in only the preparation to take a step, a spiral pattern is already in evidence in the bony structure and tissue response of pelvis and leg.

If one were to stand into the left leg, the lumbar vertebrae will side-bend left and rotate right. This facilitates the pelvis in the rotation that responds to the right leg swinging forward. Meanwhile, the thoracic spine will counter-rotate to the left. This happens to assist the torso in centering its mass over the support leg and the pelvic and the shoulder girdle in coordinating a balanced counterspiral. In other words, the spine met and continued the spiral action of the leg and the pelvis.

The bracing effect of the TLF on the lower lumbar spine and the sacroiliac joints, essential for proper load transfer between spine and legs, can only be adequately described if the caudal part of the TLF is included.[51] The fascia lata of the leg and especially the most pronounced part, the iliotibial tract, can be expanded and tensioned by the large vastus lateralis muscle. For example, when a soccer player kicks the ball while the standing leg is flexed, both the vastus lateralis and gluteus maximus will be active. The gluteus maximus couples the leg to the hipbones and to the TLF. Activation of the multifidus and the erector muscles and the subsequent tension through the erector spinal aponeurosis (all lying within the TLF envelope) develop a strong extension effect on the lower spine and a nutation effect on the sacrum.

2.1.6. *Crimping of Collagen and Auxetic Behavior*

Auxetic materials are those, which show counter-intuitive reaction to the applied force meaning, in contrast to the materials, which thin transversely under axial tensile force, these materials thicken. Poisson's ratio is a measure of the transverse strain relative to longitudinal strain.[52] Evans termed the "Auxetics" from Greek word "auxetos" which means "that may be increased."[53] Figure 4 compares the conventional and the auxetic materials during loading in Y direction.

In 2015, Gatt *et al.*[55] reported that Achilles tendons exhibit this very unusual mechanical property of a negative Poisson's ratio meaning that they get fatter rather than thinner when stretched. This report is backed by *in vivo* and *ex vivo* experiments, which clearly confirm auxeticity in this living material for strains that corresponds to those experienced during most normal everyday activities. This new information, which is not limited to the human Achilles tendon, can form the scientific basis for the design of better ligament prosthesis that could replace damaged ligaments.

From a structural perspective, ligaments and tendons are hierarchical structures: triple helices of tropo-collagen form fibers, which in turn form fibrils, fascicles and eventually ligaments/tendons. They display a waveform or a crimped structure when relaxed,[56] with most recent studies describing it as helical.[57,58] Stretching ligaments at low strains results in the disappearance of this crimping.[59] This initial deformation corresponds to the "toe-region" of the stress–strain curve and is followed by the "elastic region", a zone in which, due to further stretching, the fibers and the fascicles slide against each other, eventually returning to their original shape when the load is released.

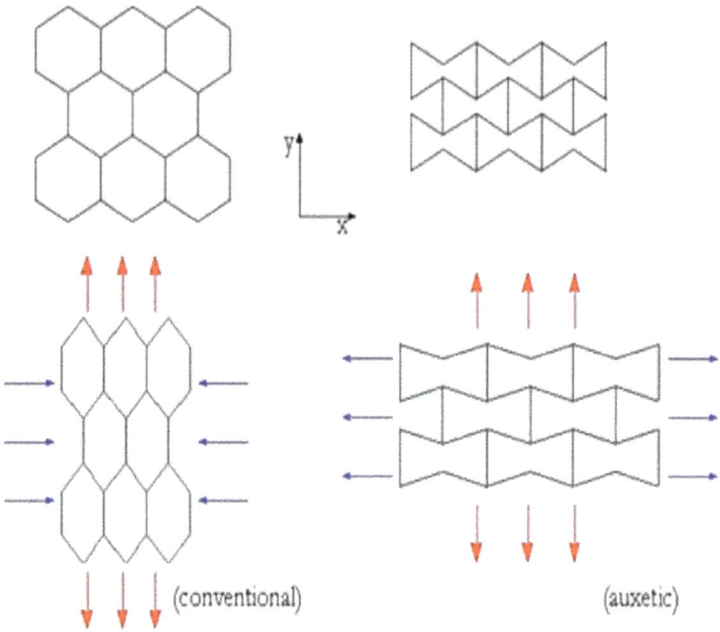

Figure 4. Loading in the Y-direction of a conventional and auxetic honeycomb structure[54]

It is beyond the scope of this work to provide an explanation for the causes of auxeticity, as this requires further in-depth studies. However, in light of the fact that auxeticity was measured in the toe-region of the stress–strain curve, where tendons/ligaments are reported to have a crimped structure,[60] it may be hypothesized that this feature of tendons is likely to play a role in the generation of this observed anomalous behavior.

This may be further corroborated when taking into consideration the work of Hansen *et al.*[59] Raspanti *et al.*[61] and Grima *et al.*[62] together. Raspanti and co-workers[61] showed that the crimps in tendons do not follow a smooth wave, but the fibrils tend to change direction abruptly resulting in large discontinuities. This crimp structure is like the crumpled paper model, which was used by Grima *et al.*[62] to describe auxetic behavior in graphene having defects. Further to this, Hansen and co-workers[59] showed that upon elongation, the crimp structure in tendons straightens from the outside to the center of the fascicle.

Taken together, these observations do suggest that upon loading, the crimp structure deforms in a way similar to a crumpled paper resulting in the observed negative Poisson's ratio. Obviously, such auxeticity in one of the planes is necessarily accompanied by a positive Poisson's ratio in the orthogonal plane, a property, which is not only characteristic of tendons but also of other systems such as ligaments, which exhibit auxeticity as a result of unfolding of wavy structures including graphene and crushed papers.

Furthermore, auxeticity in these bio-structures is most probably an evolved trait. This is because negative Poisson's ratios may give tendons/ligaments a number of advantages, which result in better functionality. For example, tendons have some viscoelastic character,[63] i.e. the presence of auxeticity may also enhance their damping capability by changing stresses and deformations present within the tendon as a function of time.[64]

Structural hierarchy and heterogeneity are inherent features in biological materials, but their significance in affecting the system behaviors is yet to be fully understood. The multilevel architectures can confer unique properties to the structure. Hierarchical structures are found in practically all complex systems, particularly naturally occurring ones and can give extremal values of unexpected properties such as negative Poisson's ratios.[65] Re-entrant foam structure is an example of "structural networks,"[66–71] that manifest a negative Poisson's ratio, whereas their components at the molecular or microscale level have positive Poisson's ratios. Among structural networks are molecular networks,[71] hierarchical structures,[65] composites[72] and hinged structures.[69,70] Negative Poisson's ratios were also observed in some materials near phase transitions.[74]

2.1.7. *Gladyschev's Principle of Substance Stability and Thermodynamics*

Living systems can be regarded as quasi-closed systems, in which quasi-equilibrium processes take place during certain scales of times.[74]

In fact, nature tends to the maximum of relative stability of structures at all hierarchical levels and sublevels of living systems. During the formation, or self-assembly, of the most thermodynamically stable structures at the highest hierarchical level (j), e.g. the supramolecular level, in accordance with the second law, spontaneously uses predominantly the least thermodynamically stable structures belonging to a lower level, for example, the molecular level (j–1). This principle is proved on a quantitative basis as applied to the molecular and to the supramolecular structural levels of biological tissues.

Physical substantiation of the principle stems from the known statement that nature tends to Gibbs energy minima. Gladyshev[74] specified the statement and asserted that nature tends to minima of specific Gibbs energies of formation of individual allotted structures at all hierarchical levels. This assertion means that nature tends to maximum stability of locally individual structures at all hierarchical levels.

As it was already mentioned, the directional action of the principle results from that the specific Gibbs energy of formation of hierarchical structures tends to a minimum. It should be stressed again that this tendency also agrees with the statement that the above structures tend to maximum stability. This successive thermodynamic self-organization (condensation or self-assembly) at the *i*th level is accompanied by chemical transformations and metabolism. These dynamic processes are very close to equilibrium.

2.2. *Enthesis*

The development of an artificial prosthesis for reconstruction/repair of ACL injuries is of increasing interest due to the need for viable tissue and reduced surgically related co-morbidity. An optimal prosthesis design is still elusive; therefore, an improved understanding of the bone–soft tissue interface is extremely urgent because the mechanism of the failure of tendon/ligament surgeries is not yet well comprehended on a molecular level.

In 2017, Wu *et al.*[75] used Raman spectral mapping to analyze, at the micron level, the chemical composition and corresponding structure of the bone-soft tissue interface. Line-mapping procedure was performed on the ACL bone insertion sites. The results suggest that different sources of interface show different boundaries, even if they seem to have the same components. Compared to the common histology results, it provided intact molecular information that can easily distinguished some relative component change.

Surgical treatment is often required and allows for possibly complete recovery; however, structural/mechanical failure rates at the surgical site of the graft have been often reported.

The tendon-to-bone insertion combines two different tissues via a gradual transition in composition, in mechanical properties, and in structure. The surgical repair outcomes are poor until now since these do not mimic the natural attachment. To date, more and more researchers focus on this area to try to identify the mechanical and the physiological functions and to compose the biomaterials that mimic the Nature structure of insertion.[76] Some researches use osteo-tendinous scaffolds, which contain opposing gradients of mineral content that resemble the Nature insertion.[77] Liu, Thomopoulos *et al.*;[78] showed that stress concentrations can be reduced by a biomimetic grading of material properties. However, the best design should be based on the full understanding of the target components.

These data can be used (1) to understand how the structure of the components change; (2) to compare the components' changes based on these structures. So, all that data can be used to imitate the biomimetic prosthesis to fulfill the ideal concept that was introduced by Hench *et al.* (2002).[79] Those data not only affirmed the former results of the randomized clinical trial (RCT) bone interface, but also provided the major information of the gradient of the insertion. In addition, those data not only deliver the ratio of the different components' changes, but also testified that the diverse interface vary in gradients. All those give the following prosthesis designer powerful evidence to make the real biomaterials for the synthetic ligament.

2.3. *Neurology of the Ligament*

The ligaments of the human body have long been considered as passive structures, and all types of reconstruction by grafts or by prostheses restore only the mechanical role of the ligament. Gladly, with the identification of specific intra-ligamentous sensory organs, their sensory role has been discussed. It is likely that the neurophysiological proprioceptive functions of ligaments are as important as their biomechanical role in maintaining joint stability.[80] In 1992, Yahia *et al.*[81] performed a study on the presence of mechanoreceptors within the substance of canine cruciate ligaments. The authors used the modified gold-chloride technique and identified Pacinian, Vater-Pacini, and Ruffini end organs and Ruffini-type receptors.[81] These results were confirmed by an immunohistochemical study conducted by Rivard *et al.*[82]; Rivard *et al.*[83] Although the mechanoreceptors have been identified, their function and classification are still to be established. Recently a 3D reconstruction of these nerve endings revealed their 3D morphology.[36] This investigation could bring some information on the function and classification of the receptors present in the cruciate ligaments.

Nerves present within ligamentous substance originate from nerves innervating muscles.[81] This idea, although well documented, has not been incorporated in the broad concept of prosthetic treatment. The peripheral nerves have significant self-repair capabilities. After an injury, the nerve ending goes through a specialized biological process aimed at creating the required conditions to regenerate. However, it is a slow process that can occasionally go wrong. Spontaneous repair of the peripheral nerves is possible thanks to Schwann cells, which cover the nerve fibers with an insulating layer of myelin. This greasy layer protects nerves and increases the transmission speed of nerve impulses. In 2018, Gomis-Coloma *et al.*[84] have discovered how the nerve (axon) induces the production of the myelin layer by the Schwann cell, so that communication is properly restored after damage. These findings may also be important to improve the mechanoreceptor regeneration in ligament grafts.

Natural ligaments are protected by a reflex: Tension present in the ligament is sensed by the mechanoreceptors and this tension stimulates reflex inhibition of the muscles knee joint. Since this role is absent in the prosthetic ligament, this is another reason for the failure of the prostheses presently existing on the market or under study.

Proprioceptive incorporation is a big challenge in biomimetic prostheses: How existing "Pacini corpuscles" or "Ruffini endings" can be incorporated into a prosthesis, or how can their role be replaced to prevent early failure of the synthetic ligament? For the time being, the only solution is to keep the remnants of the torn ligament and to combine their use to the use of a graft. However, the main obstacle with autografts is that they require big tunnels (around 10 mm) which destroy completely the remnants and their attachments.

2.3.1. *ACL Remnant*

A satisfactory outcome of ACL reconstruction depends not only on the tightness or on the strength of the graft but also on the quality of proprioceptive restoration. Mechanoreceptors of ACL are supposed to play considerable roles in the proprioceptive feedback system of knee. Mechanoreceptors in joint capsules and ligaments work through a feedback system to control the reflex activity of the muscles acting around the joint, thereby preventing abnormal movements of the joint. Since Schultz *et al.*[85] first reported the existence of mechanoreceptors in human ACL, it was subsequently established that the receptors included not just Pacinian, Ruffini or Golgi tendon type bodies, but also numerous nerve endings distributed all over the ACL.[81,86]

Although mechanoreceptors have been postulated to be an important component of neurophysiological feedback mechanisms, whether they can regenerate in the grafts after the excision of native tissues is not yet clear. Denti *et al.*[87] reported that in experimental sheep, ACL reconstruction with autologous patellar tendon resulted in the presence of mechanoreceptors in the reconstructed ACL. Mechanoreceptors were absent in cases where artificial grafts were used alone after complete removal of native remnants.

A 2017 study carried out by Sha *et al.*[88] aimed to observe the survival condition and the quantitative variation of mechanoreceptors in the tibial remnant of the ruptured ACL in human knees. Residual mechanoreceptors were found in the tibial remnants of ruptured ACL in human knees and were identified clearly by using immunohistochemistry staining.

Ruffini-like corpuscles were the most primary mechanoreceptors in the ACL remnant. It was believed that the residual mechanoreceptors have a long-term survival and a strong viability after the ACL torn. The remnant may provide a source for a faster reinnervation of the graft and a more favorable milieu for the restoration of proprioceptive function if it is preserved during ACL reconstruction.

In a 2017 study, Chun *et al.*[89] verified the presence of mechanoreceptors in both remnant ACL tissue and Achilles allografts by using immunohistochemistry staining with monoclonal antibodies against S-100 and immunocytochemical assessment with monoclonal antibodies against Nestin to visualize mechanoreceptor-positive cells.

Although the nerve regeneration process was studied largely in the context of nerve transections, very few studies have been aimed at developing strategies to improve it in the context of ligament healing or reconstruction.[90]

The molecular and the cellular mechanisms regulating neovascularization and axon regrowth after peripheral nerve (PN) injury are poorly understood. However, Wang *et al.* suggest that angiogenesis and neurogenesis are closely linked[91] and are likely modulated by the innate immune response to PN injury.[92] Macrophages are hypothesized to respond to direct endothelial cell migration and to the formation of new blood vessels in hypoxic tissues. In turn, newly formed blood vessels have been shown to guide Schwann cells and hence axon regrowth across P*N* injuries.[93,94] In support of these observations, alternatively activated, anti-inflammatory (M2-like) macrophages are linked to improved PN remodeling and positive outcomes,[95] so anti-inflammatory signaling can increase Schwann cell differentiation and migration[96] and axon growth.[92] Moreover, PN-specific ECM bioscaffolds can increase M2-like macrophage polarization and Schwann cell migration.[97]

Studies have shown that nerve wraps can release bioactive factors directly into wrapped nerves that can positively modulate both peripheral and central nerve regeneration.[98,99]

Carbon nanotubes (CNTs) are other types of conducting polymers, which have electrical conductivity. Functionalized CNTs are useful for promoting neural signal transport and help dendrite elongation and cell adhesion.[100] One of the ways to functionalize CNTs include substitution reactions such as replacement of carbon atoms from the tube wall by boron or nitrogen.[100] In a study by Bosi *et al.*,[101] dissociated embryonic rat hippocampal neurons on a mat of multi-walled CNTs (MWNTs) were deposited onto a polyethyleneimine (PE*I*) covered glass. In this condition, neurons could grow and elongate their neurites in all directions.[101]

In 2009, the group of Dr. Yahia[102] patented a biocompatible and biodegradable CNTs-based fiber capable of stimulating and sustaining cell proliferation and nerve regeneration. The biocompatible and biodegradable CNTs-based fiber comprise at least one CNT; a biodegradable copolymer; and a coagulating polymer. These biodegradable CNTs could be incorporated into synthetic ligaments to allow mechanoreceptors regeneration.

2.3.2. *Anterolateral Ligament and Combined Intra- and Extra-articular Reconstruction*

The anterolateral ligament (ALL) is the newest anatomical finding in the orthopedic world of medicine to date. The presence of the ALL in the different anatomical studies ranges from 83 to 100%, and it has been postulated that the ALL plays a significant role in knee rotatory stability, mainly in tibial internal rotation.[103] Rotational stability control is a topic that attracts the attention of experts in the field of ACL reconstruction (ACLR) surgery. It remains uncertain whether the current arthroscopic ACLR techniques are sufficient to provide rotational stability in all cases of this ligament injury, and it is not fully understood how the different patterns of ACL injuries behave.[104]

Dr. Steven Claes and Dr. Johan Bellemans[105] are two orthopedic surgeons from the University Hospital of Leuven that have spent 4 years researching pivot shifts in the knee and why they still seem to occur even after the ACL had been successfully operated on. As it happens, the theory that an extra ligament could exist on knee has been suggested around since 1879 when a French surgeon named Paul Segond[106] documented his findings. The Belgian surgeons from

Leuven further examined this hypothesis in order to solve the mystery as to the continuing complaint of joint pivot shifts, and they managed to confirm positively the theory (Figure 5).[103]

A 2018 study showed that isolated ACLR and double-bundle reconstruction do not provide sufficient control over the pivot shift.[107] The residual pivot shift rate after isolated single-bundle ACL reconstruction ranges from 10% to 20%. Furthermore, the lack of knee rotational control appears to act as a causal factor for new chondral and meniscal lesions.[108] Double-bundle reconstruction, which also reconstructs the posterolateral bundle of the ACL, was expected to improve rotational control but published results are not conclusive. However, in a 2015 meta-analysis of RCTs, it was shown that anterolateral reconstruction (ALR) is effective for reducing the rates of residual pivot shift and re-tear when compared to isolated ACL reconstruction.[109] Biomechanical studies confirm the benefit of ALR in

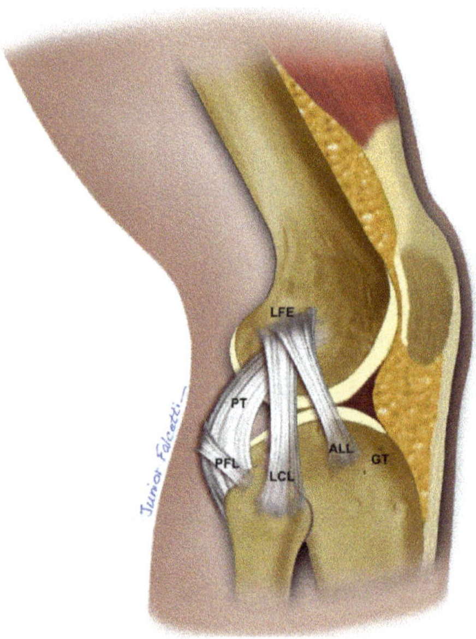

Figure 5. Anatomy of the anterolateral ligament described in previous studies. LFE lateral femoral epicondyle, ALL anterolateral ligament, GT Gerdy's tubercle, PT popliteus tendon, PFL popliteal–fibular ligament[103]

controlling medial tibial rotation. The ALL is an anatomical structure that provides a link between the pivot shift and the possibility of controlling it through the mechanical action of ALR.

When compared to historical ACL reconstruction data, combined intra- and extra-articular reconstruction does not increase the complication rate or further stiffen the joint.[110] At a mean follow-up of 6.8 years, it provides better control over the pivot shift; along with a low re-tear rate and low rate of secondary meniscus damage. These findings confirm that initial meniscus damage contributes to the development of osteoarthritis (OA) and show that combined ACL/ALL reconstruction helps to protect the cartilage when the menisci are healthy.

Finally, while the indications must still be refined, ALR can be proposed to young patients undergoing ACL reconstruction who participate in high-intensity pivot sports, have a high-grade pivot shift or who have a failed ACL reconstruction.[109]

3. Improving the Design

3.1. *Techniques for Creating the Femoral Tunnel*

An increase in the indications of independent techniques for femoral drilling in ACLR has been observed represented by the transportal or inside-out technique (TP), outside-in (OI), and OI retrograde. In 2013, the Canadian Orthopedic Association reported that 68% of surgeons used independent techniques for femoral drilling and only 31% used the transtibial technique (TT). Despite this technical change in ACLR in the past decade, there is still doubt about its objective and subjective clinical superiority, as well as the biomechanical advantages of the different techniques used.[104]

In fact, the techniques, TT, TP or others, that are used to drill the tunnels, do not appear to be the key factor for success. The key point is that the tunnel has to be drilled in the right place and in the right direction.[111]

Study of ACLR failures shows that half of them are due to technical faults. This is true for all types of transplants and especially for those involving synthetic materials, which are less tolerant than autogenous tissues.

As a whole, the ACL is not isometric. The AM bundle is taut in extension and is relaxed for a 90° knee flexion while the PL bundle is taut in flexion and is relaxed in extension. However, some transitional fibers are close to isometry.

In Figure 6, anatomical and radiological studies have been performed on cadavers' knees and per-operatively. The femoral isometric zone (F) is located at the center of the femoral attachment in between the AM and the PL bundles and is the center of a 140° circular arc, which is formed on every human knee by the posterior border of the lateral condyle. The radius of this circle varies from 17 to 26 mm. On average, point F is located at 59% of the antero-posterior length of the condyle, measured on a line parallel to the Blumensaat line and is starting from the top of the posterior condyle. It is remarkable that this arc of a circle of 140° corresponds to the human knee average range of motion. By geometrical definition, the center of this arc is

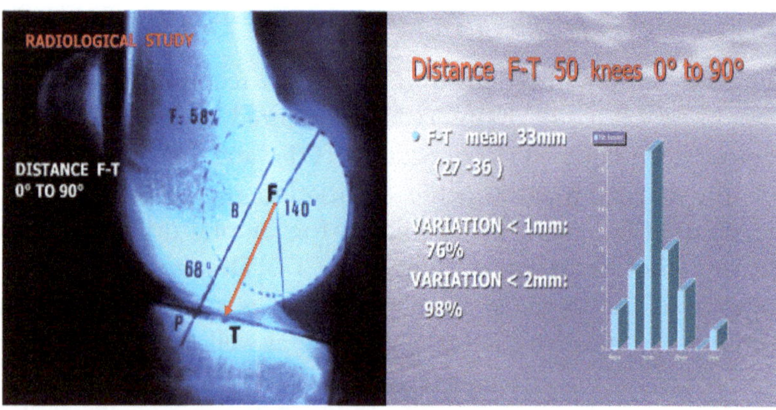

Figure 6. Anatomical and radiological studies on 50 normal knees have been performed on cadavers' knees and per-operatively: The femoral isometric zone (F) is located at the center of the femoral attachment in between the AM and the PL bundles and is the center of a 140° circular arc. The distance between the femoral center and the tibial center F-T does not vary of more than 2 mm in 98% of the cases from extension to flexion

the only point that stays at the same distance from the periphery of the posterior condyle during full motion, making logical that there is no change in length nor tension of the fibers, which are attached to this point.

Same measures were done on the tibial side. They show that the center of the tibial attachment (average 19 mm long) corresponds to the center of the total antero-posterior length of the tibial plateau as it appears on a lateral X-ray (see Figure 6), or 42% from the front of the medial plateau. The distance between the femoral center and the tibial center does not vary of more than 2 mm in 98% of the cases from extension to flexion. This strongly suggests that the fibers inserted at this place are close to isometric. This has been confirmed in 2013 by an independent computer study by Dabirrahmani *et al.*[112]

In consequence, it appears that:

1. Each knee is different as the radius of the femoral circle varies with patients. It means that per-operatively the same landmarks should not be used for everyone as far as isometry is concerned. It is easy to have a pre-operative X-ray lateral view to determine where the center of that specific arc of a circle is for this specific patient.
2. The usual techniques of drilling the femoral tunnel close to the posterior wall favors the reconstruction of the AM bundle. Nonetheless, it is very inappropriate when using synthetic fibers. It explains why, a few years ago, it appeared the need to make a double bundle reconstruction with autogenous transplants to improve the stability for each position of the knee.
3. It is as efficient but way easier and safer to perform a one-bundle technique from the center of the circle, especially with synthetic ligaments as well as with autogenous transplants. In fact, quite often, the wall between the two tunnels is very thin and fragile and the two tunnels quickly become a one big tunnel that may cause some difficulties in case of revision.

As photographed in Figure 7 the anatomic view of the ACL of a right knee, with the knee in full extension on the left side and then in flexion at 120° on the right side, it is obvious that the PL bundle and

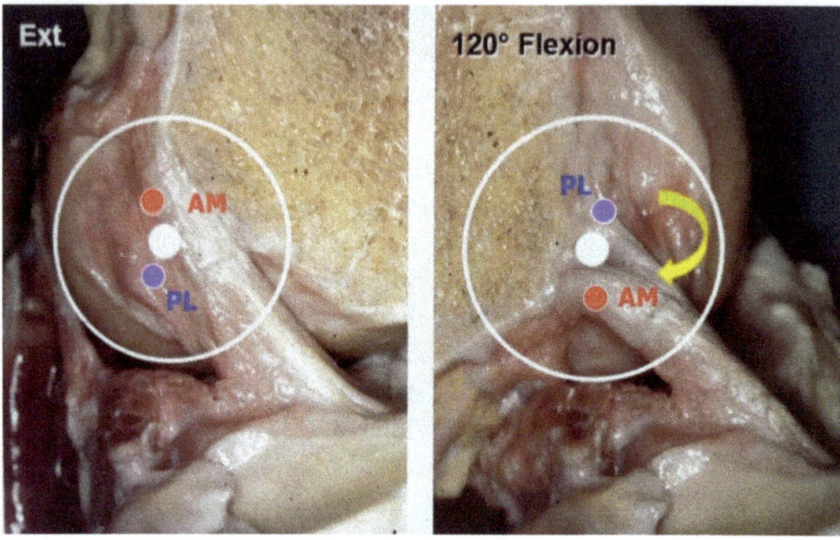

Figure 7. Anatomic view of the ACL of a right knee, with the knee in full extension on the left side and then in flexion at 120° on the right side

the AM bundle cannot be and that they are not isometric. In fact, they rotate clockwise around the center of the femoral attachment. It is clear that there is a huge change in length of each bundle between flexion and extension. This change in length is not compatible with synthetic fibers. The center is the isomeric zone and it must be the center of the femoral tunnel when performing a single bundle reconstruction.

As shown in Figure 8, the posterior condyle is a perfect arc of a circle of 140° and the center of the ACL attachment is the center of this circle. This strongly suggests that the center of the tunnel should be placed at this precise point. Here, before X-ray, the lateral condyle has been surrounded by a metallic wire and a drill is bit inserted from the center of the ACL attachment until it is flush to the lateral wall.

It is a controversial subject but more and more authors in recent studies come to the same conclusion. Nonetheless, some famous and fair knee surgeons came to think differently. Dr. Frank Noyes[113] himself said: "I am afraid we may have trained a generation of surgeons' improper surgical technique." Moreover, Dr. Freddie Fu said:

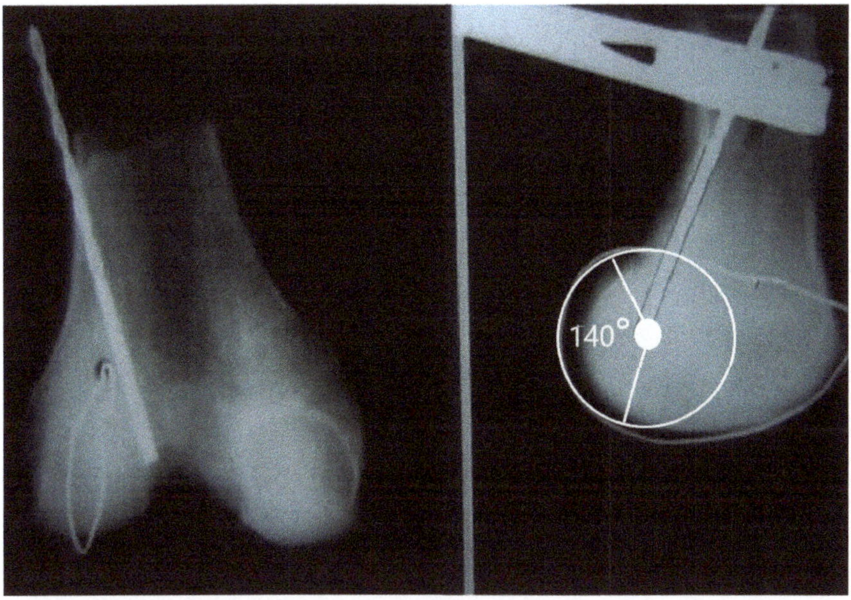

Figure 8. Posterior condyle is a perfect arc of a circle of 140° and the center of the ACL attachment is the center of this circle

"I have done over 3000 ACL reconstructions. Maybe the last 500 were correct."

In 2010, Yuki Kato *et al.*[109] published in Knee Surgery, Sports Traumatology, Arthroscopy, a study on the effect of tunnel position for anatomic ACL single bundle reconstruction on knee biomechanics in a porcine model (see Figure 9). When positioning the entrance of the tunnels in the middle of the femoral and of the tibial ACL attachments (here called MID-MID), they found that this position provided the best stability and more closely restored normal knee kinematics. "MID-MID" had similar results as double bundle reconstruction.

3.2. *Direction of Insertion Tunnels*

Another problem with ACL prostheses is that the angle between the ligament and its insertion tunnels causes combined torsion, bending,

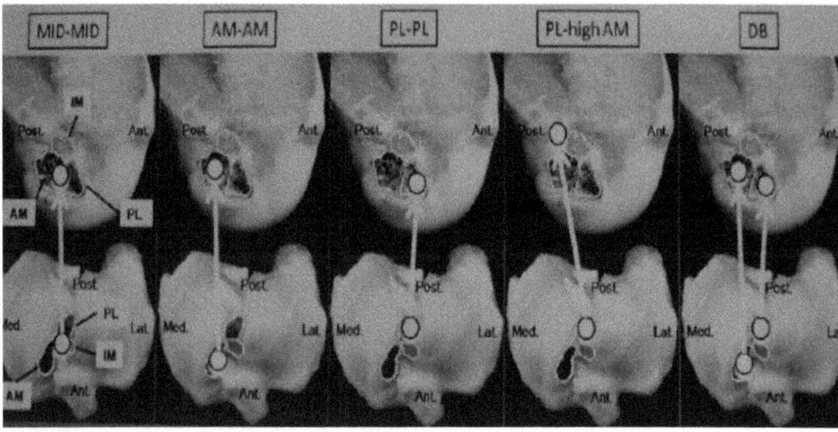

Figure 9. Effect of tunnel position for anatomic ACL single bundle reconstruction on knee biomechanics in a porcine model. MID-MID position provided the best stability and more closely restored normal knee kinematics. "MID-MID" had similar results as double bundle reconstruction[109]

and elongation loading at the ligament insertion tunnel junction. This combined loading not present in the natural ligament may be part of the reason that prosthetic ligaments fail prematurely *in vivo*. Therefore, to design a successful prosthetic ligament, it is important to consider this *in vivo* loading to choose insertion sites, which minimize combined loading. The optimal insertion of a ligament graft should be one which minimizes the deformations caused by high non-functional loads. Yoshiya *et al.*[115] defined optimal orientation of the prosthetic tunnels to be such that the bending and elongation imposed on the graft through the range of motion is minimal. Moreover, the torsional deformation of the prosthesis also has to be taken into account.[116] This parameter should be added to define the optimal orientation of the insertion tunnels. In the actual reconstruction procedure, orientation of the bony tunnels is limited because of problems with surgical accessibility due to the design of OI drill guide and soft tissue around the knee. Using a mathematical model, Drouin *et al.*[116] studied the tunnel orientation, which minimizes each of the three parameters. Results showed that the optimal orientation of the bone tunnels was

20° anteriorly in sagittal and 15° laterally from the isometric point for the femur.

Drouin *et al.*,[116] Gely *et al.*,[117] studied the optimal direction for the bonny tunnels by *in vivo* measurements using a 3D geometric virtual system with sensors fixed on the knee and a magnetic field. To minimize bending, torsion, and elongation, they demonstrated that the best option was to have a perfect alignment of the femoral and of the tibial tunnels passing through the isometric femoral and tibial zones with a 50° knee flexion.

Figure 10 shows the flexion extension and longitudinal rotation axes about which the femur and tibia can be said to rotate, respectively. Drouin *et al.* found that this model greatly simplifies the interpretation of the ACL ligament deformation analyses.[116,117] For example, in Figure 10 femoral tunnel orientations parallel to the flexion extension axis are those having maximal torsion loading,

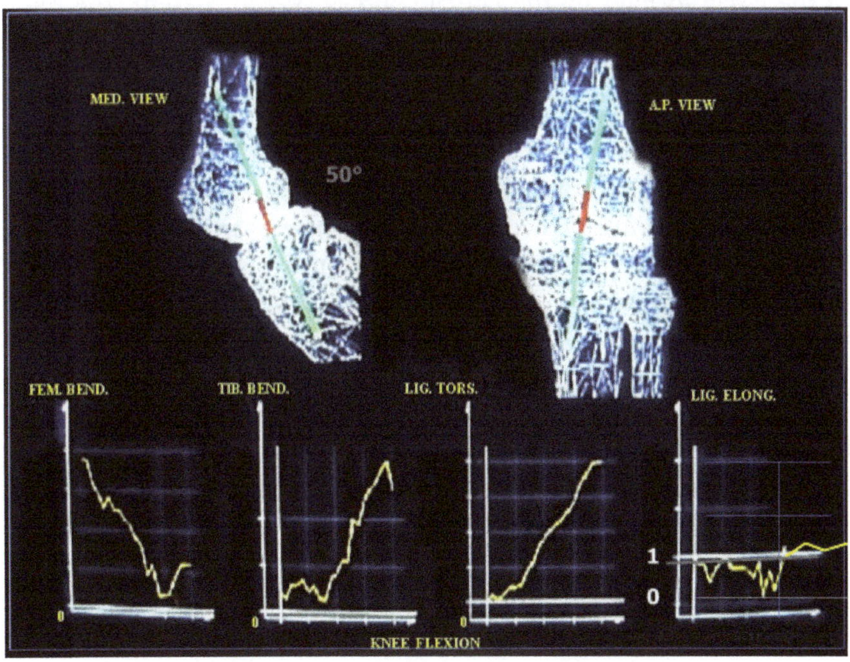

Figure 10. Orientation of tunnels[116,117]

whereas insertions perpendicular to the flexion extension axis were found to have maximal bending. This simplified relationship between complex knee movement and prosthetic deformation has implications for both graft design and surgical implantation planning.

3.3. *Proposal for a Surgical Procedure*

It is one thing to know what should be done and another thing to make it in a safe and reproducible manner. Since 1992, Laboureau proposed a technique, which complies with the requirements said before about isometry, direction of tunnels, and preservation of remnants.

First, as presented in Figure 11 the knee is in full flexion. Under arthroscopy and the help of an image intensifier giving a lateral image of the condyles, a K wire is positioned, through an antero-medial portal and flush to anterior border of the tibial plateau, at the center of the circle formed by the lateral condyle. When present, the remnants are not removed.

Second, the K-wire is pushed through the lateral condyle until it exits through the skin (see Figure 12). Then the drill is placed on the proximal side and the K-wire removed from distal to proximal until the tip is inside the notch, allowing to put the knee around 50° of flexion. Under control of the scope, the trocar tip of the K-wire is placed in the posterior part of the footprint of the stump and then it is drilled down into the tibia until it exits from the medial aspect of the tibial metaphysis.

Last, the K-wire passes through the femoral and tibial isometric points (see Figure 13). The tunnels are drilled with cannulated drill bits from OI. The tunnels are perfectly aligned with the knee around 50° of flexion. The ligament is then pulled through the tunnels and it is fixed first on the femoral side with a titanium interference screw. The isometry is controlled to avoid any over tightening whatever is the position given to the knee before tibial fixation.

This quite simple procedure allows respecting what should be the five "holy rules" of ACLR using synthetic ligaments:

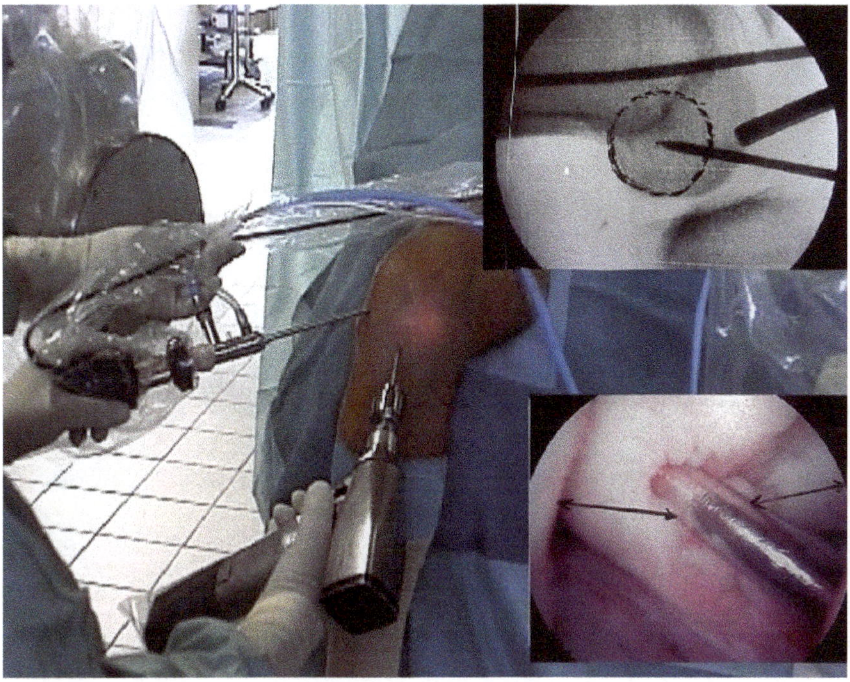

Figure 11. Knee is in full flexion. Under arthroscopy and the help of an image intensifier giving a lateral image of the condyles, a K wire is positioned, through an antero-medial portal and flush to anterior border of the tibial plateau, at the center of the circle formed by the lateral condyle. When present, the remnants are not removed

1. Isometry;
2. Alignment of tunnels;
3. Preservation of the stump for proprioception;
4. No tension to the transplant;
5. Durable and firm fixation inside the tunnels.

3.4. *Tissue and Bony Ingrowth/Biological Fixation*

It is commonly accepted that implants are set apart from the bone by an interface membrane, which, depending upon the success or the

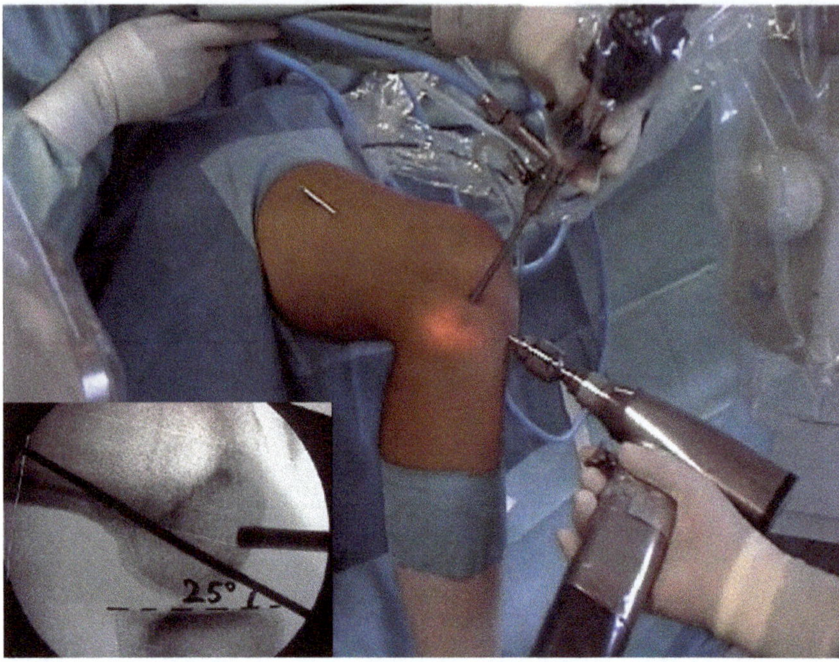

Figure 12. K-wire is pushed through the lateral condyle until it exits through the skin

failure of the reconstructive intervention, is composed of a thin connective tissue layer or a thick granulomatous-cicatrizing membrane. Success of implantation depends largely on the stability of a given device within its surroundings, whether these are hard or soft tissues. It seems that osseointegration does not take place when the carbon fiber composite ligaments (CFCL) are subjected to motion in their intraosseous tunnels and become separate from the bony bed by an interlace membrane. The condition sine qua non for osseointegration is probably the stability of the CFCL in its bony tunnel.[118]

Confirming this theory, a histomorphometric study of the tissular organization of a high-tensile polyethylene ACL prosthesis revealed widening of the intraosseous tunnels.[119] Micromotion and production of bone-resorbing factors by the organizing granulomatous tissue bone resorption seem to be responsible for the rapidly developing bone remodeling within 3 months.

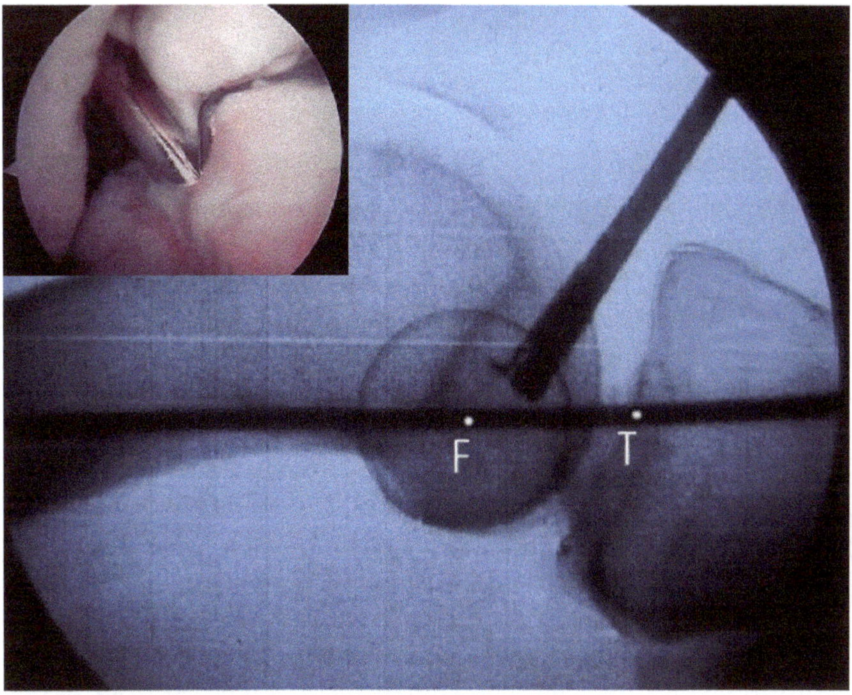

Figure 13. K-wire passes through the femoral and tibial isometric points

Marcacci *et al.* observed tissue ingrowth in the Leeds-Keio prosthetic ligament.[120] The host tissue possesses an ability to grow into the ligament and takes on the characteristics of a tissue at least partly capable of meeting its functional requirements. Fibers were oriented along the main stress planes, clearly mature in view of the presence of type I collagen, and sufficiently vascularized. Meanwhile, this study does not determine if the characteristics and strength of the tissue are comparable to those of the normal ligament.

Another study conducted by Paavolainen *et al.*[121] showed that progressive bone ingrowth in the prosthetic device permits a better pull-out behavior. They used a fixation with screws, which was strong enough to minimize the strain within the bone tunnel. This made the tissue ingrowth into the device possible. Their study is in accordance with a 1985 study of Bolton *et al.*[122] This leads to the conclusion that tissue ingrowth is an important parameter to consider in ACL replacement.

3.4.1. *Interface Tissue Engineering*

The integration of engineered ligament into bone tunnels is still concerned as a major issue. The current fixation methods do not provide the biomimetic properties of the enthesis. Tissue engineering approaches have been attempted to fabricate structures with a gradient in chemical composition and cellular contents. Two separate paradigms were established to engineer ligament enthesis. In the first approach, the insertion site was constructed upon stratified structures cultured via separate cell types.[123] These different cells would further initiate cell-mediated metaplasia and lead to natural enthesis-like tissue.[124] The second paradigm is regenerating of enthesis upon biochemically and/or mechanically stimulation of mesenchymal stem cells (MSC) to promote local cell differentiation.[125,126]

The strata constructs were composed from three phases cultured with various mature cells. The knitted mesh composed from PLGA (10:90) was cultured via fibroblast cells to mimic ligament region. The bony side, on the other hands, was constructed from sintered PLGA (85:15) and 45S5 Bioglass® microspheres followed by culturing with osteoblasts. The intermediate region, however, was comprised of sintered PLGA microspheres and it was used as an arid region.[123] This triphasic stratum enhanced proliferation of osteoblast and fibroblast and their migration into interface phase. The desired fibro-cartilaginous region, however, was not recognized through this phase.[123] This drawback was further addressed upon incorporation of chondrocytes within interface phase to regenerate fibrocartilage region within strata.[127] This fibrocartilage region, however, was not fully localized to the intended middle phase of strata.

Biochemical stimuli of MSC for promoting local differentiation was accomplished upon continuously graded scaffolds.[128] These gradients were fabricated upon incorporation of calcium phosphate components into electrospun fibers.[129–132] For instance, the nanohydroxyapatite particles were dispersed into poly(ε-caprolactone) solution and went through co-electrospinning with poly(ester urethane urea). The electrospun fibers were then treated with simulated body fluid to fabricate mineral gradient.[133] Upon proliferation of MSC cells on the graded scaffold, the formation of phenotypic gradient promoted the regeneration of ligament enthesis.[133] Despite mimicking gradient compositions of ligament interface, these structures are still in their infancy, and more investigations are required to prior to the preclinical application.

3.4.2. *Leeds-Keio*

The Leeds-Keio artificial ligament (Xiros plc., Leeds, UK), which is composed of polyethylene terephthalate (PET), has been widely used in clinical treatments. Because the fixation sites between the soft tissue and the hard tissue are mechanically the weakest regions during the early post-operative period, the rapid and robust osseointegration of artificial ligaments within bone tunnels is critical for successful ligament reconstruction. In 2011, Li *et al.*[134] demonstrated that apatite coatings on the surfaces of artificial ligaments are effective in enhancing the osseointegration of artificial ligaments within the bone tunnel. This effect was enabled because apatite is a major inorganic component of natural bone and exhibits good biocompatibility and osteoconductivity. In Li's study, an apatite coating was produced on an artificial ligament using plasma surface modification and subsequent immersion in a solution containing apatite powders.

Mutsuzaki *et al.* [135] developed an advanced biomimetic process involving a simplified alternating dipping treatment. In this process, a substrate material is precoated with amorphous calcium phosphate (ACP), which is an apatite precursor, using a simplified alternate dipping treatment followed by immersion in simulated body fluid (SBF). A continuous thin coating layer of apatite forms on the ACP-precoated substrate within 24 h in SBF. This apatite coating technique, also known as an ACP-assisted biomimetic process, provides the advantage of simplicity compared with previous biomimetic processes, which require the use of carboxymethylation, photografting, or sol–gel methods. The ACP-assisted biomimetic process was applied to a Leeds-Keio artificial ligament to prepare a thin-film apatite coating for improved osseointegration. To optimize the coating conditions, hot-pressed plate specimens from Leeds-Keio artificial ligament meshes was prepared. The plate specimens were then subjected to plasma surface modification under various conditions, followed by the alternate dipping treatment and SBF immersion. The quality of the apatite coating on the specimen and the coating adhesion to the specimen surface were evaluated as a function of the conditions (plasma power density) of the plasma surface modification. The developed plasma- and ACP-assisted biomimetic process was found to be effective in forming apatite layers on Leeds-Keio artificial ligaments.

3.4.3. *LARS*

The LARS artificial ligament was initially invented by JP Laboureau and made of *PET*. It was a "scaffold" graft but has not yet been submitted to FDA approval in the United States, and its use for the most part has occurred in Western Europe, Canada, China, Australia. LARS can be divided into two parts: the intra-articular portion and the extra-articular portion. The intra-articular portion consists of two bundles of longitudinal fibers, twisted clockwise (for right knee) or counterclockwise (for left knee) with no transverse fibers, in imitation of the ACL anatomical structure, while the extra-articular portion is knitted of longitudinal and transverse fibers to maintain together the longitudinal fibers and avoid ligament deformation. LARS has good biomechanics in terms of resisting tension, flexion, and torsion load.

The special design of the LARS ligament with open fibers in its intra-articular part was believed to be more resistant to torsional fatigue and wearing.

Li *et al.*[138] reported that composite coating of 58S bioglass and hydroxyapatite could enhance osseointegration of a PET artificial ligament in the bone tunnel. In 2011, application of the layer-by-layer hyaluronic acid chitosan coating on a PET scaffold was confirmed to be an effective procedure in inducing new collagen into the graft fibers.

In 2013, Lessim *et al.*[139] studied the effect of surface treatment of LARS ligaments using poly (sodium styrene sulphonate). The results demonstrated improvement of knee functionalities and a better adhesion of human cell lines. It was proved that the poly(sodium styrene sulphonate) grafting was a useful method in inducing fibroblast organization, and collagen and decorin deposits. Yang *et al.*[140] described a new strategy to enhance artificial ligament graft osseointegration in the bone tunnel using hydroxypropyl cellulose; the data of their study showed that the surface treatment of PET artificial ligament using hydroxypropyl cellulose might enhance graft osseointegration in the bone tunnel.

Ciobanu *et al.*[141] have developed a radical graft polymerization of polystyrene sodium sulfonate (PolyNASS) onto PET in order to enhance the interaction of the LARS ligament with fibroblasts. This method proved very efficient at accelerating their adhesion along with achieving enhanced control over the fibroblast morphology and alignment onto the PolyNaSS grafted fibers.[142]

This suggests that the PolyNASS grafting was capable of initiating bone formation, which would later on colonize the center of the ligament in a more predictable manner and hence enhance the ligament integration. This is of particular relevance as tunnel osteolysis is generally associated with the utilization of synthetic ligaments and is considered as a crucial parameter for ligament biomechanical stability.

Migonney *et al.*[143] investigated the performance of bioactive grafted PET LARS ligaments onto human osteoblasts both *in vitro* and to subsequently evaluate their osseointegration *in vivo* using an ovine relevant orthopaedic model. Taken together their results provide evidence that PolyNaSS grafting of PET ligaments, improves artificial ligament osseointegration within the bone tunnels.

4. Concluding Remarks

The advantages in using an artificial ligament are indisputable. They permit the preservation of the biological structures, a rapid functional recovery, early resumption of sports and work activities, and a shorter amount of time required for surgery. On the other hand, the clinical studies of first generations of synthetic ligaments have shown repeated synovitis reactions to the implanted material and a bad long-term functional behavior. In almost all cases, the studies reported a laxity of the knee or even a rupture of the prosthesis. This shows that artificial ligaments were not able to replace the ACL properly despite promising *in vitro* results.

Since about 10 years, publications[144] on long-term results of the latest generation of synthetic ligaments are slowly changing the minds and give us some hope. They show results that can be advantageously compared to those of classical autogenous techniques with less morbidity due to donor site problems, much faster recovery allowing to resume to normal activities including sports.

Synthetic ligaments are still having irreducible enemies who, for the majority of them, have never used the latest implants and are still sticking to the poor results of the very first trials of the years 1980 to 1990. The big initial mistake was to launch on the market ligaments which had never been seriously studied, ignoring *in vivo* stresses, biology, and even how to put them in place properly.

Since more than 25 years now, lots of improvements have been conducted. It has been understood that ligaments have to face specific stresses and that maybe the best was to try to reproduce the architecture of the natural ligament and try to place it at its anatomical position. But this anatomical position was also controversial and had first to be defined and admitted.

Nevertheless, lots of improvements have still to be done. Other materials and designs have to be tested. Lengthening of the prosthesis can be prevented by using a shape memory material, such as used by Yahia *et al.* (1993).[145] A component showing viscoelastic properties should be considered. The damping capacity of the prosthesis should be about 10–20% at physiological frequency. It is also important to develop new *in vitro* testing machines, which will give us biomechanical results close to those found by clinical analysis.

The present review of artificial ligament failure and success in the light of the biomechanics and structure of the natural ligament leads us to a biomimetic approach with an optimal design of the ligament prosthesis. Copying the structure of the natural ligament will allow us to eliminate the stress concentration which contributes to failure of the prostheses at present. Considering the biomechanical and surgical aspects determines the safety factor for the construction of the prosthesis and leads us to the development of new materials able to deal with the high demands of the biomechanics of the knee.

From these observations, new design criteria can be drawn:

- The artificial ligament should reproduce at least two of the basic structural elements of the natural ligament. It should consist of several fibers of approximately the same diameter as the fiber bundles of the natural ligament, which could share the large deformation. At least two strands should form the body of the prosthesis.
- Since it is impossible at present in daily practice to reproduce *ex nihilo* the mechanoreceptors function, the only way today is to preserve the natural stump from which it has been demonstrated that we can expect the regeneration of the mechanoreceptors. Not to remove the remnants of the torn natural ligament, ACL or PCL, should be the rule.
- It should be also important to consider a material with a greater safety factor to prevent rupture of the synthetic ligament. For structures, which have to support unpredictable loads, the safety factor should be around 2–4.

Today, the use of synthetic ligaments and tendons has slowly become "a reasonable alternative." Synthetic ACL grafts are more important than clinical nonbelievers may realize".[146] One can reasonably expect that, with the improvements due to a better knowledge of the natural physiology and the continuous research in biomechanics, biology, new materials, surgical techniques etc., synthetic implants will become a common option to treat the patients and give them easier and faster recovery. There are some promising new fibers now such as high molecular weight polyethylene (HMWPE) which have 2–3 times more tensile strength than PET and are very resistant to shearing forces.

Acknowledgments

The author would like to acknowledge the financial support from the Natural Sciences and Engineering Research Council of Canada (NSERC).

References

1. Hudson, K.; Collins, F. *JAMA,* **2015**, *313*(4), 355–356. doi:10.1001/jama.2014.10716.
2. Greenberg, S. *BMJ* **2009**, *339*, B2680. doi:10.1136/bmj.b2680.
3. Smyth, R.; Kirkham, J.; Jacoby, A.; Altman, D.; Gamble, C.; Williamson, P. *BMJ* **2011**, *342*, C7153. doi:10.1136/bmj.c7153.
4. Beauchamp, P.; Laurin, C.; Bailon, J. *Rev. Chir. Orthop. Reparatrice Appar. Mot.* **1979**, *65*(4), 197–207 (Article in French).
5. Legnani, C.; Ventura, A.; Terzaghi, C.; Borgo, E.; Albisetti, W. *Int Orthop.* **2010**, *34*(4), 465–471. doi:10.1007/s00264-010-0963-2.
6. Paulos, L. E.; Rosenberg, T. D.; Grewe, S. R.; Tearse, D. S.; Beck, C. L. *Am. J. Sports Med.* **1992**, *20*(3), 246–252. doi:10.1177/036354659202000302.
7. Wilson, W. J.; Scranton, P. E. J. *J. Bone Joint Surg. Am.* **1990**, *72*(5), 742–748.
8. Ratner, B. D. *Biomaterials.* **2007**, *28*(34), 5144–5147. doi:10.1016/j.biomaterials.2007.07.035.
9. Guidoin, M. F.; Marois, Y.; Bejui, J.; Poddevin, N.; King, M. W.; Guidoin, R. *Biomaterials.*, **2000**, *21*(23), 2461–2474.
10. Dhillon, R. S.; Schwarz, E. M.; Maloney, M. D. *Arthritis Res. Ther.* **2012**, *14*(4), 219. doi:10.1186/ar3914.
11. Hamilton, B.; Knez, W.; Eirale, C.; Chalabi, H. *Acta Orthop. Belg.* **2010**, *76*(4), 443–448.
12. Hammond, J. W.; Hinton, R. Y.; Curl, L. A.; Muriel, J. M.; Lovering, R. M. *Am. J. Sports Med.* **2009**, *37*(6), 1135–1142. doi:10.1177/0363546508330974.
13. A Hamid, M.; Mohamed Ali, M.; Yusof, A.; George, J.; Lee, L. *Am. J. Sports Med.* **2014**, *42*(10), 2410–2418. doi:10.1177/0363546514541540.

14. Reurink, G.; Goudswaard, G.; Moen, M.; Weir, A.; Verhaar, J.; Bierma-Zeinstra, S. Dutch hamstring injection therapy (HIT) study investigators. *N. Engl. J. Med.* **2014**, *370*(26), 2546–2457. doi:10.1056/NEJMc1402340.
15. Hamilton, B.; Tol, J. L.; Almusa, E.; Boukarroum, S.; Eirale, C.; Farooq, A.; Chalabi, H. *Br. J. Sports Med.*, **2015**, *49*(14), 943–950. doi:10.1136/bjsports-2015-094603.
16. Chen, T.; Jiang, J.; Chen, S. *Asia Pac. J. Sports Med. Arthrosc. Rehabil. Technol.*, **2015**, *2*(1), 15–26. doi:10.1016/j.asmart.2014.11.001.
17. Yahia, L. H.; Hagemeister, N.; Drouin, G.; Sati, M.; Rivard, C. H. *Biomimetics*, **1994**, *2*(3), 309–330.
18. Mulford, J. S.; Chen, D. *ANZ J. Surg.*, **2011**, *81*(11), 785–789.
19. CA2091833C, Jacques-Philippe Laboureau, Prosthetic ligament.
20. Nau, T.; Lavoie, P.; Duval, N. *J. Bone Joint Surg. Br.* **2002**, *84*(3), 356–360.
21. Brulez, B.; Laboureau, J.; Migonney, V.; Ciobanu, M.; Pavon-Djavid, G.; Siove, A. *U.S. Patent No. 7700147 B2.* (U.S. Patent and Trademark Office, Washington, DC, **2004**).
22. Yahia, L. H.; Drouin, G. *J. Mater. Sci.,* **1988**, *23*(10), 3750–3755. doi: 10.1007/BF00540523.
23. Woo, S. L. Y.; Young, E. P.; Kwan, M. K. *Knee Ligaments: Structure, Function, Injury, and Repair* (Raven Press, New York, **1990**).
24. Fang, F.; Lake, S. P. *Interface Focus* **2016**, *6*(1), 20150044. doi: 10.1098/rsfs.2015.0044.
25. Yahia, L. H.; Drouin, G. *J. Orthop. Res.* **1989**, *7*(2), 243–251. doi: 10.1002/jor.1100070212.
26. Girgis, F. G.; Marshall, J. L.; Monajem, A. *Clin. Orthop. Relat. Res.,* **1975**, 106, 216–231. doi:10.1097/00003086-197501000-00033.
27. Beasley, L.; Weiland, D.; Vidal, A.; Chhabra, A.; Herzka, A.; Feng, M.; West, R. *Oper. Tech. Orthopaedics* **2005**, *15*(1), 5–19. doi:10.1053/j.oto.2004.11.003.
28. Arnoczky, S. *Clin. Orthop. Relat. Res.* **1983**, 172, 19–25.
29. Amis, A.; Dawkins, G. *J. Bone Joint Surg. Br.* **1991**, *73*(2), 260–267.
30. Kurosawa, H.; Yamakoshi, K.; Yasuda, K.; Sasaki, T. *Clin. Orthop. Relat. Res.* **1991**, 265, 233–240.

31. Sapega, A.; Moyer, R.; Schneck, C.; Komalahiranya, N. *J. Bone Joint Surg. Am.* **1990**, *72*(2), 259–267.
32. Palmer, I. *Clin. Orthop. Relat. Res.* **2007**, *454*, 17–22; discussion 14. doi:10.1097/BLO.0b013e31802c7915.
33. Colombet, P.; Jenny, J.; Menetrey, J.; Plaweski, S.; Zaffagnini, S.; French arthroscopy society (SFA). *Orthop. Traumatol. Surg. Res.* **2012**, *98*(8 Suppl), S201–S210. doi:10.1016/j.otsr.2012.10.005.
34. Zantop, T.; Herbort, M.; Raschke, M.; Fu, F.; Petersen, W. *Am. J. Sports Med.* **2007**, *35*(2), 223–227. doi:10.1177/03635465062 94571.
35. Amis, A. *Knee Surg. Sports Traumatol. Arthrosc.* **2012**, *20*(4), 613–620. doi:10.1007/s00167-011-1864-7.
36. Ziegler, C.; Pietrini, S.; Westerhaus, B.; Anderson, C.; Wijdicks, C.; Johansen, S.; LaPrade, R. *Am. J. Sports Med.* **2011**, 39(4), 743–752. doi:10.1177/0363546510387511.
37. Clark, J.; Sidles, J. *J. Orthop. Res.*, **1990**, *8*(2), 180–188. doi:10.1002/jor.1100080205.
38. Burks, R. T. *Knee Ligaments: Structure, Function, Injury and Repair* (Raven Press, New York), pp. 59–77.
39. Wening, J. Y.; Zabel, A.; Lorke, D. E.; Jungbluth, K. H. Physiological approach to artiûcial replacement Paper presented at the *lst Annual Meeting, European Orthopaedic Research Society*, Paris, France, **1991**, pp. 11–12.
40. Race, A.; Amis, A. A. Mechanical properties of the two bundles of the human posterior cruciate ligament. Paper presented at the *3rd Conference of the EORS*, Paris, France, **1993**, pp. 19–20.
41. Radford, W.; Amis, A. (1990). Biomechanics of a double prosthetic ligament in the anterior cruciate deficient knee. *J. Bone Joint Surg. Br.* **1990**, *72*(6), 1038–1043.
42. Schiavone Panni, A.; Denti, M.; Franzese, S.; Monteleone, M. *Knee Surg. Sports Traumatol Arthrosc.* **1993**, *1*(1), 9–12.
43. Moewis, P.; Duda, G.; Jung, T.; Heller, M.; Boeth, H.; Kaptein, B.; Taylor, W. *PLoS One.* **2016**, *11*(7), E0159600. doi:10.1371/journal.pone.0159600.
44. Promodos, C. *The Anterior Cruciate Ligament: Reconstruction and Basic Science*, 2nd edn. (Elsevier, **2018**).

45. Fuss, F. K. Helical axis surface of the knee joint. In *Proceedings of the XIVth Congress of the International Society for Biomechanics*, Bouisset, S., Métral, S., & Monod, H. (eds.), Paris, International Society of Biomechanics, **1993**, pp. 438–439.
46. Fuss, F. K. Helical axes — kinematic analysis, interpretation, and application. In *Proceedings of the International Federation for Medical and Biological Engineering*, vol. 1, Part II Magjarevic, R., Tonkovic, S., Bilas, V., & Lackovic, I. (eds.), Croatian Medical and Biological Engineering Society, Zagreb, **2001**, pp. 620–623.
47. Fuss, F. K. Kinematics of the knee after isometric single-bundle PCL reconstruction. In *Proceedings of the 2002 Combined Orthopaedic Meeting (25th Singapore Orthopaedic Association Meeting, 22nd Asean Orthopaedic Association Meeting, 5th Combined Meeting of Spinal and Pediatric Sections APOA, 7th Meeting of Knee and Sports Medicine Section APOA, 3rd Meeting of Asia Pacific Orthopaedic Society for Sports Medicine*), CDROM edition, National University of Singapore, Singapore, **2002**.
48. Fuss, F. K.; Hamel, G.; Duval, N.; DeGuise, J.; Yahia, L. H. Altered knee kinematics after posterior cruciate ligament rupture and replacement by means of a ligament prosthesis. In *Proceedings of the 1st International Symposium on Advanced Biomaterials* (*SIBA 1997*), Yahia, L. H. (ed.), École Polytechnique, Montréal, **1997**, p. 136.
49. Fuss, F. K. *J. Anat.*, **1992**, *180*, 297–304.
50. Gracovetsky, S. *Movement, Stability and Low Back Pain: The Essential Role of the Pelvis* (Churchill Livingstone, **1997**).
51. Willard, F.; Vleeming, A.; Schuenke, M.; Danneels, L.; Schleip, R. *J. Anat.*, **2012**, *221*(6), 507–536. doi:10.1111/j.1469-7580.2012.01511.x.
52. Fung, Y. C. *Foundations of Solid Mechanics* (Prentice-Hall, Englewood, **1965**).
53. Evans, K. *Endeavour*, **1991**, *15*(4), 170–174. doi:10.1016/0160-9327(91)90123-S.
54. Ashjari, M.; Hashemi, S.; Rasoulian, A. *Material Sci. & Eng. Int. J.*, **2017**, *1*(2), 62–64. doi:10.15406/mseij.2017.01.00011.
55. Gatt, R.; Vella Wood, M.; Gatt, A.; Zarb, F.; Formosa, C.; Azzopardi, K.; Grima, J. *Acta Biomater.*, **2015**, *24*, 201–208. doi:10.1016/j.actbio.2015.06.018.

56. Rigby, B.; Hirai, N.; Spikes, J.; Eyring, H. *J. Gen. Physiol.,* **1959**, *43*(2), 265–683.
57. Reese, S. P.; Maas, S. A.; Weiss, J. A. *J. Biomech.* **2010**, *43*(7), 1394–1400. doi:10.1016/j.jbiomech.2010.01.004.
58. Vidal Bde, C.; Mello, M. L. *J. Struct. Biol.* **2009**, *167*(2), 166–175. doi:10.1016/j.jsb.2009.05.004.
59. Hansen, K. A.; Weiss, J. A.; Barton, J. K. *J. Biomech. Eng.* **2002**, *124*(1), 72–77. doi:10.1115/1.1427698.
60. Franchi, M.; Fini, M.; Quaranta, M.; De Pasquale, V.; Raspanti, M.; Giavaresi, G.; Ruggeri, A. *J. Anat.*, **2007**, *210*(1), 1–7. doi: 10.1111/j.1469-7580.2006.00666.x.
61. Raspanti, M.; Manelli, A.; Franchi, M.; Ruggeri, A. *Matrix Biol.* **2005**, *24*(7), 503–507. doi:10.1016/j.matbio.2005.07.006.
62. Grima, J. N.; Winczewski, S.; Mizzi, L.; Grech, M. C.; Cauchi, R.; Gatt, R.; Rybicki, J. *Adv. Mater.* **2015**, *27*(8), 1455–1459. doi: 10.1002/adma.201404106.
63. Peltonen, J.; Cronin, N. J.; Stenroth, L.; Finni, T.; Avela, J. *Springerplus* **2013**, *2*(1), 212. doi:10.1186/2193-1801-2-212.
64. Lakes, R. *Cell. Polym.,* **1992**, *11*, 466–469.
65. Lakes, R. *Nature,* **1993**, *361*, 511–515. doi:10.1038/361511a0.
66. Lakes, R. *Science* **1987**, *235*(4792), 1038–1040. doi:10.1126/science.235.4792.1038.
67. Hall, L.; Coluci, V.; Galvão, D.; Kozlov, M.; Zhang, M.; Dantas, S.; Baughman, R. *Science* **2008**, *320*(5875), 504–507. doi:10.1126/science.1149815.
68. Brandel, B.; Lakes, R. *J. Mater. Sci.,* **2001**, *36*(24), 5885–593. doi:10.1023/A:1012928726952.
69. Grima, J.; Jackson, R.; Alderson, A.; Evans, K. *Adv. Mater.*, **2000**, *12*(24), 1912–1918. doi:10.1002/1521-4095(200012)12:243.0.CO;2-7.
70. Ishibashi, Y.; Iwata, M. *J. Phys. Soc. Jpn.* **2000**, *69*(8), 2702–2703. doi:10.1143/JPSJ.69.2702.
71. Evans, K.; Nkansah, M. *Nature* **1991**, *353*(6340), 124. doi:10.1038/353124a0.
72. Milton, G. *Mech. Phys. Solids.* **1992**, *40*, 1105–1137.

73. Ho, D.; Park, S.; Kwon, S.; Park, K.; Kim, S. *Nat. Commun.*, **2014**, *5*(3255). doi:10.1038/ncomms4255.
74. Gladyshev, G. *Biol. Bull. Russian Acad. Sci.*, **2002**, *29*(1), 1–5. doi:10.1023/A:101320763.
75. Wu, Y.; Dong, Y., Jiang, J., Li, H., Zhu, T.; Chen, S. (2017). Evaluation of the Bone-ligament and tendon insertions based on Raman spectrum and its PCA and CLS analysis. *Scientific Reports* **2017**, *7*(38706). doi:10.1038/srep38706 (2017).
76. Saadat, F.; Deymier, A.; Birman, V.; Thomopoulos, S.; Genin, G. *J. Mech. Behav. Biomed. Mater.* **2016**, *62*, 24–32. doi:10.1016/j.jmbbm.2016.04.025.
77. Mozdzen, L.; Thorpe, S.; Screen, H.; Harley, B. *Adv. Health Mater.* **2016**, *5*(14), 1731–1739. doi:10.1002/adhm.201600181.
78. Liu, Y. X.; Thomopoulos, S.; Birman, V.; Li, J. S.; Genin, G. M. *Mech. Mater.* **2012**, *44*, 83–92. doi:10.1016/j.mechmat.2011.08.005.
79. Hench, L. L.; Polak, J. M. *Science.*, **2002**, *295*(5557), 1014–1017. doi:10.1126/science.1067404.
80. Johansson, H.; Sjölander, P.; Sojka, P. *Crit. Rev. Biomed. Eng.*, **1991**, *18*(5), 341–368.
81. Yahia, L. H.; Newman, N. M.; St-Georges, M. *Anat. Histol. Embryol.* **1992**, *21*(1), 1–8.
82. Rivard, C. H.; Yahia, L. H.; Newman, N. Immunohistochemical demonstration of sensory nerve fibers and endings in human anterior cruciate ligaments. In Paper presented at the 39th Annual Meeting, Orthopaedic Research Society, San Francisco, CA, **1993a**, pp. 15–18.
83. Rivard, C. H., Yahia, L. H., Rhalmi, S.; Newman, N. Immunohistochemical analysis of human cruciate ligAMents sensory nerve fibers and endings. In Paper presented at the SIROT, Seoul, **1993b**, p. 109.
84. Gomis-Coloma, C.; Velasco-Aviles, S.; Gomez-Sanchez, J. A.; Casillas-Bajo, A.; Backs, J.; Cabedo, H. *J. Cell. Biol.* **2018**, *217*(4), 1249–1268. doi:10.1083/jcb.201611150.
85. Schultz, R. A.; Miller, D. C.; Kerr, C. S.; Micheli, L. *J. Bone Joint Surg. Am.* **1984**, *66*(7), 1072–1076.
86. Yahia, L. H.; Newman, N. *Anat. Anz.* **1991**, *173*(4), 233–238.

87. Denti, M.; Monteleone, M.; Berardi, A.; Panni, A. *Clin. Orthop. Relat. Res.* **1994**, 308, 29–32.
88. Sha, L.; Xie, G.; Zhao, S.; Zhao, J. *Medicine (Baltimore)* **2017**, *96*(5), e6081. doi:10.1097/MD.0000000000006081.
89. Chun, K. C.; Lee, S. H.; Kim, J. W.; Jin, E. J.; Kim, K. M.; Chun, C. H. *J. Orthop. Surg. Res.*, **2017**, *12*, 93. doi:10.1186/s13018-017-0593-0.
90. Angoules, A. G. *J. Sports Med. Doping Stud.* **2013**, *3*, e136. doi: 10.4172/2161-0673.100e136.
91. Wang, H.; Zhu, H.; Guo, Q.; Qian, T.; Zhang, P.; Li, S.; Gu, X. *Front Cell. Neurosci.*, **2017**, *11*, 323. doi:10.3389/fncel.2017.00323.
92. Mokarram, N.; Merchant, A.; Mukhatyar, V.; Patel, G.; Bellamkonda, R. V. *Biomaterials* **2012**, *33*(34), 8793–8801. doi:10.1016/j.biomaterials.2012.08.050.
93. Fantin, A.; Vieira, J. M.; Gestri, G.; Denti, L.; Schwarz, Q.; Prykhozhij, S.; Ruhrberg, C. *Blood* **2010**, *116*(5), 829–840. doi:10.1182/blood-2009-12-257832.
94. Cattin, A. L.; Burden, J. J.; Van Emmenis, L.; Mackenzie, F. E.; Hoving, J. J.; Garcia Calavia, N.; Lloyd, A. C. *Cell.* **2015**, *162*(5), 1127–1139. doi: 10.1016/j.cell.2015.07.021.
95. Enam, S.; Krieger, J.; Saxena, T.; Watts, B.; Olingy, C.; Botchwey, E.; Bellamkonda, R. *Biomaterials.* **2017**, *142*, 52–61. doi:10.1016/j.biomaterials.2017.07.013.
96. Clements, M.; Byrne, E.; Camarillo Guerrero, L.; Cattin, A.; Zakka, L.; Ashraf, A.; Parrinello, S. *Neuron.* **2017**, *96*(1), 98–114.e7. doi:10.1016/j.neuron.2017.09.008.
97. Prest, T.; Yeager, E.; LoPresti, S.; Zygelyte, E.; Martin, M.; Dong, L.; Cheetham, J. *J. Biomed. Mater. Res. A.,* **2018**, *106*(2), 450–459. doi:10.1002/jbm.a.36235.
98. Suzuki, K.; Tanaka, H.; Ebara, M.; Uto, K.; Matsuoka, H.; Nishimoto, S.; Yoshikawa, H. *Acta Biomater.*, **2017**, *53*, 250–259. doi:10.1016/j.actbio.2017.02.004.
99. Van der Merwe, Y.; Faust, A.; Conner, I.; Gu, X.; Feturi, F.; Zhao, W.; Steketee, M. *EBioMedicine.*, **2017**, *26*, 47–59. doi:10.1016/j.ebiom.2017.11.017.

100. Ghasemi-Mobarakeh, L.; Prabhakaran, M.; Morshed, M.; Nasr-Esfahani, M.; Baharvand, H.; Kiani, S.; ... Ramakrishna, S. *J. Tissue Eng. Regen. Med.* **2011**, *5*(4), E17–35. doi:10.1002/term.383.
101. Bosi, S.; Fabbro, A.; Ballerini, L.; Prato, M. *Nanotechnol. Rev.*, **2013**, *2*(1), 47–57. doi: 10.1515/ntrev-2012-0067.
102. Polizu, S.; Poulin, P.; Savadogo, O.; Yahia, L. U.S. Patent No. 2009/0169594 A1. Washington, DC: U.S. Patent and Trademark Office, **2009**.
103. Ingham, S. J. M.; de Carvalho, R. T.; Martins, C. A. Q.; Lertwanich, P.; Abdalla, R. J.; Smolinski, P; Fu, F. H. *Knee Surg. Sports Traumatol Arthrosc.*, **2017**, *25*(4), 1048–1054. doi:10.1007/s00167-015-3956-2.
104. Luzo, M. V. M.; Franciozi, C. E. da S.; Rezende, F. C.; Gracitelli, G. C.; Debieux, P.; Cohen, M. *Revista brasileira de ortopedia* **2016**, *51*(4), 385–395. doi:10.1016/j.rboe.2016.05.001.
105. Claes, S.; Vereecke, E.; Maes, M.; Victor, J.; Verdonk, P.; Bellemans, J. *J. Anat.*, **2013**, *223*(4), 321–8. doi:10.1111/joa.12087.
106. Segond, P. *Recherches cliniques et expérimentales sur les épanchements sanguins du genou par entorse.* (Bureaux du "Progrès medical, Paris, **1879**).
107. Lutz, C. *Ortho. Traumatol: Surg. Res.* **2018**, *104*(1), S47–53. doi:10.1016/j.otsr.2017.03.031.
108. Stergiou, N.; Ristanis, S.; Moraiti, C.; Georgoulis, A. D. *Sports Med.* **2007**, *37*(7), 601–613. doi:10.2165/00007256-200737070-00004.
109. Rezende, F. C.; deMoraes, V. Y.; Martimbianco, A. L. C.; Luzo, M. V.; daSilveira Franciozi, C. E.; Belloti, J. C. *Clin Orth Rel Res.*, **2015**, doi:10.1007/s11999-015-4285-y.
110. Imbert, P.; Lustig, S.; Steltzlen, C.; Batailler, C.; Colombet, P.; Dalmay, F.; Lutz, C. *Ortho. Traumatol.: Surg. Res.* **2017**, *103*(8), S215–221. doi:10.1016/j.otsr.2017.09.005.
111. Laboureau, J. P.; Marnat-Perrichet, F. Isometric reconstruction of the anterior cruciate ligament: femoral and tibial tunnel placement. In *Ligaments and Ligamentoplasties* (Springer Berlin Heidelberg, Berlin, Heidelberg, **1997**), pp. 209–225. doi:10.1007/978-3-642-60428-7_10.

112. Dabirrahmani, D.; Christopher Hogg, M.; Walker, P.; Biggs, D.; Mark Gillies, R. *Comput. Biol. Med.* **2013**, *43*(12), 2287–2296. doi:10.1016/j.compbiomed.2013.10.008.
113. Noyes, F. R.; Grood, E. S. *J. Bone Joint Surg. Am.*, **1976**, *58*(8), 1074–1082.
114. Kato, Y.; Ingham, S.; Kramer, S.; Smolinski, P.; Saito, A.; Fu, F. *Knee Surg. Sports Traumatol. Arthro.* **2010**, *18*(1), 2–10. doi:10.1007/s00167-009-0916-8
115. Yoshiya, S.; Kurosaka, M.; Yamada, M.; Yamaguchi, M.; Hirohata, H.; Utsumi, T.; Iwatsubo, T. Optimal orientation of the bone tunnels in the anterior cruciate ligament reconstruction. In *37th Annual Meeting, ORS.* Anaheim, CA, **1991**.
116. Drouin, G.; Masson, M.; Yahia, L. *Biomed. Mater. Eng.*, **1991**, *1*(3), 159–165.
117. Gely, P.; Drouin, G.; Thiry, P. S.; Tremblay, G. R. *J. Biomech. Eng.*, **1984**, *106*(4), 285–294. doi:10.1115/1.3138496.
118. Boss, J. H.; Shajrawi, I.; Mendes, D. G. *J. Appl. Biomater.* **1991**, *2*(4), 241–242. doi:10.1002/jab.770020404.
119. Shajrawi, I.; Boss, J. H.; Aunullah, J.; Soudry, M.; G, M. D. Histomorphometric study of the tissular organization of a high tensile polyethylene anterior cruciate ligament prosthesis. In Paper presented at the *19th Annual Meeting of the Society for Biomaterials*, Birmingham, AL, **1993**.
120. Marcacci, M.; Gubellini, P.; Buda, R.; DEPasquale, V.; Strocchi, R.; Molgora, A. P.; Ruggeri, A. *Clin. Ortho. Rel. Res.* **1991**, *267*, 115–121. doi:10.1097/00003086-199106000-00016.
121. Paavolainen, P.; Mäkisalo, S.; Skutnabb, K.; Holmström, T. *Acta Orthopaedica* **1993**, *64*(3), 323–328. doi:10.3109/17453679308993636.
122. Bolton, C. W.; Bruchman, W. C. *Clin. Ortho. Rel. Res.* **1985**, *196*, 202–213. Retrieved from http://www.ncbi.nlm.nih.gov/pubmed/3888468.
123. Spalazzi, J. P.; Doty, S. B.; Moffat, K. L.; Levine, W. N.; Lu, H. H. *Tissue Eng.* **2006**, *12*(12), 3497–3508. doi:10.1089/ten.2006.12.3497.

124. Wang, I. E.; Shan, J. S.; Choi, R.; Oh, S.; Kepler, C. K.; Chen, F. H.; Lu, H. H. *J. Ortho. Res.* **2007**, *25*(12), 1609–1620. doi:10.1002/jor.20475.
125. Wang, X.; Wenk, E.; Zhang, X.; Meinel, L.; Vunjak-Novakovic, G.; Kaplan, D. L. *J. Control Release* **2009**, *134*(2), 81–90. doi:10.1016/j.jconrel.2008.10.021.
126. Shi, J.; Wang, L.; Zhang, F.; Li, H.; Lei, L.; Liu, L.; Chen, Y. *ACS Appl. Mater. Interfaces* **2010**, *2*(4), 1025–1030. doi:10.1021/am9007962.
127. Spalazzi, J. P.; Dagher, E.; Doty, S. B.; Guo, X. E.; Rodeo, S. A.; Lu, H. H. *J. Biomed. Mater. Res. — Part A*, **2008a**, *86*(1), 1–12. doi:10.1002/jbm.a.32073.
128. Erisken, C.; Kalyon, D. M.; Wang, H. *Biomaterials* **2008**, *29*(30), 4065–4073. doi:10.1016/j.biomaterials.2008.06.022.
129. Erisken, C.; Kalyon, D. M.; Wang, H. *J. Biomech. Eng.* **2010**, *132*(9), 091013. doi:10.1115/1.4001884.
130. Li, X.; Xie, J.; Lipner, J.; Yuan, X.; Thomopoulos, S.; Xia, Y. *Nano Lett.* **2009**, *9*(7), 2763–2768. doi:10.1021/nl901582f.
131. Zhang, X.; Bogdanowicz, D.; Erisken, C.; Lee, N. M.; Lu, H. H. *J. Shoulder Elbow Surg.* **2012**, *21*(2), 266–77. doi:10.1016/j.jse.2011.11.016.
132. Samavedi, S.; Olsen Horton, C.; Guelcher, S. A.; Goldstein, A. S.; Whittington, A. R. *Acta Biomaterialia* **2011**, *7*(12), 4131–4138. doi:10.1016/j.actbio.2011.07.008.
133. Samavedi, S.; Guelcher, S. A.; Goldstein, A. S.; Whittington, A. R. *Biomaterials* **2012**, *33*(31), 7727–7735. doi:10.1016/j.biomaterials.2012.07.008.
134. Li, H.; Ge, Y.; Wu, Y. *et al. Int. Ortho.* (*SICOT*) **2011**, *35*, 1561–1567. https://doi.org/10.1007/s00264-010-1158-6.
135. Mutsuzaki, H.; Yokoyama, Y.; Ito, A.; Oyane, A. *Int. J. Mol. Sci.* **2013**, *14*, 19155–19168.
136. Hong, Li; Yang, Wu; Yunsheng, Ge; Jia, Jiang; Kai, Gao; Pengyun, Zhang; Lingxiang, Wu; Shiyi, C. *Appl. Surf. Sci.* **2011**, *257*(22), 9371–9376, ISSN 0169-4332, https://doi.org/10.1016/j.apsusc.2011.05.110.

137. Lessim, S. *et al.* **2013**, *January*, 289–297.
138. Yang, J.; Jiang, J.; Li, Y. *et al. Int. Orthopaedics* (*SICOT*) **2013**, *37*, 515–521. https://doi.org/10.1007/s00264-012-1723-2.
139. Ciobanu, M.; Siove, A.; Gueguen, V.; Gamble, L. J.; Castner, D. G.; Migonney, V. *Biomacromolecules*, **2006**, *7*(3), 755–760. doi:10.1021/bm050694+.
140. Pavon-Djavid, G.; Gamble, L. J.; Ciobanu, M.; Gueguen, V.; Castner, D. G.; Migonney, V. *Biomacromolecules* **2007**, *8*(11), 3317–3325. doi:10.1021/bm070344i.
141. Vaquette, C.; Viateau, V.; Guérard, S.; Anagnostou, F.; Manassero, M.; Castner, D. G.; Migonney, V. The effect of polystyrene sodium sulfonate grafting on polyethylene terephthalate artificial. *Biomaterials* **2013**, *34*(29), 7048–7063, ISSN 0142-9612. https://doi.org/10.1016/j.biomaterials.2013.05.058.
142. Batty, L. M.; Norsworthy, C. J.; Lash, N. J.; Wasiak, J.; Richmond, A., 11; Feller, J. A. *Arthroscopy* **2015**, *31*, 957–968.
143. Yahia, L. H.; Hagemeister, N.; Lombardi, S.; Assad, M.; Rivard, C. H. *J. Bone Joint Surg.* **1993**, *75B*(Suppl. III), 239.
144. Lubowitz. *J. Arthro Rel. Surg.* **2015**, *31*(5), 969–970.

https://doi.org/10.1142/9789811204630_0012

Chapter 12

Comprehensive Review of the Universal Jolt Mechanism Theory for Traumatic Brain, Spine and Musculoskeletal Injuries

Tijana Ivancevic[*,||], Bojan Jovanovic[†,§], and Zoran Gojkovic[‡,¶]

[*]*Tesla Science Evolution Institute, Adelaide, Australia*
[†]*Sports Academy, Belgrade, Serbia*
[‡]*University of Novi Sad, Faculty of Medicine, Clinical Centre of Vojvodina, Clinic for Orthopedic Surgery and Traumatology, Novi Sad, Serbia*
[||]*tanya.ivancevic@gmail.com*
[§]*jovanboj@yahoo.com*
[¶]*gojkoz@gmail.com*

Abbreviations

DOF	Degrees-of-freedom
MRI	Magnetic resonance imaging
R^3	Euclidean 3D space
SE(3)	Euclidean group
SO(3)	Rotation group

1. Introduction

Briefly, the universal jolt theory of human injuries proposes that the common cause of all mechanical injuries is the Euclidean jolt, an impulsive force/loading, always eccentrically coupled to a part of body mass, which suddenly hits either human head or spine or any joint/bone and it always strikes simultaneously in several coupled degrees-of-freedom (DOFs), both translational and rotational.[1–4] Therefore, the cause of injury is never a static or a slow force, nor it goes in a single direction only.[a] Specifically, it is the *time derivative* of the *6DOF Euclidean force* with three translational components and three rotational components.

In other words, the Euclidean jolt is a sudden unnatural motion of a part of human body, which is usually caused either by an accidental external impact or by a highly dynamic human movement, which is slightly distorted (like a slipping on the ground). It is always associated with unnatural mass distribution of the human body, possibly with some added external masses, which causes sudden body mass eccentricity from the natural physiological state.

[a] Although term "jolt" may sound complicated, its basic logic is simple and similar to the 'karate chop': to brake a brick one does not apply a static force, or even a slow force, but rather as fast force as possible, which is called 'jolt'. The adjective "Euclidean" means all six motions that a rigid body can undergo in an ordinary Euclidean 3D space, namely three Cartesian translations coupled to three Eulerian rotations; this coupling between translations and rotations is explained below.

As we live in a Euclidean 3D space, formally denoted by R^3, one could think that motion of any part of human body, either caused by an accidental external impact or by a fast-voluntary human movement, "simply obeys classical 6DOF mechanics. However, these six DOFs are not independent motions as it is suggested by its standard name "degrees-of-freedom". In reality, these six motions of any rigid body in space are coupled. Firstly, three rotations are coupled in the so-called *rotation group SO(3)* (or rotation matrix, or quaternion).[5] Secondly, three translations are coupled with the rotation group to give the full Euclidean group SE(3) of rigid body motions in space, formally defined as a noncommutative product of SO(3*)* and R^3 (see Ref. [6] and the references therein).[b]

A simple way to see this is to observe someone throwing an object in the air or hitting a tennis, or a golf ball: how far and where it will fly depends not only on the standard "projectile" mechanics, but also on its local "spin" around all three axes simultaneously.[c] Every golf and tennis player knows this simple fact. Once the spin is properly defined, the *coupled Newton–Euler dynamics*[d] is obtained and its time derivative is the Euclidean jolt.

---

[b] Briefly, the gauge SE(3)-group of Euclidean micro-motions (e.g. of the brain immersed in the cerebrospinal fluid, or an intervertebral disc, or a synovial joint) contains matrices of the form $\begin{pmatrix} \mathbf{R} & \mathbf{b} \\ 0 & 1 \end{pmatrix}$, where **b** is the 3D micro-translation vector and **R** is the 3D rotation matrix, given by the product $\mathbf{R} = R_{\varphi} \cdot R\psi \cdot R_{\theta}$ of three Eulerian micro-rotations, roll = R_{φ}, pitch = R_{ψ}, yaw = R_{θ}, performed respectively about the *x*-axis by an angle ϕ, about the *y*-axis by an angle ψ, and about the *z*-axis by an angle θ,

$$R_{\varphi} = \begin{bmatrix} 1 & 0 & 0 \\ 0 & \cos\varphi & -\sin\varphi \\ 0 & \sin\varphi & \cos\varphi \end{bmatrix}, R_{\psi} = \begin{bmatrix} \cos\psi & 0 & \cos\psi \\ 0 & 1 & 0 \\ -\sin\psi & 0 & \cos\psi \end{bmatrix}, R_{\theta} = \begin{bmatrix} \cos\theta & -\sin\theta & 0 \\ \sin\theta & \cos\theta & 0 \\ 0 & 0 & 1 \end{bmatrix}$$

[c] Or, consider an irregular shaped rigid body hanging on a rope and hit it with a hammer (or, a baseball bat): it is virtually impossible to prevent it to start rotating, because every hit would be eccentric. Usually, it would both translate and rotate in/around all Cartesian three axes.

[d] Newton–Euler dynamics, formally defined in the next section, consists of three Newtonian translations *along* Cartesian axes coupled with three rotations in Euler angles (i.e. *around* Cartesian axes).

Therefore, the Euclidean jolt injury theory is based on the covariant biomechanical generalization of the classical Newton–Euler dynamics. Unlike classical engineering mechanics of multi-body systems, the *covariant force law*[7,8] for any biomechanical system proposes that forces acting on a multi-body system and causing its motions are fundamentally different physical quantities from the resulting accelerations. In simple words, forces are *massive* quantities while accelerations are *massless* quantities.[e] More precisely, the acceleration vector field includes all linear and angular accelerations of individual body segments. When they are all coupled with the total body's mass-distribution matrix of all body segments (including all masses and inertia moments and products), the result is the force co-vector field, comprising all the forces and torques acting on the individual body segments. In this way, the 6D Euclidean force for an arbitrary biomechanical system is defined.

The covariant force law states[f]:

Euclidean Force covector field = Body mass distribution
× Euclidean Acceleration vector field

Now that the 6D covariant biomechanical force on the Euclidean group SE(3) is defined, its time derivative (or, rate-of-change with respect to time) will be taken. In this way, the Euclidean jolt is found

---

[e]All vector fields are massless: velocity, acceleration and jerk — both translational (linear) and rotational (angular); all co-vector fields are massive: momentum, force and jolt — both translational and rotational.

[f]This "plain-English equation" is formally written (using the Einstein summation convention, with Greek indices labeling the three Cartesian translations and the three corresponding Euler angles around Cartesian axes):

$$F_\mu = m_{\mu\nu} a^\nu, \quad (\mu, \nu = 1, \dots, 6)$$

where F_μ denote the 6 covariant components of the external "pushing" SE(3)-force co-vector field, $m_{\mu\nu}$ represent the 6×6 covariant components of the inertia-metric tensor, while a^ν correspond to the 6 contravariant components of the internal SE(3)-acceleration vector-field.

(or, SE(3)-jolt), which is the sudden temporal change of the Euclidean force (or, SE(3)-force)[g]:

Euclidean Jolt covector field = Body mass distribution
× Euclidean Jerk vector field

And again, Euclidean jolt consists of two components: (i) coupled massless 3D linear and angular jerks (of all included body segments), and (ii) their mass distribution.[h] For the sake of simplicity, one can say that the mass distribution matrix includes all involved segmental masses and inertia moments, as well as "eccentricities" or "pathological leverages" from the normal physiological body state. In other words, there are no injuries in static or slow-motion conditions without any mass eccentricities; all injuries are caused by mutually coupled linear and angular jerks, which are also coupled with the involved human mass distribution (with a possible external mass added, which increases the overall mass eccentricity).

The Euclidean jolt causes two basic forms of discontinuous brain, spine or musculoskeletal injuries: (i) mild rotational disclinations; and (ii) severe translational dislocations (or, fractures). Ivancevic has developed the soft-body dynamics of biomechanical disclinations and dislocations, caused by the Euclidean Jolt, using the Cosserat

---

[g]Formally, the absolute (Bianchi) time-derivative $\frac{D}{dt}(.)$ of the covariant SE(3)-force F_{μ} defines the corresponding external "striking" SE(3)-jolt co-vector field:

$$\frac{D}{dt}(F_{\mu}) = m_{\mu\nu}\frac{D}{dt}(a^{\nu}) = m_{\mu\nu}\left(\dot{a}^{\nu} + \Gamma^{\nu}_{\mu\lambda}a^{\mu}a^{\lambda}\right), \qquad (1)$$

where $\frac{D}{dt}(a^{\nu})$ denotes the 6 contravariant components of the internal SE(3)-jerk vector-field and overdot ($\dot{}$) denotes the time derivative. $\Gamma^{\nu}_{\mu\lambda}$ are the Christoffel's symbols of the Levi–Civita connection for the SE(3) group, which are zero in case of pure Cartesian translations and nonzero in case of rotations, as well as in the full-coupling of translations and rotations.

[h]To emphasize the difference between massive jolts and massless jerks, consider the difference between a car crash (jolt), i.e. collision with an external mass, and a sudden brake (jerk): a sudden brake is unpleasant but survivable, even if it causes a huge deceleration, because it is massless (so, there is no momentum in it), while a car crash, even with a small speed, can be fatal because it is massive.

multipolar viscoelastic continuum model.[1-4,i] Implications of the universal jolt injury mechanism/theory are various, as follows:

- The research in traumatic brain injury (TBI) has so far identified the rotation of the brain-stem as the main cause of the TBI due to various crashes/impacts. The jolt theory contribution to the TBI research is the following: (i) rigorously defined this brain rotation as a mechanical disclination of the brain-stem tissue modeled by the Cosserat (or, microstretch)[9] multipolar soft-body model; (ii) demonstrating that brain rotation is never uni-axial but always three-axial; demonstrating that brain rotation is always coupled with translational dislocations, which is a straightforward consequence of the Euclidean jolt mechanism.[j]
- In case of spinal injury, the contribution of the universal Jolt mechanism is the following: (i) the spinal injury is always localized at the certain vertebral or intervertebral point; (ii) in case of severe translational injuries (vertebral fractures or discus herniae) they can be identified using X-ray (or, MRI or other medical imaging scans), while in case of microscopic rotational injuries (causing the back-pain syndrome) they cannot be identified using current medical imaging techniques; (iii) there is no spinal injury without one of the following two causes:
  a. Impulsive rotational + translational loading caused by either fast human movements or various crashes/impacts; and/or
  b. Static eccentricity from the normal physiological spinal form, caused by external loading.

  Any spinal injury is caused by a combination of the two points above: impulsive rotational + translational loading and mass eccentricity.

  This is a straightforward consequence of the universal jolt theory. Like in case of TBI, translational and rotational spinal injuries

[i] This multipolar viscoelastic continuum injury mechanics has been generalized in Ref. 9 to the microstretch continuum model of human fascia.

[j] In other words, these rapid rotations cannot be separately analyzed from translations in the brain, spine or synovial joint, because they are in reality always coupled.

cannot be separately analyzed because they are always coupled. Also, there are no "static injuries" without eccentricity. For example, Indian women have for centuries carried bulky loads on their heads without any spinal injuries; they just prevented any load eccentricities and any jerks in their motion.

The currently used "Principal loading hypothesis"[10] that describes spinal injuries in terms of spinal tension, compression, bending, and shear, covers only a small subset of all spinal injuries covered by the Euclidean jolt theory. To prevent spinal injuries, the spinal jolt awareness needs to be developed as an ability to control all possible impulsive spinal loadings, in all six coordinates, in particular those with mass eccentricities.

- In case of a general musculoskeletal injury, the contribution of the universal jolt theory is the following:
  (i) the injury is always localized at the certain joint or bone and caused by an impulsive loading, which hits this particular joint/bone in several coupled DOFs simultaneously;
  (ii) injury happens when most of the body mass is hanging on that joint; for example, in case of a knee injury, when most of the body mass is on one leg with a semi-flexed knee — and then, caused by some external shock, the knee suddenly "jerks" (this can happen in running, skiing, and ball games, as well as various crashes/impacts); or, in case of shoulder injury, when most of the body mass is hanging on one arm and then it suddenly jerks.

To prevent these injuries, the general musculoskeletal jolt awareness needs to be developed. For example, never overload a flexed knee and avoid any kind of uncontrolled motions (like slipping) or collisions with external objects (e.g. in case of soccer or rugby players).

2. Healthy Brain, Spine and Joint Mechanics: Coupled Newton–Euler Dynamics of Rigid Motions

To start with, consider a natural (healthy, non-pathological) fully coupled Newton–Euler SE(3) dynamics of: (i) brain's micro-motions within the cerebrospinal fluid inside the cranial cavity; (ii) any local inter-vertebral motions along the spine; and (iii) any local joint motions in the human musculoskeletal system.

The forced Newton–Euler equations on the SE(3)-group of rigid motions of the brain (within the cerebrospinal fluid), or an intervertebral joint, or a synovial joint, in the Euclidean 3-space R^3 read in vector (boldface) form:

$$\begin{aligned} \text{Newton: } \dot{p} &\equiv \mathrm{M}\dot{\nu} = \mathrm{F} + \mathrm{p} \times \omega, \\ \text{Eular: } \dot{\pi} &\equiv \mathrm{I}\dot{\omega} = \mathrm{T} + \pi \times \omega + \mathrm{p} \times \mathrm{v}, \end{aligned} \tag{2}$$

(where × denotes the vector cross product), in tensor form:

$$\begin{aligned} \dot{p} &\equiv M_{ij}\dot{\upsilon}^{j} = \mathrm{F}_i + \varepsilon^{j}_{ik}\, \mathrm{p}_j \times \omega^{k}, \ (i, j, k = 1, 2, 3) \\ \dot{\pi} &\equiv \mathrm{I}_{ij}\dot{\omega}^{j} = \mathrm{T}_i + \varepsilon^{j}_{ik}\pi_j \times \omega^{k} + \varepsilon^{j}_{ik}\mathrm{p}_i \nu^{k}, \end{aligned}$$

(where ε^{j}_{ik} is the Levi-Civita permutation symbol), and in scalar form:

$$\begin{aligned} &\text{Newton:} \quad \begin{cases} \dot{p}_1 = F_1 - m_3\upsilon_3\omega_3 + m_2\upsilon_2\omega_3 \\ \dot{p}_2 = F_2 + m_3\upsilon_3\omega_1 + m_1\upsilon_1\omega_3 \\ \dot{p}_3 = F_3 - m_2\upsilon_2\omega_1 + m_1\upsilon_1\omega_2 \end{cases} \\ &\text{Euler:} \quad \begin{cases} \dot{\pi}_1 = T_1 + (m_2 - m_3)\nu_2\nu_3 + (I_2 - I_3)\omega_2\omega_3 \\ \dot{\pi}_2 = T_2 + (m_3 - m_1)\nu_1\nu_3 + (I_3 - I_1)\omega_1\omega_3 \\ \dot{\pi}_3 = T_3 + (m_1 - m_2)\nu_1\nu_2 + (I_1 - I_2)\omega_1\omega_2 \end{cases} \end{aligned} \tag{3}$$

where $(i, j = 1, 2, 3)$

$$\mathbf{M} \equiv M_{ij} = \mathrm{diag}\{m_1, m_2, m_3\} \quad \text{and} \quad \mathbf{I} \equiv I_{ij} = \mathrm{diag}\{I_1, I_2, I_3\},$$

are simplified (diagonal) mass and inertia matrices (defining the mass–inertia distribution), with principal inertia moments given in Cartesian coordinates (x, y, z) by volume integrals (see Refs. [1–3] for technical details) and

$$\mathbf{F} \equiv F_i = [F_1, F_2, F_3] \text{ and } \mathbf{T} \equiv T_i = [T_1, T_2, T_3]$$

are gravitational and other external force and torque co-vectors,

$$\mathbf{p} \equiv p_i \equiv \mathbf{Mv} = [p_1, p_2, p_3] = [m_1 v_1, m_2 v_2, m_2 v_2]$$

and

$$\pi \equiv \pi_i \equiv \mathbf{I}\omega = [\pi_1, \pi_2, \pi_3] = [I_1\omega_1, I_2\omega_2, I_3\omega_3]$$

are linear and angular momentum co-vectors.

Equations (2)–(3) can be derived, using standard Lagrangian equations in a simplified case of purely rigid-body motions, or Kirchhoff–Lagrangian equations (see Ref. [1] for technical details) to include the surrounding fluid dynamics of the cerebrospinal or synovial fluid, from the translational + rotational kinetic energy:

$$E = \frac{1}{2}\mathrm{v}^{\mathrm{t}}\mathrm{Mv} + \frac{1}{2}\omega^{\mathrm{t}}\mathrm{I}\omega = \frac{1}{2}\mathrm{M}_{ij}\mathrm{v}^{\mathrm{i}}\mathrm{v}^{j} + \frac{1}{2}\mathrm{I}_{ij}\omega^{\mathrm{i}}\omega^{\mathrm{j}},$$

so that linear and angular momentum co-vectors are defined as

$$\mathrm{p} = p_i = \partial_\nu E \partial_{yi} E, \qquad \pi = \pi i = \partial_\omega E \partial_{\omega i} E$$

with their corresponding time derivatives, in vector form

$$\dot{\mathrm{p}} = \frac{d}{dt}\mathrm{p} = \frac{d}{dt}\partial_\nu E, \qquad \dot{\pi} = \frac{d}{dt}\pi = \frac{d}{dt}\partial_\omega E,$$

or, in tensor form

$$\dot{p}_i = \frac{d}{dt}p_i = \frac{d}{dt}\partial_{\nu i} E, \qquad \dot{\pi}_i = \frac{d}{dt}\pi_i = \frac{d}{dt}\partial_{\omega i} E,$$

or, in scalar form

$$\dot{p} = [\dot{p}_1 + \dot{p}_2 + \dot{p}_3] = [m_1\dot{\nu}_1 + m_2\dot{\nu}_2 + m_2\dot{\nu}_2],$$

$$\dot{\pi} = [\dot{\pi}_1 + \dot{\pi}_2 + \dot{\pi}_3] = [I_1\dot{\omega}_1 + I_2\dot{\omega}_2 + I_3\dot{\omega}_3].$$

3. Pathological Brain, Spine and Joint Dynamics: The SE(3)-Jolt

While healthy SE(3)-dynamics of (a brain within the cerebrospinal fluid, or any intervertebral joint, or any synovial joint) is given by the above defined coupled Newton–Euler micro-dynamics, the traumatic brain, spine or general musculoskeletal injury is actually caused by the sharp and discontinuous change in this natural SE(3) micro-dynamics, in the form of the SE(3)-jolt, causing discontinuous deformations of the brain, intervertebral disc or a synovial joint.

The SE(3)-jolt is defined as a coupled Newton + Euler jolt, which in vector form reads[k]

$$\text{SE(3)-jolt:} \begin{cases} \text{Newton jolt:} & \dot{\mathbf{F}} = \ddot{\mathbf{p}} - \dot{\mathbf{p}} \times \omega - \mathbf{p} \times \omega, \\ \text{Euler jolt:} & \dot{\mathbf{T}} = \ddot{\boldsymbol{\pi}} - \dot{\boldsymbol{\pi}} \times \omega - \boldsymbol{\pi} \times \omega - \dot{\mathbf{p}} \times \mathrm{v} - \mathbf{p} \times \dot{\mathrm{v}}, \end{cases}$$

in tensor form reads[l]:

$$\dot{F}_i = \ddot{p} - \varepsilon^j_{ik}\dot{p}_j\omega^k - \varepsilon^j_{ik}p_j\dot{\omega}^k$$
$$\dot{T}_i = \ddot{\pi} - \varepsilon^j_{ik}\dot{\pi}_j\omega^k - \varepsilon^j_{ik}\pi_j\dot{\omega}^k - \varepsilon^j_{ik}\dot{p}_j\nu^k - \varepsilon^j_{ik}p_j\dot{\nu}^k$$

and in scalar form expands as

---

[k]Note that the derivative of the cross–product of two vectors follows the standard calculus product-rule: $\frac{d}{dt}(\mathbf{u} \times \mathbf{v}) = \dot{\mathbf{u}} \times \mathbf{v} + \mathbf{u} \times \dot{\mathbf{v}}$.

[l]In this paragraph the overdots actually denote the absolute Bianchi (covariant) time-derivative (1), so that the jolts retain the proper covector character, which would be lost if ordinary time derivatives are used. However, for the sake of simplicity and wider readability, the same overdot notation is used.

$$\text{Newton jolt:}\begin{cases}\dot{F}_1 = \ddot{p}_1 - m_2\omega_3\dot{v}_2 + m_3(\omega_2\dot{v}_3 + v_3\dot{\omega}_2) - m_2v_2\dot{\omega}_3\\ \dot{F}_2 = \ddot{p}_2 - m_1\omega_3\dot{v}_1 + m_3\omega_1\dot{v}_3 - m_3v_3\dot{\omega}_1 + m_1v_1\dot{\omega}_3\\ \dot{F}_3 = \ddot{p}_3 - m_1\omega_2\dot{v}_1 + m_2\omega_1\dot{v}_2 - v_2\dot{\omega}_1 - m_1v_1\dot{\omega}_1,\end{cases}$$

$$\text{Euler jolt:}\begin{cases}\dot{T}_1 = \ddot{\pi}_1 - (m_2 - m_3)(v_3\dot{v}_2 + v_2\dot{v}_3) - (I_2 - I_3)(\omega_3\dot{\omega}_2 + \omega_2\dot{\omega}_3)\\ \dot{T}_2 = \ddot{\pi}_2 - (m_1 - m_3)(v_3\dot{v}_1 + v_1\dot{v}_3) - (I_1 - I_3)(\omega_3\dot{\omega}_1 + \omega_1\dot{\omega}_3)\\ \dot{T}_3 = \ddot{\pi}_3 - (m_1 - m_2)(v_2\dot{v}_1 + v_1\dot{v}_2) - (I_1 - I_2)(\omega_2\dot{\omega}_1 + \omega_1\dot{\omega}_2)\end{cases}$$

Here, the linear and angular jolt co-vectors are

$$\dot{\mathrm{F}} \equiv \mathrm{M}\mathrm{v} = [\dot{F}_1, \dot{F}_2, \dot{F}_3], \qquad \dot{\mathrm{T}} \equiv \mathrm{I}\dot{\omega} = [\dot{T}_1, \dot{T}_2, \dot{T}_3],$$

where

$$\ddot{\mathrm{v}} = [\ddot{\nu}_1, \ddot{\nu}_2, \ddot{\nu}_3]^t, \qquad \ddot{\omega} = [\ddot{\omega}_1, \ddot{\omega}_2, \ddot{\omega}_3]^t,$$

are linear and angular jerk vectors.

Herein, the linear and angular momenta ($\mathbf{p}$, π), forces ($\mathbf{F}$,$\mathbf{T}$) and jolts ($\dot{\mathrm{F}}$, $\dot{\mathrm{T}}$) are co-vectors (row vectors), while the linear and angular velocities ($\mathbf{v}$, ω), accelerations ($\dot{\mathrm{v}}$, $\dot{\omega}$) and jerks ($\ddot{\mathrm{v}}$, $\ddot{\omega}$) are vectors (column vectors). This fact bio-physically means that the "jerk" vector should not be confused with the "jolt" co-vector. For example in case of the TBI, the "jerk"' means shaking the head's own mass-inertia matrices (mainly in the atlanto-occipital and atlanto-axial joints), while the "jolt" means actually hitting the head with some external mass-inertia matrices included in the "hitting" SE(3)-jolt, or hitting some external massive body with the head (e.g. the ground — gravitational effect, or the wall — inertial effect). Consequently, the massless "jerk" vector represents a (translational + rotational) *non-collision effect* that can cause only weaker brain injuries, while the inertial "jolt" co-vector represents a (translational + rotational) *collision effect* that can cause hard brain injuries.

4. Microscopic Cosserat Dislocations and Disclinations Caused by the Euclidean Jolt

This section analyzes the effect of the Euclidean jolt on a human brain, or intervertebral disc, or a synovial joint — modeled in terms of Newtonian dislocations and Eulerian disclinations of a 3D anisotropic multipolar *Cosserat visco-elasto-plastic continuum*,[m,11,12] exhibiting coupled stress–strain elastic properties and irreversible deformations.

Specifically, the SE(3)-jolt $(\dot{\mathrm{F}}, \dot{\mathrm{T}})$ can cause two types of rapid discontinuous deformations in the brain, intervertebral discs and synovial joints:

1. The Newton jolt $\dot{\mathrm{F}}$ can cause both elastic (reversible) and plastic (irreversible) micro-translational Cosserat *dislocations*;
2. The Euler jolt $\dot{\mathrm{T}}$ can cause both elastic and plastic micro-rotational Cosserat *disclinations.*

To precisely define pathological dislocations and disclinations, caused by the SE(3)-jolt $(\dot{\mathrm{F}}, \dot{\mathrm{T}})$, first define the coordinate co-frame, i.e. the set of basis 1–forms $\{dx^i\}$, given in local coordinates: $x^i = (x^1, x^2, x^3) = (x, y, z)$, attached to the center-of-mass (CoM of a brain, intervertebral disc, or synovial joint). Then, in the coordinate co-frame $\{dx^i\}$ introduce the following set of the plastic SE(3)-deformations represented by exterior differential p-forms[8]:

the *dislocation current* 1-form, $\mathbf{J} = J^i dx^i$;
the *dislocation density* 2-form, $\alpha = \frac{1}{2}\alpha_{ij} dx^i \wedge dx^j$;
the *disclination current* 2-form, $\mathbf{S} = \frac{1}{2} S_{ij} dx^i \wedge dx^j$;
and the *disclination density* 3-form, $\mathbf{Q} = \frac{1}{3!} Q_{ijk} dx^i \wedge dx^j \wedge dx^k$;

where $\wedge$ denotes the exterior wedge-product. These four SE(3)-deformation forms satisfy the following set of continuity equations:

---

[m] In the authors' current work,[9] the Cosserat viscoelastic continuum model has been generalized to the microstretch continuum model for human fascia, iliopsoas and other polyarticular muscles and human lymphodynamics.

$$\dot{\alpha} = -\mathbf{dJ} - \mathbf{S}, \tag{4}$$

$$\dot{\mathbf{Q}} = -\mathbf{dS}, \tag{5}$$

$$\mathbf{d}\alpha = \mathbf{Q}, \tag{6}$$

$$\mathbf{dQ} = \mathbf{0}, \tag{7}$$

where **d** denotes the exterior derivative.

In components, the simplest, fourth equation (7), representing the *Bianchi identity*, can be rewritten as

$$\mathbf{dQ} = \partial_l Q_{[ijk]} dx^l dx^i \wedge dx^j \wedge dx^k = \mathbf{0}$$

where $\partial_i \equiv \partial/\partial x^i$, while $\theta_{[ij...]}$ denotes the skew-symmetric part of $\theta_{ij...}$.

Similarly, the third equation (6) in components reads

$$\frac{1}{3!} Q_{ijk} dx^i \wedge dx^j \wedge dx^k = \partial_k \alpha_{[ij]} dx^k \wedge dx^i \wedge dx^j; \quad \text{or}$$

$$Q_{ijk} = -6\partial_k \alpha_{[ij]} \quad \text{or } 3!$$

The second equation (5) in components reads

$$\frac{1}{3!} \dot{Q}_{ijk} dx^i \wedge dx^j \wedge dx^k = -\partial S_{[ij]} dx^k \wedge dx^i \wedge dx^j; \text{ or}$$

$$\dot{Q}_{ijk} = 6\partial_k S_{[ij]}.$$

Finally, the first equation (4) in components reads

$$\frac{1}{2} \dot{\alpha}_{ij} dx^i \wedge dx^j = (\partial_j J_i - \frac{1}{2} S_{ij})\, dx^i \wedge dx^j; \quad \text{or}$$

$$\dot{\alpha}_{ij} = 2\partial_j J_i - S_{ij}.$$

The above exterior equations can be interpreted as

- The 2-form equation (4) defines the time derivative $\dot{\alpha} = \frac{1}{2}\dot{\alpha}_{ij}dx^i \wedge dx^j$ of the dislocation density α as the (negative) sum of the disclination current **S** and the curl of the dislocation current **J**.
- The 3-form equation (5) states that the time derivative $\dot{\mathbf{Q}} = \frac{1}{3!}\dot{Q}_{ijk}dx^i \wedge dx^j \wedge dx^k$ of the disclination density **Q** is the (negative) divergence of the disclination current **S**.
- The 3-form equation (6) defines the disclination density **Q** as the divergence of the dislocation density α, that is, **Q** is the *exact* 3-form.
- The Bianchi identity (7) follows from equation (6) by *Poincaré lemma* and states that the disclination density **Q** is conserved quantity, that is, **Q** is the *closed* 3-form. Also, every 4-form in 3D space is zero.

From the above equations in *p*-forms, two important conclusions can be derived:

1. Being the derivatives of the dislocations, disclinations of the brain, intervertebral disc, or a synovial joint are higher-order tensors, and thus more complex quantities, which means that they present a higher risk for the severe mechanical injuries than dislocations — a fact which *is* supported by the literature (see review of existing TBI models given in Introduction of Ref. [1]).
2. Dislocations and disclinations of the brain, intervertebral disc, or a synovial joint are mutually coupled by the underlaying SE(3) group, which means that translational and rotational injuries of brain, spine and synovial joints cannot be separately analyzed — a fact which *is not* supported by the literature.

The Cosserat visco-elasto-plastic dislocations and disclinations have been generalized in Ref. [9] to the microstretch visco-elasto-plastic dislocations and disclinations in human fascia, iliopsoas muscle and human lymphodynamics.

5. Knee Injury Explained in Terms of the Euclidean Jolt Injury Mechanism

The knee joint comprises three articulations (see knee figure in Ref. [3]): (i) a tibio-femoral joint) between the medial and lateral condyles of the femur and tibia, (ii) patelo-femoral joint between the femur and patella, and (iii) tibio-fibular joint between tibia and fibula. The knee is double condyloid joint, with a dominant flexion/extension. As a synovial joint, the knee has strong fibrous capsule that attaches superiorly to the femur and inferiorly to the articular margin of the tibia. Given its relatively poor bony fit, the knee relies on ligaments for much of its structural stability and integrity.[10]

Knee joint injuries range from mild ligament or meniscus tearing to severe traumatic dislocations (see Ref. [13] and references therein) that fall among the most severe form of ligament injury to the lower extremity, associated with a high rate of complications.

Knee joint injuries are also frequent in sports, especially in ball games. For example, in a recently case-reported complex knee injury in a rugby league player, resulting in combined rupture of the patellar tendon, anterior cruciate and medial collateral ligaments, with a medial meniscal tear, the video-analysis suggests two points during the tackle when there was the potential for injury: the first occurred when the player was in single leg stance whilst running and received impact to his upper body from three defenders; the second occurred when the player landed on the knee and sustained a valgus and hyperflexion force under the weight of two defenders (see Ref. [3] for more details). The goal of treatment in this condition is restoration of both the extensor mechanism and knee stability.

Besides, the knee is the body part most commonly injured as a consequence of collisions, falls, and overuse occurring from childhood sports. The number of sports-related injuries is increasing because of active participation of children in competitive sports. Children differ from adults in many areas, such as increased rate and ability of healing, higher strength of ligaments compared with growth plates, and continued growth. Growth around the knee can be affected if the growth plates are involved in injuries.[14]

Literature on knee mechanics was reviewed in Ref. [15], evaluating various techniques that had been used to determine "*in vivo* loads" in the human knee joint. Two main techniques that had been used were telemetry — an experimental approach, and mathematical modeling — a theoretical approach. Telemetric analyzes had previously been used to determine the *in vivo* loading of the human hip and more recently evaluated in the determination of *in vivo* knee loads. Mathematical modelling approaches can be categorized in two ways: (i) those that use optimization techniques to solve an indeterminate system, and (ii) those that utilize a reduction method that minimizes the number of unknowns, keeping the system solvable as the number of equations of motion are equal to the number of unknown quantities (for more technical details, see Ref. [15] and references therein).

The use of a *force-controlled dynamic knee simulator* to quantify the mechanical performance of total knee replacement designs during functional activity was pioneered by Desjardins *et al.*,[16] in which dynamic *total knee replacement* (TKR) study utilized a 6DOF force-controlled knee simulator to quantify the effect of TKR design alone on TKR mechanics during a simulated walking cycle. Simultaneous prediction of implant kinematics and contact mechanics has been demonstrated using explicit *finite element* (FE) models of the *Instron/Stanmore Knee Joint Simulator, Instron, Canton, MA*[17–19] In these models, kinematic verification was performed by comparing experimental and model-predicted motion for a single implant. Both models were found to produce similar kinematic results. Estimated contact pressure distributions were also closely correlated, as long as significant edge-loading conditions were not present. Recently, an adaptive FE method for pre-clinical wear testing of TKR components was developed in Ref. [20], capable of simulating wear of a polyethylene tibial insert and to compare predicted kinematics, weight loss due to wear, and wear depth contours to results from a force-controlled experimental knee simulator. The displacement-controlled inputs, by accurately matching the experimental tibio-femoral motion, provided an evaluation of the simple wear theory. The force-controlled inputs provided an evaluation of the overall numerical method by simultaneously predicting both kinematics and wear. Proposed international standards for TKR wear simulation have been drafted, yet their methods continue to be debated.

The "gold standard" to which all TKR wear testing methodologies should be compared is measured *in vivo* TKR performance in patients. The study of Desjardins *et al.*[21] compared patient TKR kinematics from fluoroscopic analysis and simulator TKR kinematics from force-controlled wear testing to quantify similarities in clinical ranges of motion and contact bearing kinematics and to evaluate the proposed ISO force-controlled Stanmore wear testing methodology.

For human movement purposes, one can say that the safe knee motions (flexion/extension with some medial/lateral rotation in the flexed position) *are* governed by standard Euler's rotational dynamics coupled to Newton's micro-translational dynamics. On the other hand, the unsafe knee events, the main cause of knee injuries, are caused by the knee SE(3) jolts, the sharp and sudden, "delta" — (forces + torques) combined. These knee SE(3) jolts do not belong to the standard Newton–Euler dynamics. The only way to monitor them would be to measure *in vivo* the rate of the combined (forces + torques) — rise in the knee joint.

According to Ivancevic *et al.*,[3] the main cause of knee injury is the SE(3)-jolt,[n] which can cause two forms of discontinuous knee injury: (i) mild rotational disclinations and (ii) severe translational dislocations. Both the knee disclinations and dislocations, as caused by the SE(3)-jolt, are defined in Ref. [3], using the Cosserat multipolar visco-elasto-plastic continuum model.

Healthy knee dynamics is defined by coupled Newton–Euler dynamics defined in Section 2. Pathological knee dynamics is caused by the Euclidean jolt defined in Section 3.

Applying the exterior differential form equations (4)–(7) to the knee joint on can conclude that the knee dislocations and

[n] Although predominantly a hinge joint enabling a single flexion/extension cycle, it is well known that knee is actually a joint with full 6DOFs, exactly represented by the 6-parameter Euclidean group SE(3). Therefore, knee injuries are caused by the SE(3)-jolt.

disclinations are mutually coupled by the underlaying SE(3)-group, which means that translational and rotational knee injuries cannot be separately analyzed — a fact which *is not* supported by the literature. Contrary to the case of traumatic brain injury, knee dislocations are more severe than knee disclinations. This fact, despite of higher-order differential forms, is due to the fact that both human and animal knee joint is naturally designed to rotate in several directions.

While the knee SE(3)-jolt can be visualized intuitively, for the purpose of computer simulation the necessary simplified, decoupled approach (neglecting the 3D torque matrix and its coupling to the 3D force vector) is usually used. Note that decoupling is a kind of linearization that prevents chaotic behavior, giving an illusion of full predictability. In this decoupled framework of reduced complexity, the following parameters are defined: (i) the cause of knee dislocations as a linear 3D jolt vector, the time rate-of-change of a 3D force vector (linear jolt = mass × linear jerk); and (ii) the cause of knee disclinations as an angular 3-axial jolt, which is the time rate-of-change of a 3-axial torque (angular jolt = inertia moment × angular jerk). For more technical details on this decoupled computation framework, see Ref. [4].

References

1. Ivancevic, V. *Cogn. Neurodyn.*, **2009**, *3*, 281–293.
2. Ivancevic, V. *Int. J. Appl. Mech.*, **2009**, *1*(2): 387–401.
3. Ivancevic, V. *Biophys. Rev. Let.*, **2009**, *4*(3), 273–287.
4. Ivancevic, V. *Nonlin. Dyn.* **2010**, *61*(12), 123–139.
5. Wikipedia: Rotation group SO(3), **2016**.
6. Ivancevic, V.; Ivancevic, T. *New Trends in Control Theory* (World Scientific, Singapore, **2012**).
7. Ivancevic, V.; Ivancevic, T. *Human-Like Biomechanics* (Springer, Dordrecht, **2005**).
8. Ivancevic, V.; Ivancevic, T. *Geometrical Dynamics of Complex Systems* (Springer, Dordrecht, **2006**).
9. Ivancevic, T. *et al. The Evolved Athlete: A Guide for Elite Sport Enhancement, Springer Nature*, Series: Cognitive Systems Monographs (Springer Nature, Berlin, **2017**).

10. Whiting, W. C.; Zernicke, R. *Biomechanics of Musculoskeletal Injury, Human Kinetics* (Champaign, IL, **1998**).
11. Cosserat, E.; Cosserat, F.; *C.R. Acad. Sci. Paris,* **1898**, *126*, 1089–1091.
12. Cosserat, E.; Cosserat, F. *Theory of Deformable Bodies* (Hermann et Fils, Paris, **1909**).
13. Seroyer, S. T.; Musahl, V.; Harner, C. D. *Injury,* **2008**, *39*(7), 710–718.
14. Siow, H. M.; Cameron, D. B.; Ganley, T. J. *Phys. Med. Rehab.*, **2008**, *19*(2), 319–345.
15. Komistek, R. D.; Kane, T. R.; Mahfouz, M.; Ochoa, J. A.; Dennis, D. A. *J. Biomech.*, **2005**, *38*(2), 215–228.
16. DesJardins, J. D.; Walker, P. S.; Haider, H.; Perry, J. *J. Biomech.*, **2000**, *33*, 1231–1242.
17. Godest, A. C.; Beaugonin, M.; Haug, E.; Taylor, M.; Gregson, P. J. *J. Biomech.* **2002**, *35*(2), 267–275.
18. Halloran, J. P.; Easley, S. K.; Petrella, A. J.; Rullkoetter, P. *J. Biomech. Eng.* **2005**, *127*, 813–818.
19. Halloran, J. P.; Petrella, A. J.; Rullkoetter, P. *J. Biomech.*, **2005**, *38*, 323–331.
20. Knight, L. A.; Pal, S.; Coleman, J. C.; Bronson, F.; Haider, H.;, Levine, D. L.; Taylor, M.; Rullkoetter, P. J. *J. Biomech.*, **2007**, *40*, 1550–1558.
21. DesJardins, J. D.; Banks, S. A.; Benson, L. C.; Pace, T.; LaBerge, M. *J. Biomech.*, **2007**, *40*, 3458–3466.

https://doi.org/10.1142/9789811204630_0013

Chapter 13

In Silico Models for the Design of Tissue-Engineered Ligaments

Cédric Laurent[*,§], Damien Durville[†], Didier Mainard[‡], Xiong Wang[‡], and Rachid Rahouadj[*]

[*] *Université de Lorraine, CNRS, Arts et Métiers ParisTech, LEM3, F-54000 Nancy, France*

[†] *CNRS, MSSMat, UMR 8579, Ecole Centrale Paris, Grande Voie des Vignes, 92290 Chatenay-Malabry, France*

[‡] *CNRS, IMoPA, UMR 7365, Biopôle, Université de Lorraine, 9 Avenue de la Forêt de Haye, 54504 Vandeuvre-lès-Nancy, France*

[§] *cedric.laurent@univ-lorraine.fr*

Abbreviations

ACL	Anterior cruciate ligament
ACLR	ACL reconstruction
AM	Anteromedial
CATE	Computer-aided tissue Engineering
CFD	Computational fluid dynamics
CT	Computed tomography
DB	Double-bundle
ECM	Extracellular matrix
FDM	Fused deposition modeling
FE	Finite element
FISS	Flow-Induced Shear Stress
μCT	Micro-CT
MSC	Mesenchymal Stem Cells
OSS	Octahedral shear strain
PL	Posterolateral
PLCL	Copoly(lactic acid-co-(ε-caprolactone))
RP	Rapid prototyping
RVE	Representative volume element
SB	Single-bundle
SEM	Scanning electron microscopy
SLS	Selective laser sintering

1. Ligament Tissue Engineering

1.1. *Tissue Engineering*

Tissue engineering involves the development of biological substitutes to restore or replace lost tissue function.[1] It may potentially provide the patient with an immunologically tolerant substitute able to progressively turn into a biological tissue, and it has been used in the last decade for various tissues including but not limited to skin, cartilage, bone, liver, nerve or blood vessels.[2,3] Some authors have separated different approaches in tissue engineering: (1) the use of isolated cells expanded *in vitro* (2) the use of tissue-inducing substances such as growth factors and (3) the seeding and growing of cells in three-dimensional (3D) structures called scaffolds.[4] Nonetheless, most of the studies implicitly combine these three approaches for the purpose of growing specific biosubstitutes capable of replacing a damaged tissue. The role of the scaffold includes two different interrelated scales: (1) the macroscopic scale at which the scaffold should meet the anatomical dimensions of the tissue to be replaced, and should fulfill the physiological function of the native tissue during the rehabilitation period and (2) the microscopic scale at which the scaffold should promote tissue formation by providing the cells with a suited micro-environment.[5] After having selected a scaffold, common tissue engineering approaches use bioreactors so as to provide the cells with an adapted environment by controlling temperature, oxygen, pH, metabolites or biologically active molecules.[6] They are also used to transfer to cells the mechanical stimuli required for tissue formation and to overcome mass transport limitations occurring in static culture.[6–8] The tissue engineering approach which is thought to be suited begins with the seeding of reparative cells into the scaffold, then cultured in a bioreactor until enough new tissue has grown, and finally implanted at the place of the damaged tissue where it should degrade while the biological tissue is forming.[9]

1.2. *Interest for Ligament Reconstruction*

Ligament has been viewed as a potential promising application of tissue engineering principles in the early 2000's[10,11]. Particularly, most applications of ligament tissue engineering concern the anterior cruciate ligament (ACL), whose role in the knee kinematics has been largely described in the literature.[12–18] It constitutes the primary restraint against anterior tibial translation, and also limits the internal rotation of the tibia with respect to the femur. ACL is one of the most frequently injured structures of the knee joint, and the number of injury diagnoses tends to increase,[19] especially because of the increasing practice of high-risk sports for knee ligaments.

The replacement of ACL through intra-articular augmentation (i.e. ligamentoplasty) therefore constitutes a socio-economic challenge. The main critical aspects concerning ligamentoplasty are (1) the location of graft insertions (2) the graft initial tension (3) the fixation of graft and (4) the graft choice. As far as this last point is concerned, the use of autografts (mainly patellar tendon, hamstring tendon or quadriceps tendon[20]) has clearly become the gold standard. Associated with adapted rehabilitation protocols,[20,21] these techniques enable a return to full-sport participation within 6 months after reconstruction. However, they still possess some limitations such as donor site morbidity,[15,20] strength loss due to ligamentization,[19] or poor knee kinematics recovery.[22,23]

The use of synthetic grafts (Versigraft, Dacron, Gore-Tex, Leeds-Keio polyester, etc.) has been very popular in the 1980s–1990s. However, they showed very limited success due to long-term mechanical limitations,[11] including excessive joint laxity due to graft creep. In contrast, tissue engineering has been seen as a promising solution for repairing musculoskeletal tissues such as ligaments.[11,24] Indeed, due to the gradual transfer of load-bearing responsibilities from the graft to the newly formed tissue which should occur, long-term mechanical limitations reported for artificial grafts may be avoided by restricting the mechanical requirements to a short post-surgery period. However, despite a large variety of scaffolds proposed for ligament,[4,24–34] tissue-engineered solutions struggle to reach the clinics, due to the complexity and the variety of scientific fields that need to be involved and combined in order to propose a relevant biosubstitute meeting the key requirements for ligament tissue engineering. Moreover, the challenge of anchoring the proposed solutions within bone tunnels is still highly challenging. This issue of anchorage a soft tissue to bone is also of primary importance as far as tendon is concerned this will be particularly discussed in the following sections.

1.3. *Key Requirements for Ligament Tissue Engineering*

The scaffold design is of crucial interest in the tissue engineering process, as it will considerably influence both the biological activity of the cells that will adhere on, and the scaffold's capability to replace the physiological function of the native tissue during the rehabilitation period. The design of optimal scaffolds for a specific tissue engineering application has consequently always been a central point for tissue engineers.[35] It has initially been often said that Mother's Nature was the best designer and should be mimicked in the design of scaffolds.[3,36] However, the exact match of the native tissue properties by the biomimetism paradigm may not be the priority focus of tissue engineers in a first step,[37] but rather the finding of optimal structures for a given list of key requirements which are still generally unknown.[5] It seems indeed unrealistic that tissue engineering will enable to create copies of native tissues, but it may rather pretend to create biological constructs capable of restoring a lost function.[38]

1.3.1. *Scaffold morphology*

As far as ligament tissue engineering is concerned, an adapted scaffold should obviously be biocompatible and limit the risk of disease transmission and infection. As a result, no toxic products or lubricants should be used during the process of the scaffold material or architecture, and the scaffold should be easily sterilizable.[39] The scaffold should be made of a biodegradable material, whose degradation should not produce harmful material.[9,39,40] The scaffold should act as a 3D template for *in vitro* and *in vivo* tissue formation.[9] The blood vessels providing *in vivo* the tissues and cells with nutrients are lacking at the early stage of the implantation,[41] especially because of the poor environment constituted by the synovial liquid surrounding most ligaments. Scaffolds with high porosity and large interconnected pores are therefore required to facilitate cell ingrowth, nutrient inflow and waste outflow.[42–44] However, the scaffold morphology should also offer a sufficient area available for cell adhesion and a sufficient mechanical integrity, which involves an upper limit.[45] A large pore size is also required for the vascularization of the new tissue[46,47]; however, although vascularization is of a crucial interest for the repair of tissues such as liver[48] or bone,[49,50] it may be viewed as a secondary requirement for ACL which is moderately vascularized.[25] The ideal pore size range within a scaffold is different according to the cell type[51,52]; it has been sometimes approximated around 5–10 times the cell diameter.[53] In the case of ACL tissue engineering, it has been commonly accepted that the scaffold should exhibit pores with diameters more than 200–250 μm.[25,27] The pore size has been demonstrated to be more determinant that the overall porosity on the tissue formation, even if the latter obviously influences the mechanical and flow effective properties of the scaffold.[8] Despite similar porosity and pore size, two scaffolds with different microstructures may result in a different permeability and therefore they may not be similar in terms of cell seeding and nutrients transportation.[54] It has been indeed reported for instance that the accessible radius of a pore, characterized by the largest sphere that can reach the pore from the scaffold periphery, is far much relevant than pore sizes in the prediction of tissue formation.[42] Moreover, specific surface area[37,54] should also be cited as a critical aspect of scaffold morphology, since it will largely influence cell adhesion as well as the facilitated exchange of chemical substances from cells to the media. This specific surface area evolves in time due to tissue growth and scaffold degradation and should remain sufficient to ensure such exchanges.

One of the main requirement — and particularly in the case of ACL tissue engineering — is that the scaffold should maintain integrity until the new tissue regenerates, and it should enable to fulfill the function of the native tissue during the rehabilitation period.[7,55,56] Ideally, the tissue formation should progressively compensate the scaffold biodegradation towards the regeneration of a biological load-bearing tissue.[43] The kinetics of this load-bearing transfer from the scaffold to the new tissue is obviously a critical aspect of ligament tissue engineering (Figure 1), since a premature scaffold degradation may lead to a critical situation during which the physiological function of the ligament is not satisfied.

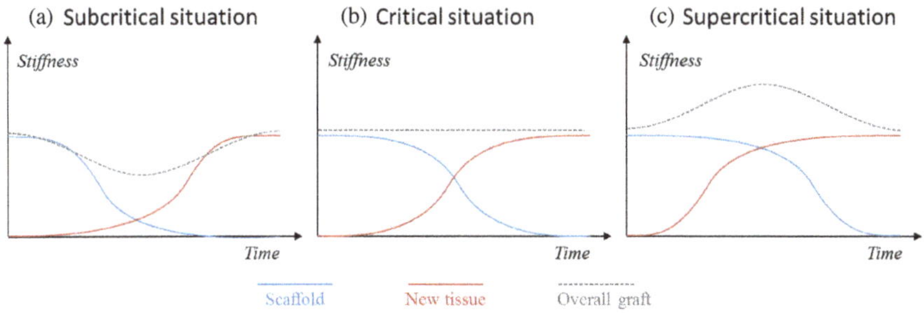

Figure 1. Potential situations depending on the rates of scaffold degradation and tissue formation. Subcritical situation (a) may lead to a physiological dysfunction, whereas supercritical (c) situation should be preferred

1.3.2. *Mechanical properties*

The question of which properties of the native tissue should be mimicked (and at which level) is complicated and open.[56] As the mechanical behavior of biological tissues are often far from simple, it is necessary to select and prioritize a subset of mechanical properties as key requirements for a tissue engineering scaffold.[57] This subset of properties may be restrained in priority to those essential to restore the normal function of the tissue during the rehabilitation period, as it is not realistic to match the exact properties of the native material. Within this framework, the mechanical requirements for the ACL scaffold may be defined at the scale of the global structure (load and stiffness) and not at the scale of a representative volume element (stress and modulus), as the aim is not to mimic the intrinsic material properties of ligamentous tissue.

These design criteria may be based on measurements of physiological loadings during daily activities rather than on the *in vitro* mechanical characterization of harvested ACL. These physiological loadings have been quantified either from the kinematical analysis of the knee under various loading by means of 3D imaging image,[58,59] or from direct *in vivo* measurements by means of sensors implantation.[60,61] Briefly, it has been shown that the ACL is commonly subjected to strains more than 4%[60] resulting in loads more than 400N[62] during daily activities. Noteworthy, the *in vivo* loading of ACL is displacement-induced rather than force-induced, and a less stiff tissue than the native ACL would consequently encounter smaller loads for a given elongation. These experimental data will be considered as a key requirement for a clinically relevant graft solution, and it should consequently orient the scaffold design step. They are more realistically reachable than the native properties of ACL, which could bear more than 1500N.

Moreover, it is crucial in a tissue engineering approach to consider the whole surgical procedure when determining these mechanical key requirements. Indeed, in the case of ACL, the ultimate failure load of current fixation techniques were estimated below 600N,[20] and it is consequently useless to design a scaffold with a superior failure load. As the physiological function of ACL consists in restraining displacements between tibia and femur, it is of great interest that the substitute offers a sufficient stiffness. However, the stiffness needed for a functional recovery of the ACL during rehabilitation activities has been seldom reported.

It may be thus considered that a suitable scaffold should offer a stiffness exceeding 100N/mm, as measured *in vitro* on harvested native ACL.[63] *In vitro* mechanical characterization of native ACL has permitted to emphasize that the ACL tensile response was non-linear with a pronounced toe region.[63] As this toe region enables a small knee laxity and results in small forces within the ACL during daily activities, it should therefore be taken into account when determining the suited mechanical response of an ACL scaffold. At last, the biomechanical behavior of the scaffold will obviously vary in time with scaffold degradation and tissue formation.[56] It is therefore crucial to point out that even if a tissue matches the suited properties at the implantation time, it does not prevent failure during the rehabilitation period, and the variations of scaffold mechanical response in time should then be considered to assess the suitability of a scaffold for ACL repair (see Section 4).

1.3.3. *Other aspects*

Several crucial clinical aspects should also take place in the list of main key requirements. As far as the anatomy is concerned, the scaffold should exhibit a geometry compatible with the site of replacement.[56,64,65] An appropriate external geometry should indeed facilitate a better fixation and a better stress distribution at the implant's interfaces[7]. In the particular case of ACL, several anatomical studies have reported 7–12 mm in width and 22–41 mm in length depending on the considered bundle.[12,14,17] It is likely that a scaffold which does not respect the maximal ACL width may lead to articular dysfunction.

Moreover, it is widely recognized that the ACL could be separated into two main bundles (anteromedial (AM) and posterolateral (PL)), whose functions and dimensions are different. While common reconstruction procedures aims at replacing the broken ACL by a single-bundle (SB) prosthesis, it has been reported that anatomic double-bundle (DB) reconstructions aiming at reconstructing separately the AM and PL bundles of the ACL offer promising results concerning the restoration of knee kinematics, particularly in the case of rotatory loads.[66–69] Consequently, it is likely that a scaffold which could be tailored to match the requirements for either SB or DB reconstructions may constitute a promising graft source. Additional surgical procedures due to the use of a tissue-engineered construct should be avoided in order to ease its clinical application.[11,56] Particularly, in the case of ACL tissue engineering, it is necessary to consider the future clinical fixation of the scaffold into bone tunnels from the beginning of the scaffold design step. At last, for any clinical applications, a scaffold should obviously be adapted to large-scale production[56] and able to maintain its properties during packaging and storage.[57]

1.4. *Rationale for Computational Approaches*

The multi-disciplinary and multiscale issues associated with tissue engineering in general and ligament tissue engineering, have convinced some research groups that computer-based tools may help to head for suited clinically relevant tissue-engineered constructs. The ideal scaffold architecture for a specific application should result from a trade-off between a list of design criteria suited for the particular tissue,[70] and a methodological approach of multi-objective design optimization may therefore be adequate.[71] Therefore, it has appeared obvious for researchers with an engineering background to use computational tools in order to help in this optimization procedure. Indeed, scaffolds were originally mainly issued from a trial-and-error approach,[72] which resulted in material- and time-consuming design steps. The interest of computational approaches in view of shortening the design process of scaffolds and so as to propose better architectures according to a list of criteria has therefore been raised by the tissue engineers.[46]

These computational approaches may be used to (1) optimize various properties of initial selected scaffold, (2) understand the cellular microenvironment, which will result from external loading, (3) optimize the process of culturing scaffolds within bioreactors, (4) understand and interpret the results of biological observations, (5) predict the evolution of tissue-engineered construct properties. These applications therefore constitute the outline of the following. The expression "computer-aided tissue engineering" (CATE) has firstly appeared in the beginning of the 2000s[2], and has gain more popularity since.[65,73–77] CATE it has been originally associated with the emerging techniques of rapid prototyping (RP) fabrication, and was used to define the computer-aided technologies that may be used in every step involved in the repair of tissues using the tissue engineering principles, including the imaging, the rapid prototyping modeling, the tissue identification, the scaffold modeling and the computed-aided surgical planning.[2] Some authors rather talk about *in silico* models to describe computational approaches aiming to understand and predict the biological evolution of tissue-engineered constructs,[78–81] but this term focus rather on the modeling of growing cells that on the scaffold itself. In the present chapter, the general term "computational approaches" is used, in order to include both these different terminologies. Given the amount of work in this challenging field, this chapter does not pretend to give a review of computer-based tissue engineering studies, but rather to present the most relevant computational approaches that have been applied or developed from the 2000s to tissue engineering and may be applied or extended in the future to the case of ligament.

2. Designing Ligament Scaffolds

2.1. *Defining Scaffold Morphology*

2.1.1. *3D imaging*

The authors of this chapter have detailed previously how the different morphological characteristics of the scaffold were important in the definition of a scaffold for a specific application. Once a scaffold has been designed, it is therefore crucial to characterize its morphology, and computational methods are often used based on 3D imaging. Indeed, global properties such as percentage porosity do not provide sufficient information about scaffold morphology.[9] Scaffold morphological properties such as pore size distribution may be assessed by scanning electron microscopy (SEM)[82] or mercury porosimetry. However, these techniques have several limitations including their destructive nature and they may not provide sufficient information about the real 3D shape of the scaffold[9]. In opposition, the capability to get a 3D digitized definition of the scaffold geometry may be used to precisely assess and optimize the morphological properties of a scaffold. The characteristics of the pores network can usually be determined using existing software associated with micro-computed tomography (μCT) acquisition.

Pore interconnectivity, porosity and pore size distribution may therefore be easily obtained by these ready-made algorithms[82–84] or using dedicated software.[42,52,85] As a non-destructive technique, the interest of μCT techniques has risen compared to common computed tomography (CT), which does not allow the accurate tissue microstructure to be imaged.[86] In return, μCT is only applicable to small samples of scaffolds unlike common CT,[87] but this drawback is progressively compensated with the evolution of imaging techniques. The resolution of μCT is restricted to a few micrometers, which may not enable nanometer structures to be visualized in opposition with SEM.[52] However, μCT offers the advantage on SEM to be non-destructive.[9] It consequently allows the same scaffold to be imaged at different time points[72,86] and it is adapted to the framework of clinical routines. μCT techniques has also been used for instance so as to image the microstructure of trabecular bone in view of generating biomimetic bone-like scaffolds by means of RP techniques,[88] or to compare morphological properties of different scaffolds.[9,89] It may also enable to characterize the 3D bone ingrowth within scaffolds.[42,72,90–93] As a result of these 3D imaging techniques, pore size distribution and interconnectivity may then be computed from the scaffold numerical description,[54,72,82,85] as well as pore anisotropy, scaffold permeability,[72] specific surface area,[54] overall porosity,[54,88,94] or connectivity density of trabecular spacing.[88]. These morphological computations may be validated by performing mercury porosimetry.[95]

2.1.2. *Rapid prototyping techniques*

In order to enable computational methods to be applied on scaffolds, its external shape and microstructure must be firstly converted into a properly meshed 3D object. This 3D mesh may result from 3D imaging, as explained above, which obviously firstly requires processing the scaffold. This is therefore not compatible with an optimization process prior to scaffold fabrication. Alternatively, the scaffold may be issued from a mathematical modeling and its geometry directly issued from a CAD definition. The final scaffold geometry could therefore be determined from the microstructure design and the target anatomical shape using Boolean operators.[96,97] This is however not needed in the case of ligament tissue engineering, where the external shape of the suited graft is well known, and maybe not of prior importance. The defined scaffold microstructures are generally complex and may not be processable by means of common scaffolding techniques.

This obstacle has been overcome from the 2000s with the development of RP techniques, which allow a precise reconstruction of 3D objects from their digitized geometry. 3D imaging may then be used in order to compare the CAD target geometry and the corresponding actual geometry obtained by RP techniques. Indeed, conventional methods for manufacturing scaffolds do not allow an accurate control of pore size, pore geometry, pore distribution or internal channels within scaffolds.[98] It has been reported that the resulting non-optimal geometries led to a poor nutrient diffusion, to restrictions in mass transport leading to a lack of tissue ingrowth into the scaffold,[49,54,99] and that they do not offer sufficient mechanical properties in the case of load-bearing applications.[100] In contrast, RP techniques enable the reproducible fabrication of versatile 3D scaffolds with a precisely controlled architecture.[39,70,83,101] Thanks to this versatility, RP techniques — also called solid free-form fabrication techniques — have emerged as powerful tools in view of designing geometries optimized for cellular activity[49,102] and have therefore been extensively used for scaffold fabrication, especially in case of bone and cartilage tissue engineering. RP is to date the only way of manufacturing the complex architectures that may result from mathematically-defined microstructures.[56]

These techniques resulting from a layer-by-layer building through material deposition can be separated into fused deposition modeling (FDM), 3D printing, stereolithography and selective laser sintering (SLS).[43,97–99,103,104] The principle, weakness and strength of different RP technologies have been reviewed and compared to conventional scaffold fabrication techniques.[43,70,98] They have all shown a great potential to process structures for tissue engineering applications.[37,88,93,104–108] As the main limitation of these RP techniques is the limited number of materials that can be used,[99] RP has also been used to create negative molds corresponding to the open pores of the obtained scaffold,[48,99] and therefore to fill the interstices with common scaffold-fabricating techniques such as solvent casting.[56,101]

Such techniques enable to optimize the scaffold's microstructure without processing it. Indeed, scaffold microstructure is obviously a key factor for cell seeding, cell proliferation, nutrients income and waste products outcome. The scaffold microstructure also influences the way in which macroscopic loading or flow conditions are transmitted to the cells. Rationally-designed scaffold morphology may be needed in such a way that the macroscopic loadings of flows result in homogeneous local stimuli, and thus a homogeneous distribution of tissue.[109] In opposition with common scaffold fabrication techniques, rationally designed microstructures may allow the cells to penetrate deep inside the scaffold[54] and enable to generate gradients of cell distribution using inhomogeneous scaffold microstructures.[7,110] Indeed, biological tissues exhibit gradients enabling the whole tissue or organ to behave normally,[36] which have been called functional gradients. As a consequence, the need for functionally graded scaffolds has been raised.[7,107]

The term "functionally graded" is related to structures such as bone or cartilage, whose natural microstructure and/or composition are clearly inhomogeneous from the outer to the inner layers.[7] For instance, architecture with cone-shaped channels and a diameter gradient has been proposed.[41] It offers large pore size at the periphery of the scaffold and smaller pores in inner regions, and it has been shown to facilitate oxygen supply and consequently cell viability and proliferation. It may indeed overcome the mass transport restrictions due to the occupation of the exterior of the scaffold by growing tissue.[45,49,111,112] The need for gradients and/or stratified multiphasic scaffolds has been also reviewed in the particular case of interfaces tissue engineering,[113] which is a very challenging but crucial field of tissue engineering in view of the integration of tissue-engineered implants.

2.1.3. *A multilayer braided scaffold as a good candidate for ligament*

Rapid prototyping techniques, even if very promising for several tissue engineering applications (mainly bone or cartilage), are not the most adapted to structures such as tendon or ligament because of their low tensile properties. Considering the demanding mechanical requirement that need to be fulfilled in ligament tissue engineering, researchers have preferred textile architectures such as twisted,[10] knitted,[33] braided[4] structures, or aligned parallel fibers.[34]

Among the various types of available structures, the authors of the present chapter have selected an assembly of concentric circular braided layers[29,85,114] for the following reasons: (1) it is deformable in the low strain range but exhibits high stiffness and strength for large strains, which mimics the behavior of the native tissue, (2) it is able to offer the required network of interconnected pores, (3) it is largely tailorable in terms of morphology and mechanics by playing with the number of layers of the structure, the fiber diameters and the braiding angle of each layer, (4) it is adapted to computed-based approaches because of its predictable geometry resulting from the braiding process, (5) it offers a pore size gradient which facilitates the transport of nutrients and wastes from the heart of the scaffold to its periphery.

Among the variety of available biomaterials, copoly(lactic acid-co-(ε-caprolactone)) (PLCL) was selected for the following reasons: (1) it offers an excellent biocompatibility associated with a slow degradation rate,[115] (2) it allows both the brittle behavior of PLLA and the low stiffness of PCL to be compensated,[116] (3) it is tailorable by varying the lactic acid/ε-caprolactone proportions in the copolymer.[117] PLCL fibers with different lactic acid/ε-caprolactone proportions were then tested and compared in terms of elastic modulus, strain to rupture and creep, and as a result, fibers made of P(LL85/CL15) were chosen as a relevant trade-off between the low modulus of caprolactone and the low deformability of lactide.

The processing step should not affect the material properties and should allow reproducible and predictable structures to be formed.[43] Consequently, a custom process was designed in order both to extrude homogeneous PLCL fibers from the raw material and to form multilayer braids from these fibers in a reproducible manner. The fiber diameter, number of layers and braiding angles were kept variable in order to adjust the different morphological and mechanical properties of the as-made scaffold. As a result, tailorable multilayer braided scaffolds were obtained from very small amount of raw material. Then, computer-based methods inspired from reported algorithms[42] was used to characterize a priori the morphology of the braided scaffold, from a numerical description of its geometry based on the analysis of fiber trajectories during the braiding process (Figure 2).

The characterization of the morphology was based on a numerical description of the scaffold issued from the analysis of fiber trajectories during the braiding process.[118,119] The geometry of this virtual scaffold was validated by comparing its cross-sections with cross-sections of actual scaffolds.[85] The morphology was characterized by the pore size distribution within the virtual scaffold and the interconnectivity of pores. Computed pore size distribution were at last validated by comparison with mercury porosimetry.[85] Ultimately, from these algorithms a geometry able to fulfill the requirements for ligament tissue engineering in terms of pore size and interconnectivity was selected. Particularly, the scaffold offers a clear positive pore size gradient from the core to the periphery, which is thought to be beneficial for mass transport properties.[41]

As reminded above, the question of anchoring tissue-engineered ligament within the joint is still unresolved and constitutes a real clinical challenge. Indeed, the properties of ligament anchorage are often much lower than the graft properties,[19] and the native progressive interface between ligament and bone limits stress concentration. Recent studies aim at proposing an anchorage strategy together with a tissue-engineered ligament,[120] in order to reproduce the progressive anatomical transition between bone and ligament.[121] It may be therefore interesting to extend the previous approach to the design of bone–ligament scaffolds: for instance, the multilayer braided ligament scaffold may be embedded with a polymer foam issued from the solvent-casting method as widely reported.[122] The porosity gradient reported in the braided scaffold may be also extended to the porous foam, by progressively increasing the size of porogen particles from the core to the periphery of the scaffold. μCT reconstructions are thus required to visualize and compute the actual morphology of the bone–ligament–bone construct, as illustrated below (Figure 2) in the case of a first trial of a bone–ligament construct made of a braid embedded into a polymeric foam.

2.2. *Optimizing Scaffold Properties*

The ability to generate structures with desired mechanical properties is essential for the understanding of their involvement on tissue formation,[123] and in order to propose clinically relevant scaffolds for a given application. Among the variety of scaffold microstructures that have been proposed in the literature, a large range of static and dynamic mechanical properties have been found to be achievable so

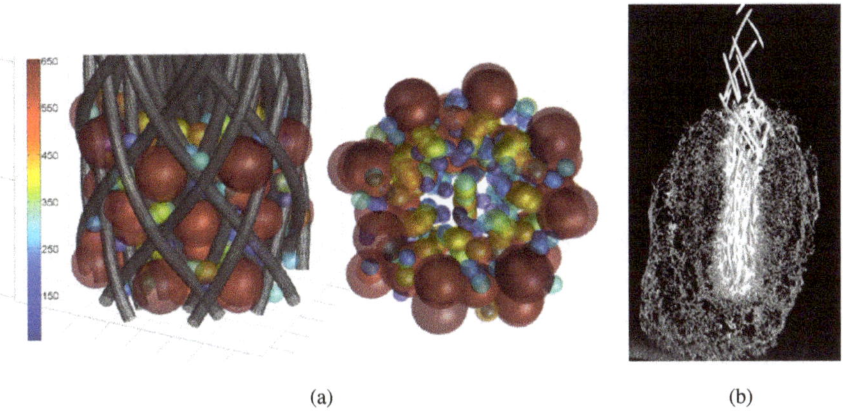

Figure 2. (a) Computer-based characterization of the morphology of a braided scaffold for ligament tissue engineering. (b) 3D reconstruction of a prototype of bone–ligament construct from μCT **acquisition**

as to satisfy the specific requirements associated with the target tissue.[37] However, quantifying the macroscopic properties resulting from given microstructure and external shape by using an experimental approach involves costly protocols and long-term experiments,[8] whereas numerical approaches may enable to predict these properties. The comparison between properties reachable by the scaffold and biomechanical published data are then of great interest.[106]

Two main numerical methods are generally used in order to predict (and thus optimize) scaffold mechanical properties. The first one uses the finite element (FE) method to predict scaffold mechanical macroscopic properties starting from its numerical description as obtained above. The FE method has been widely used in biomechanics, either to analyze the stress, strain and displacement fields in the skeleton, to design orthopedic devices or analyze biological mechanisms.[87] The FE method has the advantage to be adapted to non-homogeneous structures, such as scaffold geometries acquired using 3D reconstruction techniques.[124] Starting from a properly meshed object and adapted boundary conditions, it enables to compute several physical quantities at each discrete points of the digitized scaffold. Consequently, FE methods have been widely used to assess the mechanical behavior of different scaffolds and consequently their biomechanical optimality on the basis of the mechanical behavior of their constitutive material, their microstructure and their external shape.[49,86,93] Iterative algorithms can then be set in order to optimize the scaffold by playing on microstructure and/or material properties.[86] By using FE methods and μCT acquisitions, significant correlations have been demonstrated between the simulated mechanical properties of a CAD scaffold and experimental data, then emphasizing the ability to design scaffolds with predictable properties in a nondestructive manner.[99]

The second widespread method aims at optimizing and predicting the properties of periodic scaffolds starting from the definition of a unit cell by means of homogenization techniques. A CATE approach may be used in order to create various structures resulting from the repetition of cellular units (issued either from a library[100] or from 3D imaging[64]), which serve as building blocks to create a final scaffold fitting an expected external shape.[7,96,97] A library of well-characterized unit blocks[100] as well as specific CAD software[35] have been proposed to help the design of complex scaffolds for given external shape and microstructure. Starting from a mathematical definition of scaffold microstructure and the external shape issued from imaging techniques, CAD of porous scaffolds has therefore been proposed for numerous tissues.[97] Homogenization techniques are powerful tools to predict scaffold properties such as diffusivity, or mechanical and flow properties at the tissue level.[8,125] They allow multiscale analysis of continuum problems to be performed, by giving relationships between macroscopic properties and mechanical micro-environment within a representative volume element (RVE) assuming a scaffold periodicity.[56,71,96,123,125–127]

One of the main assumptions of these homogenization procedures is the separation of micro- and macro-scales,[123] which requires that the unit-cell is significantly smaller than the overall construct. Asymptotic homogenization eventually combined with FE implementation may be used so as to select the building blocks that lead to the most suited effective scaffold properties and to study the effect of process parameters on the global scaffold properties.[64] Both the direct and inverse homogenization techniques may be used.[128] The first one consists in determining the macroscopic properties of a periodic scaffold starting from a given unit cell and by means of homogenization theory,[102] while in the second technique, a topological optimization is used to iteratively determine the optimal material distribution within a unit cell that leads to the desired macroscopic properties,[5,128] generally starting from non-porous unit blocks. The optimization of scaffold topology should include multi-objective optimization problems, as for instance a stiffness-based design may involve unreachable pores if the diffusivity requirements are not taken into account.[129] To summarize, unit-cell based scaffold design may be seen as a powerful tool in the design of periodic scaffolds with given targeted effective properties. The problem is then once again raised of the criteria that should be taken into account for the optimization scheme.

Such homogenization techniques are only valid in the case of regular periodic structure, which is not the case for the multilayer braided scaffold presented above. Therefore, a finite element approach was applied to this geometry in order to predict macroscopic properties resulting from a set of process parameters. It is thought that in the case of ligaments, that are constantly subject to torsion and stretch during daily activities, the macroscopic loading is the prevalent cause of the mechanical stimuli sensed at the cellular scale, in opposition to the case of bone or cartilage where shear strain and fluid velocity have been shown to be correlated to tissue formation.[130] Therefore, a FE modeling of the dry scaffold was developed, assuming that biological fluid will not have a significant influence on the mechanical stimuli and on the macroscopic response of the scaffold.

A recent FE code dedicated to textiles[131] was used in order to (1) predict and optimize the tensile response of the scaffold (2) establish the relations between external loading and mechanical stimuli at the fiber scale (3) compute the scaffold geometries corresponding to different states of stretching. Details of the code used in this study have been previously reported,[131] and its application to the multilayer braided scaffold has been presented,[29] as well as its validation using μCT.[132] Briefly, the approach aims at reproducing the nonlinear behavior of textile materials by simulating the relative motions between fibers, individually modeled by an enriched kinematical beam model accounting for cross-sectional strains within a large deformation framework. The nonlinear stress–strain response of isolated PLCL fibers is approximated by an elastoplastic constitutive law consisting in a linear elastic part followed by a Chaboche-type hardening, whose parameters have been determined by using the least squares method from tensile tests on P(LL85/CL15) fibers for a given strain rate.

The process of contact detection consists in (1) the determination of proximity zones where contacts are likely to occur within the global assembly of beams (2) the creation of intermediate geometries defined as the average of fibers axes (3) the generation of contact elements at discrete locations on these intermediate geometries by using planes orthogonal to these geometries. The contact–friction interactions are then modeled in the form of a regularized penalty law in the normal direction and a Coulomb's law for tangential friction.

As far as the definition of boundary conditions are concerned, rigid bodies attached to both ends of each layer of the multilayer braid are used to prescribe loads or displacements to each layer, while isolated fibers bound to these rigid bodies by means on average conditions are allowed to rearrange. As the initial configuration of the scaffold cannot be known *a priori*, the definition of an arbitrary initial configuration is firstly used, in which trajectories of fibers are described by helices and fibers are therefore interpenetrated within the same layer. This interpenetration is gradually reduced by means of contact conditions starting from the braiding pattern of the construct. As a result of this nonlinear iterative process, a non-interpenetrated configuration of the braid is obtained as the equilibrium configuration of the assembly of fibers which satisfies the braiding pattern of the scaffold. Once this first initial configuration has been computed, a series of boundary conditions which aims at reproducing the braiding tension needed to tighten fibers during the braiding process and the pre-tension applied before the scaffold testing is prescribed. The layers are free to rearrange each other in such a way that the pitch length of each layer results from the satisfaction of mechanical equilibrium. The tensile — and/or torsion — test is then simulated by prescribing an increasing displacement — and/or rotation — to one edge of each layer of the scaffold.

The employed FE approach allowed the *a priori* unknown initial geometry of the braided scaffold to be computed, starting from an arbitrary configuration which depends on the process parameters. This geometry has been found to match the actual scaffold geometry by comparing their cross-sections.[29] Computed tensile responses for different scaffold configurations have been compared to experimental tensile tests performed on the corresponding actual scaffolds.[29] It has been shown that the FE simulations were able to predict the non-linear response of the braided construct in terms of toe region, yield load and stiffness, notwithstanding a slight overestimation of the scaffold stiffness. This overestimation has been mainly explained by the fact that the simulated scaffold is made of identical fibers with average properties, which does not reflect the variability of fibers whose yield induce experimentally the yield of the entire construct. As in Figure 3, one of the rehabilitation exercise that has been reported to induce maximal *in vivo* strains in the ACL[60] has been simulated, namely isometric quads contraction, modeled by prescribing a 4.4% stretch on the scaffold.

Besides, further work is currently performed to simulate the mechanical behavior of two separate scaffolds in the case of double-bundle (DB) ACL reconstruction, which has been reported to result

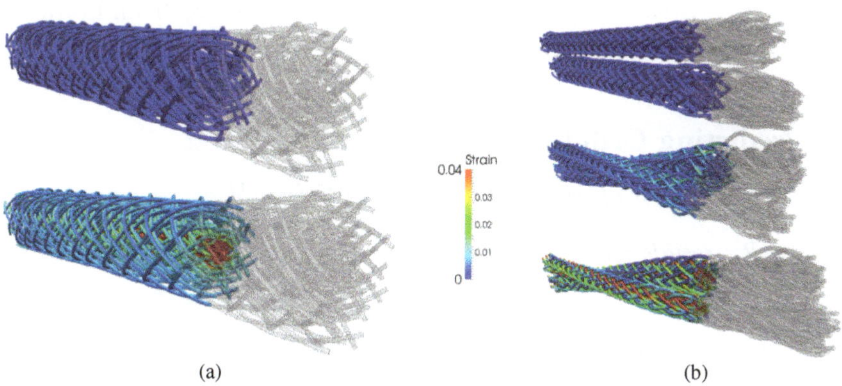

Figure 3. (a) Finite element simulation of an isometric contraction applied on a braided scaffold. (b) Example of finite element simulation of a double-bundle scaffold. The color field corresponds to equivalent octahedral shear strain

in a better restoration of the knee kinematics.[133] It involves complex boundary conditions based on clinical data to be prescribed, and may enable to draw conclusions about the mechanical suitability of a DB reconstruction and to propose adapted scaffold configurations in this particular case. An example of loading situations that can be prescribed to a DB ligament is illustrated above (Figure 3).

As mentioned above, it may be crucial to include the fixation device in the beginning of the design process, in order to provide surgeons with a ready-to-use substitute. It may be therefore interesting to extend the previous computational approach to the case of a bone–ligament construct, and to evaluate *a priori* the mechanical properties of the bone-ligament interface. As far as the bony part is concerned, a solution consists in creating porous foam as illustrated above. However, such processes do not enable to compute precisely micro-mechanical stimuli, as long as the geometry of pores is not fully predictable. Alternatively, rapid prototyping techniques may enable to provide with a porous bony fixation, starting from a geometry issued from CAD software. As an illustration, a design of bone–ligament construct is proposed below. Macroscopic mechanical properties of both braided ligamentous part and 3D-printed bony part may then be obtained from FE method, and the mechanical properties of bone–ligament construct may thus be assessed and optimized from homogenized properties, as Figure 4.

3. Predicting Cellular Micro-Environment

3.1. *Prediction of Micro-Mechanical Stimuli*

3.1.1. *Rationale for characterizing micro-mechanical environment*

In the previous section, the authors focused on the capability of some numerical tools to predict the effective properties of the scaffold and thus to propose optimal microstructures without requiring a classical trial-and-error approach. However, global mechanical properties of the scaffold do not provide information about the local mechanical stimuli at the cellular scale, which is necessary to understand the

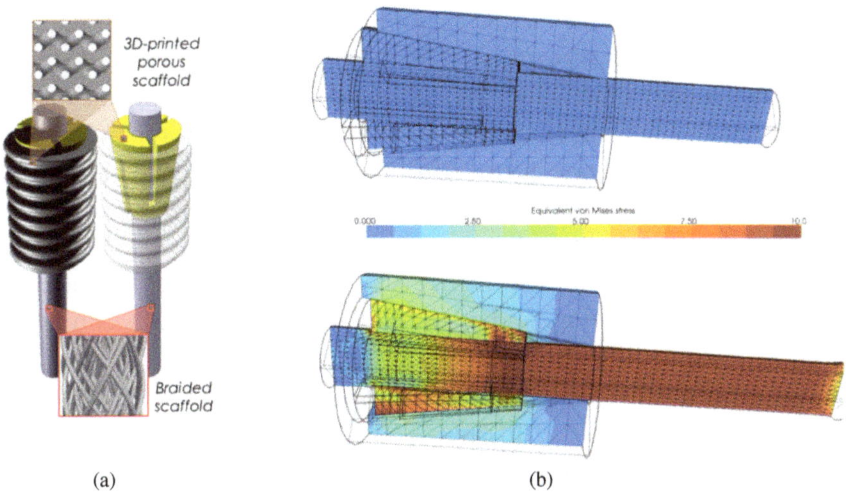

Figure 4. (a) Computer-aided design of a bone–ligament construct made of a braided ligamentous part and a 3D-printed bony part. (b) Finite element simulation of the mechanical properties of bone-ligament properties from homogenized properties

biological activity of such scaffolds.[109,130,134] Direct measurements of the local stimuli due to a macroscopic loading on a complex scaffold architecture are difficult, if not impossible, to perform. Computational methods constitute therefore a useful tool in the determination of local mechanical environment, by relating the external environment of the overall scaffold and the mechanical stimuli acting at the cell level.[112,135] With such micro–macro relationships, it may then be possible to determine the macroscopic loading which leads to the best suited micromechanical stimuli for a specific application[136] or the local stimuli that will be sensed by the cells once the scaffold will be implanted.

Indeed, cells in the metabolism are constantly subject to mechanical stimuli due to external physiological loading (e.g. bone), substrate stretching resulting from physiological movement (e.g. ligament) and/or fluid flow within the tissues (e.g. blood vessels). These mechanical stimuli are sensed by the cells and turned into biochemical responses, by means of mechanisms collectively designated as mechano-transduction.[137,138] These mechano-biological processes are thought to allow tissues to be fit for their mechanical function. For instance, it has been shown that if an increase of the substrate stiffness results in a lower strain felt by the cells (i.e. the loading is force-controlled and not displacement-controlled), the environment will be more favorable to bone formation, and otherwise a soft or fibrous tissue will be maintained.[139]

Experimental studies have reported that the local mechanical environment of cells influences their shape and migration direction,[140] their collagen secretion and extracellular matrix (ECM) composition,[141,142] their differentiation[141] and proliferation.[143] Therefore, the simple seeding of cells within a porous scaffold is often insufficient to promote a suited tissue formation,[70] and a micro-mechanical environment is required. These macroscopic external loadings which cause the local stimuli may be induced *in vitro* by mechanical stimulation or *in vivo* by functional demands.[112] The mechanical stimuli sensed by the cells is influenced by scaffold material properties, scaffold architecture, cells location within the scaffold (as the spatial distribution of stimuli is not homogeneous), and by the characteristics of the macroscopic loading and flow conditions prescribed throughout the dynamic bioreactor.[136] Even if not fully understood, these micro-mechanical requirements should be considered from the beginning of the tissue engineering strategy and the scaffold design step. Indeed, the scaffold, together with the internal fluids, serves as a structure, which links macroscopic loads (at the tissue scale) to micro-mechanical stimuli (at the cellular scale). Therefore, the knowledge of the required mechanical stimuli for a specific tissue engineering application may help the design of the scaffold microstructure and/or the determination of the suited culture conditions.[144]

Generally, micro-mechanical stimuli at the cellular scale due to either substrate deformation or fluid flow can be quantified in a given scaffold using FE methods and computational fluid dynamics (CFD), respectively. Therefore, computational approaches are suited in order to understand and optimize the mechano-biological phenomenon that may lead to a functional tissue-engineered substitute. The two next paragraphs briefly present some applications of these two computational methods (FE and CFD) for characterizing micro-mechanical stimuli. For both methods, a properly meshed description of the 3D scaffold is required and has been generally obtained via the previously described imaging techniques.

3.1.2. *Application of Finite Element method*

Finite Element Method (FE) associated with images from μCT have been especially applied on scaffolds for bone, in order to quantify the micro-mechanical stimuli (i.e. stress and strain fields) induced by different loadings (compressive loading,[47,124,145] both compressive loading and fluid flow,[136] or uniaxial strain[146]). The computed mechanical stimuli may then be related to bone formation, enabling to assess the ultimate evolution of a scaffold once implanted.[147] Such computations may be also further used in order to predict bone remodeling phenomena.[148] It has been shown that, depending of the scaffold architecture, the cells may be locally subject to stresses several orders of magnitude higher than the prescribed macroscopic stress,[136] even if local mechanical stimuli have been usually found lower than the prescribed macroscopic loading.[145] Even in the case of a compression test, it has been shown that many parts of the scaffold can be subject to tension due to structural effects.[145]

FE have also been used in order to understand biological observations, such as the influence of the hydrogels composition on the mechano-transduction signals.[149] Although cellular strain has commonly been equated to the local surface strain by assuming that the cells are perfectly attached to the surface of the scaffold, it has been shown that the cells do not necessarily adhere to a single surface but may bridge different scaffolds struts.[146] This assumption has been found to have a tendency to undervalue cellular strains, as it has been shown for instance that 76% of cells were attached to multiple struts of a bone scaffold.[146] This may be particularly the case for the braided scaffold presented above for ligament tissue engineering, in which it has been observed that cells clearly form bridges between fibers in the first days of culture.[150] Moreover, the contractile forces that the cells prescribe to their substrate are not taken into account in these studies. Nevertheless, it is thought that these cells-generated forces aim at creating a strain-rich environment, which is not necessary if an external loading is applied.[130] As noted above, FE requires the mechanical properties of the constitutive material to be identified. As the aim is to quantify micro-mechanical stimuli, the elastic properties of the constitutive material have been often determined in such a way that the simulated macroscopic properties of the scaffold match experimental results.[145]

3.1.3. *Application of Computer Fluid Dynamics*

Computer Fluid Dynamics (CFD) techniques allow to compute the complete 3D flow fields within a scaffold under fluid flow inlet.[6,151] The validation of flow-induced shear stress computations by experimental measurements of flow properties within pores is a very delicate — if not impossible — task.[152–154] The transport of nutrients within scaffolds has however been modeled and validated by local measurements in order to assess cellular nutrient utilization; among other results, it enables to determine what nutrients are potentially limiting.[112]

For instance, the diffusion of oxygen within different scaffold architectures has been modeled, and it has permitted to draw conclusions about the interest of pore size gradients to facilitate nutrient supply.[41] While theoretical methods can only provide mean values of flow-induced stimuli that do not reflect the real shear stress distribution within the scaffold microstructure,[152] the computation of local flow within an accurate scaffold geometry using CFD methods has been reported to give precise local information.[152,154] The distribution of fluid velocity and fluid shear stress in response to a perfusion fluid flow has been computed generally in combination with μCT acquisition[47,124,130,136,151,155] within different types of structures such as bone scaffolds prepared via solvent casting/particle leaching technique[156], trabecular bone[155] or CAD-based scaffolds.[110]

CFD methods have also been used to assess the effect of pore size and accessibility on the scaffold permeability and shear stresses,[42] or the effect of some scaffold parameters and culture conditions on the shear stress distribution[110,152] and flow velocity.[110] They have noteworthy enabled to confront these shear stresses to cell densities[110] and tissue differentiation.[136] CFD may then be used in view of improving the bioreactor for a given scaffold on the basis of fluid flow requirements[6] (see Section 3.2). The tissue ingrowth within scaffolds should be numerically taken into account by considering time-dependent boundary conditions, which remains a challenging task.[6] Indeed, the tissue formation influences the biological activity by changing both the biochemical and mechanical environment.[157] It may be modeled by coating the scaffold with an increasing layer for an increased cultivation period.[153] However, the cell proliferation is influenced by various biochemical factors which should not result in a homogeneous layer increase. By taking into account morphological variations due to cellular ingrowth or scaffold degradation, it has been suggested that the scaffold should be subject to a decreasing flow rate over time, so as to maintain a physiological range of micro-mechanical stimuli.[124,136] It is of interest to note that in such CFD modeling, the deformability of the scaffold due to flow conditions has been neglected which may lead to errors.[153]

As a result, the combination of both FEM and CFD towards a more accurate prediction of mechanical stimuli including the interrelated effects of dynamic stretching, strain rate or flow conditions, is likely to constitute the next future advances in computational approaches for tissue engineering. Indeed, whereas a lot of studies aiming at assessing the mechanical stimuli induced by an external loading neglect the fluid–structure interactions,[134,145] cyclic strain inevitably involves a fluid movement, and these two types of mechanical stimuli are then interrelated. The mechanical stimuli at the cellular scale may indeed be significantly influenced by the fluid phase which is present in the scaffold pores.[47] However, as the consideration of fluid–structure interactions has a substantial computational cost, one may therefore assume the influence of this media flow to be minimal for low strain rates.[134] Whereas this computational cost could be drastically reduced by restricting the simulations to two dimensions, models based on 2D cell culture have failed to represent the biological activity within a 3D structure, due to the lack of contextual cues.[157,158]

As the computer capacity does seldom allow performing an analysis of an entire scaffold, studies are often performed on RVE considered as representative of the whole structure.[55,134,144,145,154,158] They enable the regional variance of micro-mechanical stimuli to be assessed.[134,144] However, numerical approaches may also be applied by assuming a homogeneous porous media that obeys a Darcy's law so as to ease the computational cost. It has for instance been used to assess and optimize the efficiency of seeding procedures in a time-saving way compared to experimental approaches[159] (see Section 3.2).

3.1.4. *Application of the braided ligament scaffold*

As far as ligament tissue engineering is concerned, they are few reported studies predicting the micro-mechanical stimuli that may appear in a ligament scaffold due to external loading. Indeed, such studies firstly require a numerical description of the scaffold, which is not easily obtainable with common textile techniques used for scaffold fabrication. However, it has been illustrated previously that numerical developments have permitted from 2010 to define a braided scaffold, obtain a proper numerical definition of its morphology,[85] and implement it within a FE code so as to predict its properties.[29,114] Such simulations thus enable to assess the relationship between prescribed external loading and local micro-mechanical stimuli, and thus provide with crucial information to interpret the results of dynamical culture.

As an illustration, the distribution of local Octahedral Shear Strain (OSS) at the surface of the braided scaffold during common physiological exercises (squats) has been represented in Figure 5. The authors clearly observe that local strains are lower that global prescribed strain due to structural effects. Moreover, it appears that some parts of the scaffold are very poorly stimulated (mainly at the periphery of the scaffold, see Figure 3) due to the progressive recruitment of fibers during the stretching of the scaffold. It gives important information concerning the interpretation of further tissue growth or differentiation within the scaffold. Indeed, it may be thought that cellular response will be heterogeneous within the scaffold due to both this gradient of mechanical stimuli and the gradient in morphology (see Figure 2).

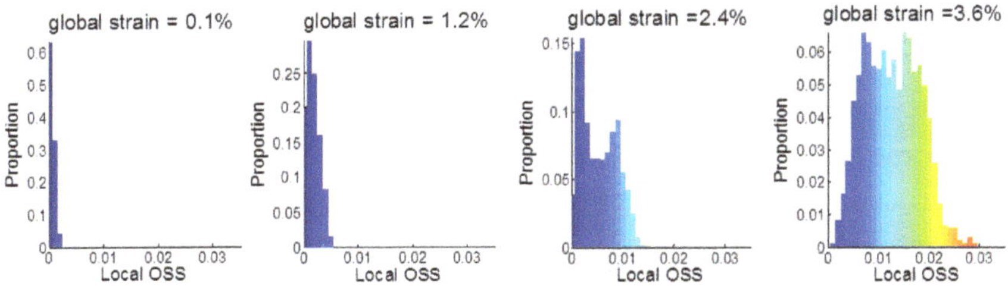

Figure 5. Evolution of the local distribution of Octahedral Shear Strain (OSS) during a common physiological loading (squats, modeled by a 3.6% prescribed longitudinal strain[60]

3.2. *Optimizing Cell Structure and Bio*

The scaffold material should ideally attract the cells, and facilitate cell adhesion, motility and proliferation, which may need an appropriate surface chemistry and good hydrophilicity.[7,39,44,112] For instance, coating a scaffold with suitable protein may be viewed as a good way to compensate material hydrophobicity,[7] as well as the combination of several materials with antagonist properties.[103] Noteworthy, recent works have particularly specified that the progressive delivery of cells, genes and/or proteins should also be seen as major requirements for a scaffold.[56,128,157] One of the aims is to send signals to the metabolism that allow the inflammation reaction to be overcome.[72] Moreover, the choice of an adapted cell source as well as efficient *in vitro* cell expansion and cell seeding are obviously essential steps toward the success of tissue engineering.[112]

A cell source adapted to the clinical application of tissue engineering principles should provide easily available cells with a high potential to proliferate and synthesize ECM.[160] The choice of a relevant cell source for each specific application is a crucial first step of the tissue engineering approach, as the use of different cell types may highly influence the outcome of tissue engineered product.[161] Although fibroblasts may constitute a promising cell source for ligament of tendon,[160,162] mesenchymal stem cells (MSC) have been generally preferred in tissue engineering strategies because of their higher potential to proliferate and to synthesize ECM.[161] As a result, the clinical procedure would consist in harvesting these MSC from the patient's bone marrow after the diagnosis of a ligament rupture, and then in expanding MSC using a culture passage.[8]

These cells should then be seeded into the scaffold, and the seeding procedure should minimize cell injury, minimize cell seeding time, and result in a homogeneous and reproducible cell distribution.[159] It has been suggested that internal seeding of cells is suitable in terms of cells distribution and amount.[111] Indeed, a homogeneous spatial distribution of cells, combined with a supply of nutrients and a removal of waste products which limit local restrictions, are required in order to avoid the accumulation of ECM in the periphery of the scaffold.[112] Inhomogeneous ECM formation leads indeed to pores obstruction and consequently to increasing transport restrictions, resulting in even more ECM inhomogeneity.

Computational approaches may largely help to find the best solutions for efficient cell seeding in a given scaffold, since it enables to simulate the fluid flow within a scaffold,[6,151,152,154,159] the diffusion of biochemical products during regeneration,[81] or the tissue growth and its impact on fluid flow[163]. As in Figure 6, from the definition of a properly meshed geometry as obtained previously for the braided scaffold for ligament tissue engineering, CFD tools may be used to simulate the diffusion of tracers (representing the proliferation of cells or the diffusion or nutrients/waste products) within the scaffold, so as to optimize the parameters of cell seeding or fluid flow (pressure, fluid velocity, etc.).

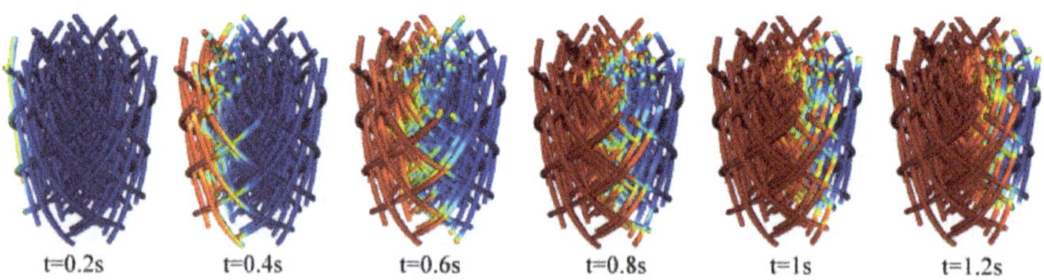

Figure 6. Illustration of CFD applied to a braided scaffold for ligament tissue engineering: diffusion of a tracer within the scaffold

Once the cells adhere on scaffold, the seeded scaffold should be cultured within the scaffold under dynamic culture conditions, since required mass transport properties may be fulfilled by means of flow conditions prescribed by a dynamic bioreactor. Nevertheless, once implanted within the body, the absence of this controlled flow may lead to poor blood supply and thus to a limited tissue survival[112] especially in the case of ACL repair, where external vascularization is not expected. Even if the mechanical stimuli at the cellular scale may be controlled by varying the flow conditions alone within the bioreactor, it has been shown that external mechanical stimulations have the benefit to involve both solid and fluid stimuli (see previous section), the latter being adjustable by varying the strain rate.[47]

The use of a dynamic bioreactor which prescribes cyclic loading has thus been raised, and particularly in the case of ACL tissue engineering as far as cyclic strain has been shown to increase the proliferation of fibroblasts and their ECM production.[143] Noteworthy, the cellular response under mechanical stimuli not only depends on their magnitude but also of their frequency,[86] whose ideal value still needs to be determined. Culturing scaffold in perfusion bioreactors allow the necrosis of the scaffold core due to poor nutrients delivery to be overcome.[152,154] Indeed, cells are often numerous in the periphery of a scaffold due to better seeding and nutrient providing. As they grow, they may obstruct the pores and restrict the nutrient providing for cells in the center of the scaffold.[45,84,112] A dynamic fluid environment has therefore been preferred in tissue engineering so as to optimize nutrients transportation as well as to mimic the dynamic environment present within the body.[152,153,164] As the same flow rate within two morphologically different scaffolds results in different flow-induced shear stresses, CFD methods may be used in view of identifying the flow conditions and scaffold architectures which are best suited for a specific tissue-engineering application.[155]

Even if it is clear that such micro-mechanical stimuli are required, their ideal amplitude, frequency and direction have not been clearly established, especially since the mechano-responsiveness of cells is subject to variation among individuals.[135] Numerous mechanisms are involved during the dynamic culture of a scaffold within a bioreactor, and they are often difficult to separate experimentally.[112] Several studies have reported discrepancies amongst data concerning the suited flow-induced shear stress, which may be due to differences in the scaffold dimensions, microstructure and material and to the different flow conditions prescribed.[109] Consequently, while flow-induced shear stresses greater than 0.5 Pa have been sometimes shown to stimulate cells using 2D parallel flow experiments,[165,166] other studies have reported that shear stress exceeding 5 mPa were detrimental to cell viability.[47] This emphasizes the misunderstanding of the overall implied mechanisms as well as the need to complete the actual models and experiments.

Consequently, the use of computational approaches is crucial in order to understand the precise microenvironment transferred to the cells when a scaffold is subject to dynamic loading of flow perfusion within a bioreactor. It enables to draw conclusions concerning the best-suited microenvironment, and consequently to define the culture parameters (amplitude of mechanical loading, flow velocity, etc.) that will permit to obtain the most relevant tissue-engineered construct.

3.3. *Mechanobiological Models*

The prediction of mechanical stimuli at the scaffold surface using the methods cited above may enable to predict the cellular activity under given culture conditions if combined with mechanobiological models. Indeed, computational models may enable to compare different predictions of the biological response with experimental observations, thereby contributing to the understanding of complex biological mechanisms and reducing the cost of experimental research.[50,158] As a lot of biological mechanisms are involved during the culture of cells seeded into a bioreactor, computational methods may be viewed as essential tools to determine the prevalent mechanisms.[87,112] They could allow the effect of bioreactor design and culture conditions to be assessed prior to their design in order to avoid time-consuming experiments,[164] and may allow the understanding of the mechanotransduction mechanisms to be improved by comparing model predictions with experimental data.

Particularly, the mechanisms underlying the cellular differentiation have drawn the attention of tissue engineers, as they are known to depend drastically on the mechanical environment. Models have been compared and confronted to *in vivo* observations in the case of fracture healing, which is known to depend on the mechanical micro-environment.[139,167] Numerous recent studies have started from a work of Prendergast *et al.*[168] to formulate the stimulus for cell differentiation based on cell distortion, i.e. a combination of both the OSS and the flow-induced shear stress (FISS)[136] or the fluid velocity[55,71,109,144,169] that are directly related in the case of a Newtonian fluids. Substrate strain and fluid flow are assumed to control the formation of either fibrous tissue for high magnitudes of these two parameters or bone for low magnitudes.[168]

Particularly, computational methods have been used to evaluate the predictive potential of different mechano-regulation algorithms, especially in the case of bone fracture healing under axial load[169] and torsional rotation[167] due to available experimental data. Generally, mechano-regulation models are used to predict the tissue differentiation within the scaffold, which induces variations of the local material properties and consequently variations of the local stimuli, and so forth until an equilibrium is reached.[144,158,169] While several mechano-regulation algorithms have been reviewed, the still opened question is to determine which one reflects the best the biological mechanisms.[87] By comparing different proposed algorithms, it has been shown that the deviatoric strain (i.e. OSS mentioned above) was the most significant mechanical stimuli during bone fracture healing[167,170]. Indeed, deviatoric strain alone allowed the fracture healing patterns to be simulated, whereas flow velocity or pore pressure — alone or combined — did not lead to such results. It has nevertheless been suggested that none of the several tested algorithms were able to predict the healing patterns[167] in the case of ovine tibia healing, although the algorithm regulated by both deviatoric strain and fluid velocity was found to be the closest to experimental data.[139]

Several studies aiming at predicting the tissue ingrowth and/or at optimizing scaffold microstructure or culture conditions have therefore been reported.[130,144] For instance, by combining the predicted

OSS and FISS with mechano-biological models, multiscale FE modeling of different scaffolds has permitted to select the most suited CAD-based microstructures for bone and cartilage.[109] Some studies also assumed that the tissue formation was governed by some nutrient concentration rather than by mechanical stimuli. In this case, the tissue formation, and particularly the matrix synthesis, has been directly related to the computed nutrients distributions such as oxygen profiles.[112] However, the tissue ingrowth actually depends on numerous factors and may hardly be related to a single nutrient distribution. The process of cell proliferation has been also modeled in the form of a diffusion phenomenon modeled by Fick's law.[8,125,139,147,158] Some authors have therefore considered diffusivity within the scaffold as a crucial design criterion for tissue formation and mass transport properties.[123] However, it has also been suggested that random walk models may be a better way to explicitly model the cell proliferation and migration of different cell populations.[55] As the animal experimental studies are site-specific and species-specific, specific bone chambers which induce bone growth and enable bone samples to be harvested regularly have been developed to constitute a source of experimental data.[158] It has especially enable to demonstrate that mechano-regulatory models may predict the tissue growth and differentiation, and that the flow-induced stimuli may not have a high influence on the predicted tissue patterns.[158]

The currently available models suffer from several limitations that are inevitable considering the complexity and multi-disciplinary nature of the tissue formation and differentiation. For instance, phenomena such as growth factor influence, cell death and cell mitosis were generally neglected.[158] Moreover, the reported studies were mainly limited to short-term behavior because of the complex interactions and mechanisms involved, such as morphological, mechanical and chemical variations due to the scaffold biodegradation, tissue formation and cell–cell interactions.[129,157] These models also neglect the inter-variability of cells mechano-sensitivity which would require the integration of genetics into the models used.[135] Consequently, computational methods for the modeling of tissue formation do not currently allow precise and reliable predictions. For the moment, these methods may not be used as a predictive tool at the scaffold design step, but rather as a comparative tool to help the understanding of experimental observations and the identification of the prevalent mechanisms involved in the tissue formation or cell spreading. It is however likely that future advances in both experimental data and more complex mathematical modeling will soon allow a better understanding of those mechanisms.

In the case of ligament tissue engineering, such mechano-biological models may be of primary interest concerning the reconstruction of a progressive bone–ligament interface. Indeed, the gradients in mechanical properties and cellular nature within the bone–ligament interface are known to improve the mechanical properties of bone–ligament construct, by minimizing stress concentration. It may thus be interesting to predict the ability of a bone–ligament scaffold (such as the one proposed previously, see Figure 4) to promote the formation of a progressive transition going from fibrous tissue to bony tissue, with a progressively mineralized fibro-cartilage. As in Figure 7, the results of finite element simulations of bone–ligament construct were used in order to predict the cellular differentiation due to micromechanical environment. In this illustration, the initial arbitrary configuration was supposed to be the post-implantation phase, in which stem cells are seeded in the braided scaffold, and osteoblasts are present around the bony part of the scaffold. Then, cells proliferation was modeled using the common Fick's law, introducing diffusion coefficients for each cell type (to be identified based on biological

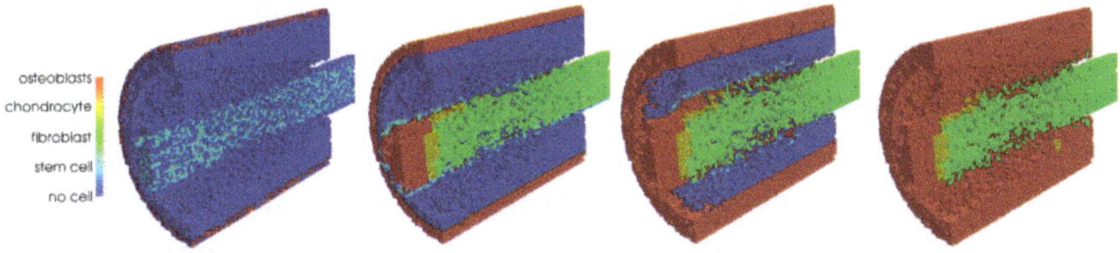

Figure 7. Example of mechanobiological model implemented in the finite element simulations of bone–ligament construct. The model provide with information concerning the evolution (from left to right) of cellular type within the bone–ligament scaffold, due to simulated mechanical stimuli

observations). After each proliferation step, the cell type was actualized depending on the OSS resulting from the FE simulations presented above (Figure 4). The algorithm was stopped when cells fully proliferated: it can be observed that due to mechanical stimuli, a slight zone of cartilage appears between bone and fibrous tissue, if the well-known mechano-biological model of Prendergast *et al.*[168] is used. Obviously, this example only constitutes an illustration of the interest of computational approaches for bone–ligament tissue engineering and must be widely corroborated by biological observations.

4. Predicting the Evolution of Tissue

The scaffold should ideally degrade at a rate matching the rate of tissue formation.[11,46] However, the ideal degradation rate of a scaffold is an issue as it depends on the tissue formation it induces, which in return depends of the scaffold material and architecture. Tissue formation and scaffold degradation are therefore strongly interrelated, especially since the formation of a tissue layer on the scaffold surface may prevent further degradation.[125] Moreover, *in vitro* characterization of the degradation behavior of scaffolds may significantly differ from *in vivo* assessments which are often necessary.[30] For instance, the biodegradation of several commonly-used biomaterials may lead to a reduction of the local pH and negative metabolic effects,[40,103] which are difficult to reproduce *in vitro*. Fast degradation rates have been reported to have a dramatically negative effect on tissue formation.[8] Therefore, it has been often considered that the degradation rate should be as slow as possible to ensure a long term success,[8] and that a material with a controllable degradation rate may be suitable so as to choose the best material from biological observations.[39,102]

Some studies tried to assess numerically the variations in time of scaffold effective properties by updating the elastic modulus values in a FE modeling of the scaffold.[171] Moreover, μCT techniques may enable to image both the scaffold and the mineralized bone in a non-destructive manner. Consequently, the combination of the scaffold and mineralized bone that has formed may be imaged at different time points, and FE methods may predict the variations of scaffold properties due to tissue formation.[42] It has been used for instance to assess the variations of the Young modulus of bone–scaffold constructs during cyclic loading.[91] Moreover, reported homogenization approaches have been initially limited by the assumption that the tissue formation or scaffold degradation did not participate to the effective properties,[5] limiting the viability of the results to the short-term period. However, recent studies dealing with topological optimization have taken into account the variations in time of the effective properties of the scaffold due to both the scaffold degradation and the tissue formation.[8,71] Using a voxel-based FE approach (i.e. scaffold meshing is directly issued from the discretization of the space within small unit cubes) material resorption due to polymeric hydrolysis and tissue formation have been modeled by simply removing or adding voxels.[125,129] These microscopic phenomena require a multiscale modeling, as the local degradation influences the scaffold effective properties, which results in different mechanical stimuli and then in variations in tissue formation.[8]

In the case of ligament tissue engineering, while numerous scaffolds have been proposed and their initial mechanical behavior characterized and optimized, the question of the evolution properties of these scaffolds during its degradation in the first phase of the rehabilitation protocol has been poorly assessed. However, this point is crucial since (1) accumulated plastic strain within the scaffold during this period may lead to unsuited graft laxity (2) the potential loss of mechanical properties in this period due to scaffold degradation must be compensated by tissue growth (3) variation of mechanical properties of the scaffold may lead to a variation of cellular microenvironment, which is known to influence the cellular activity.[172–174] To answer these issues, collecting experimental data may be complex due to the long period during which this transition takes place (several weeks to several months). Both *in vivo*[115,175–178] and *in vitro*[179–183] studies are reported concerning the degradation of scaffolds for different applications, but the assessments of the evolution of their mechanical properties inevitably involves large (and costly) experimental campaigns. Results issued from *in vivo* experiments are crucial, but the results are often limited to observations of histological cross-sections that only provide poor information concerning the evolution of scaffold properties. Moreover, the evolution of mechanical properties are usually restricted to apparent properties (compressive modulus, ultimate strength, etc.) and limited to the elastic range. The question of how these results can be confronted and used to assess the suitability of a scaffold for a given clinical application is then crucial.

The prediction of scaffold macroscopic properties as illustrated in Section 2.2 may enable to assess their variations over time by considering both the scaffold biodegradation and the tissue formation, thus avoiding long-term studies to be performed and allowing a best initial scaffold configuration to be determined.[87] However, the problem of scaffold's fate over time depends on numerous interdependent parameters that are complex to model in such numerical studies. In the reported dedicated FE model for braided scaffold, the numerical model starts from elasto-plastic properties of single fibers: consequently, the evolution of scaffold response could be predicted by integrating changes in individual fiber properties within this code. Several models based on damage[184–187] have been developed in order to take into account the variation of polymer mechanical properties during hydrolytic degradation. Such models may thus be used in order to quantify the effect of polymer degradation on scaffold mechanical properties.

As an illustration, the evolution of elasto-plastic behavior of isolated fibers due to hydrolytic degradation over a ten-weeks period has been assessed from tensile tests. FE simulations starting from these evolving properties have therefore been performed in order to: (1) assess the evolution of mechanical properties during scaffold degradation, including the accumulation of plastic strain (2) quantify the effect of degradation on the microenvironment at the cellular scale.

A clear decrease of the Young's modulus has been observed, thus involving a decrease in scaffold stiffness, as illustrated in Figure 8. The other properties such as yield strain, strain at rupture or maximal stress, were less intuitive and were fitted on experimental data based on a Chaboche-type elasto-plastic hardening,[29] introducing damage parameters as proposed in Refs. [184,185]. The resulting evolution

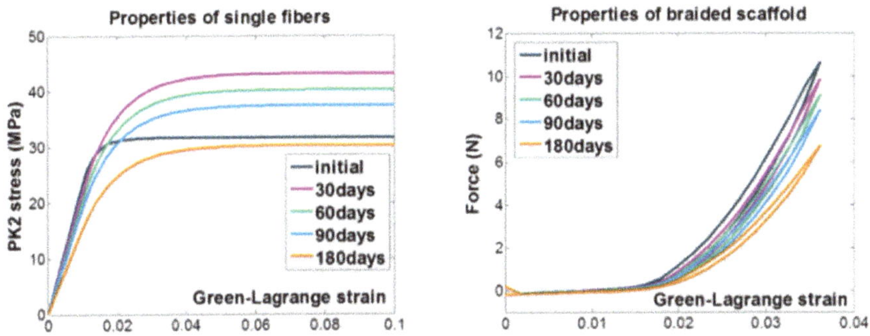

(a) (b)

Figure 8. (a) Simulated evolution of single fibers from tensile test on isolated fibers (b) resulting simulated scaffold response from FEM

of force–strain response of the braided scaffold due to polymer degradation is illustrate below (Figure 8) from FE simulations. Due to structural effects, the scaffold does not enter into the plastic zone for the prescribed physiological loading (3.6% of global strain), even if the fibers would individually deform plastically for such a strain. These preliminary results have also enabled to assess the evolution of cellular microenvironment during such degradation. It was found that the global distribution of OSS is not significantly affected by the degradation in the first two months, due to the fact that the load was controlled in displacement rather than in force.

Obviously, this work was performed with no consideration of the effect of growing tissue on the predicted scaffold mechanical properties, which constitutes the next step of such an approach. This progressive load transfer from scaffold to growing tissue is indeed one of the most important challenges to be risen in tissue engineering, as it is practically impossible to measure separately the participation of scaffold and growing tissue in the overall mechanical properties of the tissue-engineering ligament due to interrelated effects.

Such models including both scaffold evolving properties and tissue growth, together with the computational approaches detailed in the previous sections, may enable in the future to propose scaffolds with required properties both at the implantation time and after physiological loading due to the rehabilitation procedure. It may also provide tissue engineers with crucial information concerning the micro-environment which is the most suited in order to head for the most relevant bio-substitute for a given clinical application.

References

1. Vacanti, C. A.; Vacanti, J. P. *Orthop. Clin. North Am.* **2000**, *31*(3), 351.
2. Sun, W.; Lal, P. *Comput. Methods Programs Biomed.* **2002**, *67*(2), 85.
3. Rajagopalan, S.; Robb, R. A. *Med. Image Anal.* **2006**, *10*(5), 693.
4. Laurencin, C. T.; Freeman, J. W. *Biomaterials* **2005**, *26*(36), 7530.
5. Hollister, S. J.; Maddox, R. D.; Taboas, J. M. *Biomaterials* **2002**, *23*(20), 4095.
6. Hutmacher, D. W.; Singh, H. *Trends Biotechnol.* **2008**, *26*(4), 166.
7. Leong, K. F.; Chua, C. K.; Sudarmadji, N.; Yeong, W. Y. *J. Mech. Behav. Biomed. Mater.* **2008**, *1*(2), 140.
8. Sanz-Herrera, J. A.; García-Aznar, J. M.; Doblaré, M. *Acta Biomater.* **2009**, *5*(1), 219.
9. Jones, J. R.; Poologasundarampillai, G.; Atwood, R. C.; Bernard, D.; Lee, P. D. *Biomaterials* **2007**, *28*(7), 1404.
10. Altman, G. H.; Horan, R. L.; Lu, H. H.; Moreau, J.; Martin, I.; Richmond, J. C.; Kaplan, D. L. *Biomaterials* **2002**, *23*(20), 4131.
11. Vunjak-Novakovic, G.; Altman, G.; Horan, R.; Kaplan, D. L. *Annu. Rev. Biomed. Eng.* **2004**, *6*, 131.
12. Bicer, E. K.; Lustig, S.; Servien, E.; Selmi, T. A. S.; Neyret, P. *Knee Surg. Sports Traumatol. Arthrosc.* **2010**, *18*(8), 1075.
13. Dargel, J.; Gotter, M.; Mader, K.; Pennig, D.; Koebke, J.; Schmidt-Wiethoff, R. *Strateg. Trauma Limb Reconstr.* **2007**, *2*(1), 1.
14. Duthon, V. B.; Barea, C.; Abrassart, S.; Fasel, J. H.; Fritschy, D.; Ménétrey, J. *Knee Surg. Sports Traumatol. Arthrosc.* **2005**, *14*(3), 204.
15. Karmani, S.; Ember, T. *Curr. Orthop.* **2003**, *17*(5), 369.
16. Woo, S. L.-Y.; Abramowitch, S. D.; Kilger, R.; Liang, R. *J. Biomech.* **2006**, *39*(1), 1.
17. Zantop, T.; Petersen, W.; Sekiya, J. K.; Musahl, V.; Fu, F. H. *Knee Surg. Sports Traumatol. Arthrosc.* **2006**, *14*(10), 982.
18. Zantop, T.; Schumacher, T.; Diermann, N.; Schanz, S.; Raschke, M. J.; Petersen, W. *Arch. Orthop. Trauma Surg.* **2006**, *127*(9), 743.

19. Unwin, A. *Orthop. Trauma* **2010**, *24*(2), 100.
20. Karmani, S.; Ember, T. *Curr. Orthop.* **2004**, *18*(1), 49.
21. Grinsven, S. van; Cingel, R. E. H. van; Holla, C. J. M.; Loon, C. J. M. van. *Knee Surg. Sports Traumatol. Arthrosc.* **2010**, *18*(8), 1128.
22. Gao, B.; Zheng, N. (Nigel). *Clin. Biomech.* **2010**, *25*(3), 222.
23. Moraiti, C. O.; Stergiou, N.; Vasiliadis, H. S.; Motsis, E.; Georgoulis, A. *Gait Posture* **2010**, *32*(2), 169.
24. Leong, N. L.; Petrigliano, F. A.; McAllister, D. R. *J. Biomed. Mater. Res. A* **2013**.
25. Cooper, J. A.; Lu, H. H.; Ko, F. K.; Freeman, J. W.; Laurencin, C. T. *Biomaterials* **2005**, *26*(13), 1523.
26. Lu, H. H.; Cooper Jr., J. A.; Manuel, S.; Freeman, J. W.; Attawia, M. A.; Ko, F. K.; Laurencin, C. T. *Biomaterials* **2005**, *26*(23), 4805.
27. Freeman, J. W. *Afr. J. Biotechnol.* **2009**, *8*(25).
28. Freeman, J. W.; Woods, M. D.; Cromer, D. A.; Ekwueme, E. C.; Andric, T.; Atiemo, E. A.; Bijoux, C. H.; Laurencin, C. T. *J. Biomech.* **2011**, *44*(4), 694.
29. Laurent, C. P.; Durville, D.; Mainard, D.; Ganghoffer, J.-F.; Rahouadj, R. *J. Mech. Behav. Biomed. Mater.* **2012**, *12*, 184.
30. Fan, H.; Liu, H.; Wong, E. J. W.; Toh, S. L.; Goh, J. C. H. *Biomaterials* **2008**, *29*(23), 3324.
31. Fan, H.; Liu, H.; Toh, S. L.; Goh, J. C. H. *Biomaterials* **2009**, *30*(28), 4967.
32. Chen, X.; Qi, Y.-Y.; Wang, L.-L.; Yin, Z.; Yin, G.-L.; Zou, X.-H.; Ouyang, H.-W. *Biomaterials* **2008**, *29*(27), 3683.
33. Vaquette, C.; Kahn, C.; Frochot, C.; Nouvel, C.; Six, J.-L.; De Isla, N.; Luo, L.-H.; Cooper-White, J.; Rahouadj, R.; Wang, X. *J. Biomed. Mater. Res. A* **2010**, *94A* (4), 1270.
34. Gentleman, E.; Livesay, G. A.; Dee, K. C.; Nauman, E. A. *Ann. Biomed. Eng.* **2006**, *34*(5), 726.
35. Starly, B.; Lau, W.; Bradbury, T.; Sun, W. *Comput.-Aided Des.* **2006**, *38*(2), 115.
36. Cai, S.; Xi, J. *Comput.-Aided Des.* **2008**, *40*(10–11), 1040.
37. Moroni, L.; de Wijn, J. R.; van Blitterswijk, C. A. *Biomaterials* **2006**, *27*(7), 974.
38. Mironov, V.; Visconti, R. P.; Kasyanov, V.; Forgacs, G.; Drake, C. J.; Markwald, R. R. *Biomaterials* **2009**, *30*(12), 2164.

39. Almeida, H. de A.; da Silva Bártolo, P. J. *Med. Eng. Phys.* **2010**, *32*(7), 775.
40. Cheung, H.-Y.; Lau, K.-T.; Lu, T.-P.; Hui, D. *Compos. Part B Eng.* **2007**, *38*(3), 291.
41. (Ahn, G.; Park, J. H.; Kang, T.; Lee, J. W.; Kang, H.-W.; Cho, D.-W. *J. Biomech. Eng.* **2010**, *132*(10), 104506.
42. Jones, A. C.; Arns, C. H.; Hutmacher, D. W.; Milthorpe, B. K.; Sheppard, A. P.; Knackstedt, M. A. *Biomaterials* **2009**, *30*(7), 1440.
43. Leong, K. F.; Cheah, C. M.; Chua, C. K. *Biomaterials* **2003**, *24*(13), 2363.
44. Park, S.; Kim, G.; Jeon, Y. C.; Koh, Y.; Kim, W. *J. Mater. Sci. Mater. Med.* **2008**, *20*(1), 229.
45. Murphy, C. M.; Haugh, M. G.; O'Brien, F. J. *Biomaterials* **2010**, *31*(3), 461.
46. Fedorovich, N. E.; Alblas, J.; Hennink, W. E.; Öner, F. C.; Dhert, W. J. A. *Trends Biotechnol.* **2011**, *29*(12), 601.
47. Milan, J.-L.; Planell, J. A.; Lacroix, D. *Biomaterials* **2009**, *30*(25), 4219.
48. Jiankang, H.; Dichen, L.; Yaxiong, L.; Bo, Y.; Bingheng, L.; Qin, L. *Polymer* **2007**, *48*(15), 4578.
49. Chan, K. S.; Liang, W.; Francis, W. L.; Nicolella, D. P. *J. Mech. Behav. Biomed. Mater.* **2010**, *3*(8), 584.
50. Peiffer, V.; Gerisch, A.; Vandepitte, D.; Van Oosterwyck, H.; Geris, L. *Biomech. Model. Mechanobiol.* **2011**, *10*(3), 383.
51. Oh, S. H.; Park, I. K.; Kim, J. M.; Lee, J. H. *Biomaterials* **2007**, *28*(9), 1664.
52. Fierz, F. C.; Beckmann, F.; Huser, M.; Irsen, S. H.; Leukers, B.; Witte, F.; Degistirici, Ö.; Andronache, A.; Thie, M.; Müller, B. *Biomaterials* **2008**, *29*(28), 3799.
53. Landers, R.; Pfister, A.; Hübner, U.; John, H.; Schmelzeisen, R.; Mülhaupt, R. *J. Mater. Sci.* *37*(15), 3107.
54. Melchels, F. P. W.; Barradas, A. M. C.; van Blitterswijk, C. A.; de Boer, J.; Feijen, J.; Grijpma, D. W. *Acta Biomater.* **2010**, *6*(11), 4208.
55. Byrne, D. P.; Lacroix, D.; Prendergast, P. J. *J. Orthop. Res.* **2011**, *29*(10), 1496.
56. Hollister, S. J. *Adv. Mater.* **2009**, *21*(32–33), 3330.

57. Butler, D.; Goldstein, S.; Guilak, F. *J. Biomech. Eng.* **2000**, *122*(6), 570.
58. Hosseini, A.; Gill, T. J.; Li, G. *J. Orthop. Sci.* **2009**, *14*(3), 298.
59. Li, G.; DeFrate, L. E.; Rubash, H. E.; Gill, T. J. *J. Orthop. Res.* **2005**, *23*(2), 340.
60. Beynnon, B. D.; Fleming, B. C. *J. Biomech.* **1998**, *31*(6), 519.
61. Fleming, B. C.; Beynnon, B. D. *Ann. Biomed. Eng.* **2004**, *32*(3), 318.
62. Toutoungi, D.; Lu, T.; Leardini, A.; Catani, F.; O'Connor, J. *Clin. Biomech.* **2000**, *15*(3), 176.
63. Jones, R.; Nawana, N.; Pearcy, M.; Learmonth, D.; Bickerstaff, D.; Costi, J.; Paterson, R. *Clin. Biomech.* **1995**, *10*(7), 339.
64. Fang, Z.; Starly, B.; Sun, W. *Comput.-Aided Des.* **2005**, *37*(1), 65.
65. Sun, W.; Starly, B.; Nam, J.; Darling, A. *Comput.-Aided Des.* **2005**, *37*(11), 1097.
66. Plaweski, S.; Grimaldi, M.; Courvoisier, A.; Wimsey, S. *Knee Surg. Sports Traumatol. Arthrosc.* **2011**, *19*(8), 1277.
67. Shen, W.; Jordan, S.; Fu, F. *J. Orthop. Surg. Hong Kong* **2007**, *15*(2), 216.
68. Kondo, E.; Merican, A. M.; Yasuda, K.; Amis, A. A. *Am. J. Sports Med.* **2011**, *39*(2), 279.
69. Yasuda, K.; Tanabe, Y.; Kondo, E.; Kitamura, N.; Tohyama, H. *Arthrosc.- J. Arthrosc. Relat. Surg.* **2010**, *26*(9), S21.
70. Liu Tsang, V.; Bhatia, S. N. *Adv. Drug Deliv. Rev.* **2004**, *56*(11), 1635.
71. Chen, Y.; Zhou, S.; Li, Q. *Biomaterials* **2011**, *32*(22), 5003.
72. Lacroix, D.; Planell, J. A.; Prendergast, P. J. *Philos. Trans. Math. Phys. Eng. Sci.* **2009**, *367*(1895), 1993.
73. Laurent, C. P.; Durville, D.; Vaquette, C.; Rahouadj, R.; Ganghoffer, J.-F. In *Biomechanics of cells and tissues*, **2013**, Vol. 9, pp. 1–44.
74. Giannitelli, S. M.; Accoto, D.; Trombetta, M.; Rainer, A. *Acta Biomater.* **2014**, *10*(2), 580.
75. In *Computer-Aided Tissue Engineering*; Liebschner, M. A. K., Ed.; Humana Press Inc: Totowa, **2012**; Vol. 868, pp. 1–360.
76. Wettergreen, M. A.; Bucklen, B. S.; Sun, W.; Liebschner, M. A. K. *Ann. Biomed. Eng.* *33*(10), 1333.
77. Sun, W.; Darling, A.; Starly, B.; Nam, J. *Biotechnol. Appl. Biochem.* **2004**, *39*(1), 29.

78. Semple, J. L.; Woolridge, N.; Lumsden, C. J. *Tissue Eng.* **2005**, *11*(3–4), 341.
79. Galbusera, F.; Cioffi, M.; Raimondi, M. T. *Biomed. Microdevices* **2008**, *10*(4), 547.
80. Spencer, T. J.; Hidalgo-Bastida, L. A.; Cartmell, S. H.; Halliday, I.; Care, C. M. *Biotechnol. Bioeng.* **2013**, *110*(4), 1221.
81. Carlier, A.; van Gastel, N.; Geris, L.; Carmeliet, G.; Van Oosterwyck, H. *PLoS Comput. Biol.* **2014**, *10*(11), e1003888.
82. Lee, K.-W.; Wang, S.; Dadsetan, M.; Yaszemski, M. J.; Lu, L. *Biomacromolecules* **2010**, *11*(3), 682.
83. Elomaa, L.; Teixeira, S.; Hakala, R.; Korhonen, H.; Grijpma, D. W.; Seppälä, J. V. *Acta. Biomater.* **2011**, *7*(11), 3850.
84. Silva, M. M. C. G.; Cyster, L. A.; Barry, J. J. A.; Yang, X. B.; Oreffo, R. O. C.; Grant, D. M.; Scotchford, C. A.; Howdle, S. M.; Shakesheff, K. M.; Rose, F. R. A. J. *Biomaterials* **2006**, *27*(35), 5909.
85. Laurent, C. P.; Ganghoffer, J.-F.; Babin, J.; Six, J.-L.; Wang, X.; Rahouadj, R. *J. Biomech. Eng.* **2011**, *133*(6), 65001.
86. Jaecques, S. V. N.; Van Oosterwyck, H.; Muraru, L.; Van Cleynenbreugel, T.; De Smet, E.; Wevers, M.; Naert, I.; Vander Sloten, J. *Biomaterials* **2004**, *25*(9), 1683.
87. Boccaccio, A.; Ballini, A.; Pappalettere, C.; Tullo, D.; Cantore, S.; Desiate, A. *Int. J. Biol. Sci.* **2011**, *7*(1), 112.
88. Tellis, B. C.; Szivek, J. A.; Bliss, C. L.; Margolis, D. S.; Vaidyanathan, R. K.; Calvert, P. *Mater. Sci. Eng. C* **2008**, *28*(1), 171.
89. Melchels, F. P. W.; Bertoldi, K.; Gabbrielli, R.; Velders, A. H.; Feijen, J.; Grijpma, D. W. *Biomaterials* **2010**, *31*(27), 6909.
90. Baas, E.; Kuiper, J. H.; Yang, Y.; Wood, M. A.; El Haj, A. J. *J. Biomech.* **2010**, *43*(4), 733.
91. Roshan-Ghias, A.; Lambers, F. M.; Gholam-Rezaee, M.; Müller, R.; Pioletti, D. P. *Bone* **2011**, *49*(6), 1357.
92. Tuan, H. S.; Hutmacher, D. W. *Comput.-Aided Des.* **2005**, *37*(11), 1151.
93. Williams, J. M.; Adewunmi, A.; Schek, R. M.; Flanagan, C. L.; Krebsbach, P. H.; Feinberg, S. E.; Hollister, S. J.; Das, S. *Biomaterials* **2005**, *26*(23), 4817.
94. Khoda, A. K. M. B.; Ozbolat, I. T.; Koc, B. *J. Biomech. Eng.-Trans. Asme* **2011**, *133*(1), 11001.

95. Karageorgiou, V.; Kaplan, D. *Biomaterials* **2005**, *26*(27), 5474.
96. Hollister, S. J. *Nat. Mater.* **2006**, *5*(7), 590.
97. Yoo, D. J. *Biomaterials* **2011**, *32*(31), 7741.
98. Yeong, W.-Y.; Chua, C.-K.; Leong, K.-F.; Chandrasekaran, M. *Trends Biotechnol.* **2004**, *22*(12), 643.
99. Saito, E.; Kang, H.; Taboas, J. M.; Diggs, A.; Flanagan, C. L.; Hollister, S. J. *J. Mater. Sci. Mater. Med.* **2010**, *21*(8), 2371.
100. Wettergreen, M. A.; Bucklen, B. S.; Starly, B.; Yuksel, E.; Sun, W.; Liebschner, M. A. K. *Comput.- Aided Des.* **2005**, *37*(11), 1141.
101. Hutmacher, D. W.; Sittinger, M.; Risbud, M. V. *Trends Biotechnol.* **2004**, *22*(7), 354.
102. Chen, Y.; Zhou, S.; Cadman, J.; Li, Q. *Biotechnol. Bioeng.* **2010**, *107*(4), 737.
103. Li, J.; Zhang, L.; Lv, S.; Li, S.; Wang, N.; Zhang, Z. *J. Biotechnol.* **2011**, *151*(1), 87.
104. Melchels, F. P. W.; Feijen, J.; Grijpma, D. W. *Biomaterials* **2010**, *31*(24), 6121.
105. Becker, S. T.; Bolte, H.; Krapf, O.; Seitz, H.; Douglas, T.; Sivananthan, S.; Wiltfang, J.; Sherry, E.; Warnke, P. H. *Oral Oncol.* **2009**, *45*(11), e181.
106. Eshraghi, S.; Das, S. *Acta Biomater.* **2010**, *6*(7), 2467.
107. Sudarmadji, N.; Tan, J. Y.; Leong, K. F.; Chua, C. K.; Loh, Y. T. *Acta Biomater.* **2011**, *7*(2), 530.
108. Zein, I.; Hutmacher, D. W.; Tan, K. C.; Teoh, S. H. *Biomaterials* **2002**, *23*(4), 1169.
109. Olivares, A. L.; Marsal, È.; Planell, J. A.; Lacroix, D. *Biomaterials* **2009**, *30*(30), 6142.
110. Melchels, F. P. W.; Tonnarelli, B.; Olivares, A. L.; Martin, I.; Lacroix, D.; Feijen, J.; Wendt, D. J.; Grijpma, D. W. *Biomaterials* **2011**, *32*(11), 2878.
111. Chung, C. A.; Ho, S.-Y. *Ann. Biomed. Eng.* **2010**, *38*(4), 1655.
112. Sengers, B. G.; Taylor, M.; Please, C. P.; Oreffo, R. O. C. *Biomaterials* **2007**, *28*(10), 1926.
113. Dormer, N. H.; Berkland, C. J.; Detamore, M. S. *Ann. Biomed. Eng.* **2010**, *38*(6), 2121.
114. Laurent, C. P.; Latil, P.; Durville, D.; Rahouadj, R.; Geindreau, C.; Orgéas, L.; Ganghoffer, J.-F. *J. Mech. Behav. Biomed. Mater.* **2014**, *40*, 222.

115. Jeong, S. I.; Kim, B.-S.; Kang, S. W.; Kwon, J. H.; Lee, Y. M.; Kim, S. H.; Kim, Y. H. *Biomaterials* **2004**, *25*(28), 5939.
116. Vilay, V.; Mariatti, M.; Ahmad, Z.; Pasomsouk, K.; Todo, M. *J. Appl. Polym. Sci.* **2009**, *114*(3), 1784.
117. Hiljanen-Vainio, M. P.; Orava, P. A.; Seppälä, J. V. *J. Biomed. Mater. Res.* **1997**, *34*(1), 39.
118. Potluri, P.; Rawal, A.; Rivaldi, M.; Porat, I. *Compos. Part Appl. Sci. Manuf.* **2003**, *34*(6), 481.
119. Sun, X.; Sun, C. *Compos. Struct.* **2004**, *65*(3–4), 485.
120. Ma, J.; Smietana, M. J.; Kostrominova, T. Y.; Wojtys, E. M.; Larkin, L. M.; Arruda, E. M. *Tissue Eng. Part A* **2012**, *18*(1–2), 103.
121. Place, E. S.; Evans, N. D.; Stevens, M. M. *Nat. Mater.* **2009**, *8*(6), 457.
122. Vaquette, C.; Frochot, C.; Rahouadj, R.; Wang, X. *J. Biomed. Mater. Res. B Appl. Biomater.* **2008**, *86B* (1), 9.
123. Kang, H.; Lin, C.-Y.; Hollister, S. *J. Struct. Multidiscip. Optim.* **2010**, *42*(4), 633.
124. Sandino, C.; Planell, J. A.; Lacroix, D. *J. Biomech.* **2008**, *41*(5), 1005.
125. Sanz-Herrera, J. A.; Doblaré, M.; García-Aznar, J. M. *J. Biomech.* **2010**, *43*(13), 2480.
126. Jean, A.; Engelmayr Jr., G. C. *J. Biomech.* **2010**, *43*(15), 3035.
127. Norato, J. A.; Johnson, A. J. W. *J. Biomech. Eng.-Trans. Asme* **2011**, *133*(9), 91003.
128. Hollister, S. J.; Lin, C. Y. *Comput. Methods Appl. Mech. Eng.* **2007**, *196*(31–32), 2991.
129. Sturm, S.; Zhou, S.; Mai, Y.-W.; Li, Q. *J. Biomech.* **2010**, *43*(9), 1738.
130. Stops, A. J. F.; Heraty, K. B.; Browne, M.; O'Brien, F. J.; McHugh, P. E. *J. Biomech.* **2010**, *43*(4), 618.
131. Durville, D. *Comput. Mech.* **2012**, *49*(6), 687.
132. Laurent, C. P.; Latil, P.; Durville, D.; Rahouadj, R.; Geindreau, C.; Orgéas, L.; Ganghoffer, J.-F. *J. Mech. Behav. Biomed. Mater.* **2014**, *40*, 222.
133. Desai, N.; Alentorn-Geli, E.; van Eck, C. F.; Musahl, V.; Fu, F. H.; Karlsson, J.; Samuelsson, K. *Knee Surg. Sports Traumatol. Arthrosc. Off. J. ESSKA* **2016**, *24*(3), 862.
134. Stops, A. J. F.; Harrison, N. M.; Haugh, M. G.; O'Brien, F. J.; McHugh, P. E. *J. Mech. Behav. Biomed. Mater.* **2010**, *3*(4), 292.

135. Prendergast, P. J.; Checa, S.; Lacroix, D. In *Computational Modeling in Biomechanics*; De, S., Guilak, F., K, M. M. R., Eds.; Springer Netherlands, **2010**; pp. 353–372.
136. Sandino, C.; Lacroix, D. *Biomech. Model. Mechanobiol.* **2011**, *10*(4), 565.
137. Ingber, D. E. *FASEB J.* **2006**, *20*(7), 811.
138. Chen, C. S. *J. Cell Sci.* **2008**, *121*(20), 3285.
139. Lacroix, D.; Prendergast, P. J. *J. Biomech.* **2002**, *35*(9), 1163.
140. Raeber, G. P.; Lutolf, M. P.; Hubbell, J. A. *Biomech. Model. Mechanobiol.* **2007**, *7*(3), 215.
141. Altman, G. H.; Horan, R. L.; Martin, I.; Farhadi, J.; Stark, P. R. H.; Volloch, V.; Richmond, J. C.; Vunjak-Novakovic, G.; Kaplan, D. L. *Faseb J.* **2001**, *15*(14), 270.
142. Chiquet, M.; Renedo, A. S.; Huber, F.; Flück, M. *Matrix Biol.* **2003**, *22*(1), 73.
143. Webb, K.; Hitchcock, R. W.; Smeal, R. M.; Li, W.; Gray, S. D.; Tresco, P. A. *J. Biomech.* **2006**, *39*(6), 1136.
144. Milan, J.-L.; Planell, J. A.; Lacroix, D. *Biomech. Model. Mechanobiol.* **2010**, *9*(5), 583.
145. Lacroix, D.; Chateau, A.; Ginebra, M.-P.; Planell, J. A. *Biomaterials* **2006**, *27*(30), 5326.
146. Stops, A. J. F.; McMahon, L. A.; O'Mahoney, D.; Prendergast, P. J.; McHugh, P. E. *J. Biomech. Eng.-Trans. Asme* **2008**, *130*(6), 61001.
147. Sanz-Herrera, J. A.; García-Aznar, J. M.; Doblaré, M. *Comput. Methods Appl. Mech. Eng.* **2008**, *197*(33–40), 3092.
148. Ganghoffer, J.-F.; Rahouadj, R.; Boisse, J.; Forest, S. *J. Non-Equilib. Thermodyn.* **2016**, *41*(1), 49
149. Appelman, T. P.; Mizrahi, J.; Seliktar, D. *J. Biomech. Eng.-Trans. Asme* **2011**, *133*(4), 41010.
150. Laurent, C. P.; Vaquette, C.; Martin, C.; Guedon, E.; Wu, X.; Delconte, A.; Dumas, D.; Hupont, S.; Isla, N. D.; Rahouadj, R.; Wang, X. *Processes* **2014**, *2*(1), 167.
151. Cinbiz, M. N.; Tigli, R. S.; Beskardes, I. G.; Gumusderelioglu, M.; Colak, U. *J. Biotechnol.* **2010**, *150*(3), 389.
152. Boschetti, F.; Raimondi, M. T.; Migliavacca, F.; Dubini, G. *J. Biomech.* **2006**, *39*(3), 418.

153. Lesman, A.; Blinder, Y.; Levenberg, S. *Biotechnol. Bioeng.* **2010**, *105*(3), 645.
154. Maes, F.; Van Ransbeeck, P.; Van Oosterwyck, H.; Verdonck, P. *Biotechnol. Bioeng.* **2009**, *103*(3), 621.
155. Porter, B.; Zauel, R.; Stockman, H.; Guldberg, R.; Fyhrie, D. *J. Biomech.* **2005**, *38*(3), 543.
156. Voronov, R.; VanGordon, S.; Sikavitsas, V. I.; Papavassiliou, D. V. *J. Biomech.* **2010**, *43*(7), 1279.
157. Owen, S. C.; Shoichet, M. S. *J. Biomed. Mater. Res. A* **2010**, *94A* (4), 1321.
158. Geris, L.; Andreykiv, A.; Oosterwyck, H. V.; Sloten, J. V.; Keulen, F. van; Duyck, J.; Naert, I. *J. Biomech.* **2004**, *37*(5), 763.
159. Adebiyi, A. A.; Taslim, M. E.; Crawford, K. D. *Biomaterials* **2011**, *32*(34), 8753.
160. Petrigliano, F. A.; McAllister, D. R.; Wu, B. M. *Arthrosc. J. Arthrosc. Relat. Surg.* **2006**, *22*(4), 441.
161. Ge, Z.; Goh, J.; Lee, E. *Cell Transplant.* **2005**, *14*(8), 573.
162. Deng, D.; Liu, W.; Xu, F.; Yang, Y.; Zhou, G.; Zhang, W. J.; Cui, L.; Cao, Y. *Biomaterials* **2009**, *30*(35), 6724.
163. Guyot, Y.; Papantoniou, I.; Chai, Y. C.; Bael, S. V.; Schrooten, J.; Geris, L. *Biomech. Model. Mechanobiol.* **2014**, *13*(6), 1361.
164. Singh, H.; Teoh, S. H.; Low, H. T.; Hutmacher, D. W. *J. Biotechnol.* **2005**, *119*(2), 181.
165. Bakker, A. D.; Soejima, K.; Klein-Nulend, J.; Burger, E. H. *J. Biomech.* **2001**, *34*(5), 671.
166. McGarry, J.; Klein-Nulend, J.; Mullender, M.; Prendergast, P. J. *FASEB J.* **2004**, *18*(15), 482.
167. Isaksson, H.; van Donkelaar, C. C.; Huiskes, R.; Ito, K. *J. Orthop. Res.* **2006**, *24*(5), 898.
168. Prendergast, P. J.; Huiskes, R.; Søballe, K. *J. Biomech.* **1997**, *30*(6), 539.
169. Lacroix, D.; Prendergast, P. J.; Li, G.; Marsh, D. *Med. Biol. Eng. Comput.* *40*(1), 14.
170. Isaksson, H.; Wilson, W.; van Donkelaar, C. C.; Huiskes, R.; Ito, K. *J. Biomech.* **2006**, *39*(8), 1507.
171. Bawolin, N. K.; Li, M. G.; Chen, X. B.; Zhang, W. J. *J. Biomech. Eng.-Trans. Asme* **2010**, *132*(11), 111001.

172. Rathbone, S. R.; Glossop, J. R.; Gough, J. E.; Cartmell, S. H. *J. Mech. Behav. Biomed. Mater.* **2012**, *11*, 82.
173. Skardal, A.; Mack, D.; Atala, A.; Soker, S. *J. Mech. Behav. Biomed. Mater.* **2013**, *17*, 307.
174. Wang, J. H.-C.; Yang, G.; Li, Z. *Ann. Biomed. Eng.* **2005**, *33*(3), 337.
175. Carey, L. E.; Dearth, C. L.; Johnson, S. A.; Londono, R.; Medberry, C. J.; Daly, K. A.; Badylak, S. F. *Biomaterials* **2014**, *35*(29), 8297.
176. Jeong, S. I.; Kim, B.-S.; Lee, Y. M.; Ihn, K. J.; Kim, S. H.; Kim, Y. H. *Biomacromolecules* **2004**, *5*(4), 1303.
177. Saito, E.; Liu, Y.; Migneco, F.; Hollister, S. J. *Acta Biomater.* **2012**, *8*(7), 2568.
178. Wang, Y.; Rudym, D. D.; Walsh, A.; Abrahamsen, L.; Kim, H.-J.; Kim, H. S.; Kirker-Head, C.; Kaplan, D. L. *Biomaterials* **2008**, *29*(24–25), 3415.
179. Liu, Y. S.; Huang, Q. L.; Kienzle, A.; Müller, W. E. G.; Feng, Q. L. *Mater. Sci. Eng. C* **2014**, *38*, 227.
180. Shirazi, R. N.; Ronan, W.; Rochev, Y.; McHugh, P. *J. Mech. Behav. Biomed. Mater.* **2016**, *54*, 48.
181. Wang, Y.; Yang, X.; Gu, Z.; Qin, H.; Li, L.; Liu, J.; Yu, X. *Mater. Sci. Eng. C* **2016**, *66*, 185.
182. Zhang, Q.; Jiang, Y.; Zhang, Y.; Ye, Z.; Tan, W.; Lang, M. *Polym. Degrad. Stab.* **2013**, *98*(1), 209.
183. Zhao, L.; Zhang, Z.; Song, Y.; Liu, S.; Qi, Y.; Wang, X.; Wang, Q.; Cui, C. *Mater. Des.* **2016**, *108*, 136.
184. Vieira, A. C.; Guedes, R. M.; Tita, V. *J. Biomech.* **2015**, *48*(12), 3478.
185. Vieira, A. C.; Guedes, R. M.; Tita, V. *Int. J. Solids Struct.* **2014**, *51*(5), 1164.
186. Vieira, A. C.; Guedes, R. M.; Tita, V. *Compos. Struct.* **2012**, *94*(11), 3149.
187. Vieira, A. C.; Vieira, J. C.; Ferra, J. M.; Magalhães, F. D.; Guedes, R. M.; Marques, A. T. *J. Mech. Behav. Biomed. Mater.* **2011**, *4*(3), 451.

https://doi.org/10.1142/9789811204630_bmatter

Index

S

T

U

Lightning Source UK Ltd.
Milton Keynes UK
UKHW021842140421
381970UK00001B/39

9 789811 204623